Statistics for Biology and Health

For further volumes:
http://www.springer.com/series/2848

Anthony B. Miller
Editor

Epidemiologic Studies in Cancer Prevention and Screening

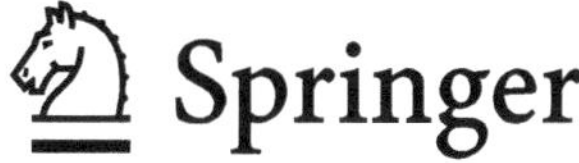

Editor
Anthony B. Miller
Dalla Lana School of Public Health
University of Toronto
Toronto, ON, Canada

ISSN 1431-8776
ISBN 978-1-4614-5585-1 ISBN 978-1-4614-5586-8 (eBook)
DOI 10.1007/978-1-4614-5586-8
Springer New York Heidelberg Dordrecht London

Library of Congress Control Number: 2012951334

Printed on acid-free paper

Springer is part of Springer Science+Business Media (www.springer.com)

Preface

Of the five components of cancer control, prevention, early detection (including screening) treatment, rehabilitation and palliative care, prevention is regarded as the most important. Yet the knowledge available to prevent many cancers is incomplete, and even if we know the main causal factors for a cancer, we often lack the understanding on how to put this knowledge into effect. Further, with the long natural history of most cancers, it could take many years to make an appreciable impact upon the incidence of cancer.

Because of these facts, many have come to believe that screening has the most potential for reduction of the burden of cancer. Yet, as we have tried to apply the knowledge gained on screening for cancer, we have come to recognize that screening can have major disadvantages, and achieve little at substantial cost, thus reducing the resources that are potentially available for both prevention and treatment.

Thus the time seems right for a comprehensive overview of the evidence base for both cancer prevention and screening. The main aim of the book is to provide a realistic appraisal of the evidence for both cancer prevention and cancer screening, combined with an accounting of the extent programs based upon available knowledge have had an impact in the population.

The issues are that the evidence base for many approaches to cancer prevention does not include an assessment of the extent prevention programs have had an impact, and in the case of screening, a failure of recognition that much of the evidence available is from trials conducted many years ago, and with advances in cancer treatment, the contribution of screening may be far less than many would have us believe.

Thus the book has the following objectives:

1. To present a rigorous and realistic evaluation of the evidence for population-based interventions in prevention of and screening for cancer, with particular relevance to those believed to be applicable now, or on the cusp of application.
2. To evaluate the relative contributions of prevention and screening.
3. To discuss how, within the health systems with which the authors are familiar, prevention and screening for cancer can be enhanced.

You will find as you go through the book some overlap between the chapters and some disagreements as to conclusions or interpretation of data. Overlap is often instructive as are disagreements, as they identify areas where further research may be needed to provide the necessary evidence base for action.

I trust you will enjoy reading the book. I should be grateful, if you detect errors, if you could bring them to my attention.

Toronto, ON, Canada Anthony B. Miller

Cancer Prevention and Screening

Publisher: Springer Science+Business Media, LLC, New York: Senior Editor, Marc Strauss

Editor: Anthony B. Miller, MD, Professor Emeritus, Dalla Lana School of Public health, University of Toronto, Canada

Contents

Contributors

Dennis J. Ahnen Denver Department of Veterans Affairs Medical Center, University of Colorado School of Medicine, Denver, CO, USA

S/M Gastroenterology, Gastroenterology Administration, Denver, CO, USA

Philippe Autier International Prevention Research Institute (iPRI), Lyon, France

Chemin du Saquin, Espace Européen, batiment G, Ecully (Lyon), France

Aaron Blair Occupational and Environmental Epidemiology Branch, Division of Cancer Epidemiology and Genetics, National Cancer Institute, Bethesda, MD, USA

F. Xavier Bosch Head, Cancer Epidemiology Research Program (CERP), Catalan Institute of Oncology (Institut Català d'Oncologia - ICO) & Bellvitge Biomedical Research Institute (IDIBELL), Avda. Gran Via 199-203 08907 L'Hospitalet de Llobregat (Barcelona), Barcelona, Spain

Otis W. Brawley American Cancer Society, Emory University, Atlanta, GA, USA

Nathalie Broutet Department of Reproductive Health and Research, World Health Organization, Geneva 27, Switzerland

Robert Burton School of Public Health and Preventive Medicine, Monash University, Melbourne, Vic, Australia

Department of Epidemiology and Preventive Medicine, Epidemiology & Preventative Medicine Monash Medical School Building, The Alfred Hospital, Level 6 The Alfred Centre (Alfred Hospital), Melbourne, Vic, Australia

Cynthia Callard Physicians for a Smoke-free Canada, Ottawa, ON, Canada

Roy Cameron School of Public Health and Health Systems and Propel Centre for Population Health Impact, University of Waterloo, West Waterloo, ON, Canada

Neil Collishaw Physicians for a Smoke-free Canada, Ottawa, ON, Canada

Marilys Corbex Institute of Tropical Medicine, Antwerp, Belgium

Paul Demers Occupational Cancer Research Centre, Cancer Care Ontario, Toronto, ON, Canada

Michelle C. Dunn Surveillance Research Program Division of Cancer Control and Population Sciences, National Cancer Institute, Bethesda, MD, USA

Jennifer Enns Family Medicine Research Unit, Faculty of Medicine, University of Manitoba, Winnipeg, Canada

Eric J. Feuer Surveillance Research Program Division of Cancer Control and Population Sciences, National Cancer Institute, Bethesda, MD, USA

Christine M. Freidenreich Department of Population Health Research, Alberta Health Services - Cancer Care, Calgary, AB, Canada

J. Dik F. Habbema Department of Public Health, Erasmus MC University Medical Center Rotterdam, The Netherlands

Matti Hakama Tampere School of Public Health, Cancer Registry of Finland, University of Tampere, Tampere, Finland

William Hocking Marshfield Center, Marshfield, WI, USA

Karin Hohenadel Occupational Cancer Research Centre, Cancer Care Ontario, Toronto, ON, Canada

William Hryniuk CAREpath, Toronto, ON, Canada

W. Philip T. James London School of Hygiene and Tropical Medicine, International Association for the Study of Obesity, London, UK

Alan Katz Family Medicine Research Unit, Faculty of Medicine, University of Manitoba, Winnipeg, Canada

Jon Kerner Canadian Partnerships Against Cancer, Toronto, ON, Canada

Barnett S. Kramer Division of Cancer Prevention, National Cancer Institute, Bethesda, MD, USA

Annie Langley Department of Population Health Research, Alberta Health Services - Cancer Care, Calgary, AB, Canada

David T. Levy Pacific Institute for Research and Evaluation, University of Baltimore, Baltimore, MD, USA

Brigid M. Lynch Department of Population Health Research, Alberta Health Services - Cancer Care, Calgary, AB, CANADA

James Marshall Department of Cancer Prevention and Population Sciences, Roswell Park Cancer Institute, Buffalo, NY, USA

Loraine Marrett Prevention and Cancer Control, Cancer Care Ontario, Toronto, ON, Canada

Anthony B. Miller Dalla Lana School of Public Health, University of Toronto, Toronto, ON, Canada

Swati G. Patel Fellow in Gastroenterology, University of Colorado School of Medicine, Aurora, CO, USA

Julietta Patnick NHS Cancer Screening Programmes, Sheffield, UK

Mary Reid Department of Medicine, Roswell Park Cancer Institute, Buffalo, NY 14263, USA

Kurt Straif Section of IARC Monographs, International Agency for Research on Cancer, Lyon, France

Natasha K. Stout Department of Population Medicine, Harvard Medical School and Harvard Pilgrim Health Care Institute, Boston, MA, USA

Hideo Tanaka Division of Epidemiology and Prevention, Aichi Cancer Center Research Institute, Osaka, Japan

David B. Thomas Fred Hutchinson Cancer Research Center, Seattle, WA, USA

Andreas Ullrich Department of Chronic Diseases and Health Promotion (CHP), World Health Organization Cancer Control Programme, Geneva 27, Switzerland

Paolo Vineis Centre for Environment and Health, School of Public Health, Imperial College, Medical School, London, UK

Cheng-Har Yip Department of Surgery, University of Malaya, Kuala Lumpur, Malaysia

Part I
Prevention of Cancer

Chapter 1
Health Promotion Approaches to Reducing Cancer Incidence

Roy Cameron and Jon Kerner

1.1 Introduction

Modifiable risk factors for cancer and other preventable chronic diseases (e.g., heart, lung, and diabetes) are prevalent worldwide. It is urgent to reduce the incidence of these diseases to enhance health, to support health care system sustainability, and to promote global development and prosperity. Hence, the WHO is spearheading a United Nations noncommunicable disease (NCD) initiative (The World Bank Human Development Network 2011).

The Ottawa Charter for Health Promotion (World Health Organization 1986) characterizes health promotion as "the process of enabling people to increase control over, and to improve, their health" (p. 1). To that end, the charter emphasizes the importance of (1) building healthy public policy, (2) creating supportive environments, (3) strengthening community actions, (4) developing personal skills, and (5) reorienting health services. These means to achieving health are highly applicable to reducing cancer incidence. This chapter provides an overview how progress is being made and can be accelerated.

Health promotion interventions can reduce disease at national, state, and community levels. For instance, in Finland a comprehensive, sustained program led to a 65 % reduction in annual coronary heart disease mortality among middle-aged men between baseline (1967–1971) and 1995 and reduced lung cancer mortality by almost 60 % (Puska 2002). Risk factor reduction led to 50–72 % of the drop in coronary heart disease mortality in Finland between 1982 and 1997; 23 % of the drop was due to

R. Cameron (✉)
School of Public Health and Health Systems and Propel Centre for Population Health Impact, University of Waterloo, 200 University Avenue, West Waterloo, ON N2L 3G1, Canada
e-mail: cameron@healthy.uwaterloo.ca

J. Kerner
Canadian Partnerships Against Cancer, Toronto, ON, Canada

A.B. Miller (ed.), *Epidemiologic Studies in Cancer Prevention and Screening*, Statistics for Biology and Health 79, DOI 10.1007/978-1-4614-5586-8_1,

Dietary and lifestyle factors	CVD	Type 2 diabetes	Cancer	Dental disease	Fracture	Cataract	Birth defects	Obesity	Metabolic syndrome	Depression	Sexual dysfunction
Avoid smoking	**↓**	**↓**	**↓**	**↓**	↓	**↓**		**↑**			**↓**
Pursue physical activity	**↓**	**↓**	**↓**		**↓**			**↓**	**↓**	↓	↓
Avoid overweight	**↓**	**↓**	**↓**		**↑**	**↓**			**↓**		↓
Diet											
Consume healthy types of fats[a]	**↓**	**↓**							↓		
Eat plenty of fruits and vegetables	**↓**		↓		↓	↓	↓	↓			
Replace refined grains with whole grains	↓	↓						**↓**	**↓**		
Limit sugar intake[b]	↓	↓		↓				↓	**↓**		
Limit excessive calories								↓	**↓**		
Limit sodium intake	↓										

Original Source: Authors' summary of a review by the WHO and FAO 2003; Bacon and others 2003; Fox 1999; IARC 2002.

Adapted from: Willett et al. 2006.

Note: **Bold** = convincing; Standard = probable relation; ↑ = increase in risk; ↓ = decrease in risk.

a. Replace trans and saturated fats with mono- and polyunsaturated fats, including a regular source on N-3 fatty acids.

b. Includes limiting sugar-based beverages.

Fig. 1.1 Convincing and probable relationships between dietary and lifestyle factors and chronic diseases

improved treatment (Laatikainen et al. 2005). California's tobacco control program led to a 6 % drop in lung cancer incidence within the first decade (averting some 11,000 cases), with no comparable decrease in comparison jurisdictions (Barnoya and Glantz 2004). During the 2 years after Toronto banned smoking in public indoor spaces, hospital admissions for cardiovascular and respiratory conditions fell 39 % and 33 %, respectively, in this city, but not in surrounding communities (Naiman et al. 2010).

It is critical to be strategic in addressing health promotion for NCD prevention. A first strategic decision involves selecting intervention targets. Tobacco use, physical inactivity, and unhealthy eating are major sources of cancer risk and thus current strategic priorities (e.g., Willett et al. 2006, World Bank: see Fig. 1.1 from Willett).

A second strategic decision involves defining the approach to intervention. This chapter overviews three intervention strategies that can work in concert: (1) "scaling up" face-to-face clinical intervention with individuals; (2) using high-reach, low-cost delivery systems (e.g., print, electronic) to influence large numbers of people at risk; and (3) altering environments (social, physical, policy) to promote population health. The emphasis here is on the latter two approaches, particularly the third strategy, which is at the heart of health promotion. All three strategies are described to provide perspective and to illustrate how linkage and synergy is created across the strategies. Each approach is presented at a high level.

Major influential organizations provide ready access to evidence and resources pertinent to action. These sources of regularly updated evidence (Appendix Table A.1.1) are provided to promote resources of ongoing value.

The final section of this chapter concerns capacity to create and execute coherent prevention strategies. Lessons learned from tobacco control inform the NCD agenda (Green et al. 2006). Hence, examples from tobacco control are often used as illustrations. A core lesson is that appropriate research methods must guide action at system and population levels. What is often most valuable is not definitive "proof" that an intervention works, but rather ongoing integration of evidence from multiple sources (traditional research, evaluation, surveillance) to guide continuous improvement of interventions and systems as they are implemented in specific, ever evolving contexts (see Fig. 1.2). This framing pervades this chapter.

1.2 Strategies

1.2.1 Strategy 1: Scaling Up Face-to-Face Intervention Within the Health Care System

Face-to-face intervention with individuals or small groups can have population level impact if efficacious interventions are widely implemented. The US Preventive Services Task Force synthesizes pertinent evidence and disseminates guidelines for providers, especially for primary care (Appendix Table A.1.1).

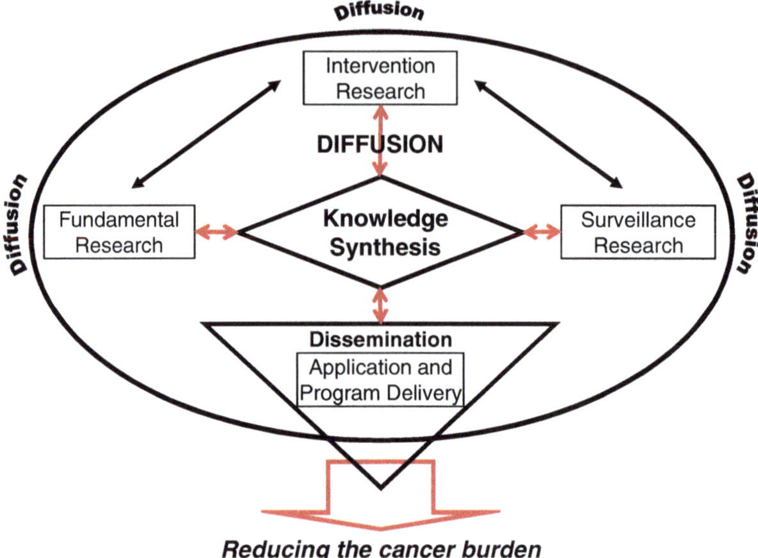

Fig. 1.2 Dynamic model of cancer research and diffusion and dissemination

The evidence is typically from randomized controlled trials so treatment effects can be interpreted with confidence. Recently, the importance of directly assessing the generalizability of findings across providers, settings, and patients has been emphasized (Glasgow et al. 1999). This approach reflects the established "pipeline" research model (Greenwald et al. 1990).

To go beyond helping individual patients and contribute to reduced disease incidence, additional research approaches are needed. Spoth's (2008) framework shifts research toward a paradigm of public health impact. It describes a translational research agenda with four domains: (1) effectiveness of interventions, (2) extensiveness of their population coverage, (3) efficiency of interventions, and (4) engagement of eligible populations or organizations. Strategic research in each domain provides evidence to enhance the population level impact of preventive maneuvers across health care systems. Observational studies to identify attributes of primary care practices that facilitate delivery of health promotion maneuvers may also guide practice managers and policymakers seeking to improve practice and system-level prevention impact (Hogg et al. 2009).

Health care systems can help reduce disease incidence, but this strategy has limitations. Scaling up clinical preventive maneuvers to levels required for population level impact is costly and constrained by system capacity. For instance, Yarnall et al. (2003) estimated that an average family physician would need about 7.4 h per working day to implement all recommendations of the US Preventive Services Task Force, aside from time needed to address all other patient issues. There are typically even tighter constraints in systems serving vulnerable populations (e.g., the poor, aboriginal populations, racial/ethnic minorities, the geographically isolated). In some settings, use of all practice staff may surmount constraints (Peckham et al. 2011).

Use of lay volunteers to deliver face-to-face prevention programs (e.g., smoking cessation) also could expand capacity to provide "clinical" programs in a context of constrained resources. But to be "scaled up" and sustained, such programs would require a host organization (e.g., a nongovernment organization – NGO) to provide capacity to recruit, train, organize, and monitor volunteers. This would impose major opportunity costs (e.g., by diverting resources from advocacy for public policies) that may or may not be defensible. Little is known about the costs and benefits of this approach given the historical emphasis on efficacy studies and absence of evidence to inform decisions about program design, delivery, and cost (Manske et al. 2004).

1.2.2 Strategy 2: High-Reach, Low-Cost Programs Directed at Individuals at Risk

Behavior change programs based on print, telephone, and electronic media can contribute to population level impact given their high reach and relatively low cost.

Such programs are used, for instance, to support smoking cessation. Government-funded telephone-based quitlines serve states and provinces in North America, based on evidence of efficacy (Stead et al. 2007). The North American Quitline Consortium (NAQC) now facilitates continual improvement of the lines using ongoing evaluation and surveillance data. NAQC sponsored development of the Minimal Data Set (Campbell et al. 2007) to enable standardized evaluation for comparative studies of relative costs and impacts of various service models. Such studies can support accountability requirements, guide continual improvement, and assess outcomes in an evolving context (e.g., as the population of smokers changes). This adds direct value to those who fund, provide, or use these services.

Surveillance studies show that most cessation lines reach a low percentage of smokers in the populations they serve. Since it is more feasible to enhance the population level impact of the lines (i.e., the total number of smokers who quit or cut down) by increasing reach versus the quit rate (McDonald 1999), increasing reach is now a priority of the Consortium. If new promotions increase the proportion of smokers who use lines (assessed via surveillance), ongoing evaluation research can assess changes in quit rate as the population of smokers served broadens. It is not just a matter of "proving efficacy" and scaling up an intervention but continuing to use evaluation and surveillance studies to guide system-level decisions and improve population level impact.

Social media are being used to promote health behavior change, including smoking cessation (Shahab and McEwen 2009; Free et al. 2009). These programs, and the platforms that support them, evolve very rapidly. By the time a traditional research study is completed and reported, the program and technology may both be obsolete. In this context, developmental evaluation (Patton 2010) may be ideal for enabling service providers and researchers to jointly engage in ongoing development, improvement, and testing of programs, platforms, and promotional strategies.

Face-to-face and high-reach, low-cost strategies can be combined. For instance, to extend the reach of quitlines, the North American Quitline Consortium is seeking to enhance linkage between health care providers and quitlines. This could enable more providers to address smoking with more patients since they can limit their role to referral and not spend time on intervention delivery.

Integration of clinical and high-reach/low-cost approaches to create an efficient, coherent service system was envisioned by Abrams et al. (1996). The model calls for matching smokers to services based on an initial assessment of their needs, then referring them to progressively more intensive (and costly) services as needed in a "stepped care" approach. This would use resources efficiently and provide smokers with a coherent, staged set of services, with systematic follow-up with more intensive intervention as needed after failed quit attempts. Ongoing evaluation can guide development and improvement of such systems, which are now being proposed (e.g., Smoke-Free Ontario – Scientific Advisory Committee 2010).

1.2.3 Strategy 3: Environmental Change to Influence Entire Populations

Environments (social, physical, and policy) profoundly influence behavior, although this influence is grossly underestimated (Ross and Nisbett 1991). This empirically demonstrated effect of environments exerting widespread and sustained influence on behavior provides a compelling empirical rationale for environmental intervention, the foundation of the health promotion approach (Potvin and Jones 2011).

Geoffrey Rose (1992) provided a core conceptual foundation for this orientation. Rose distinguished between variability in risk of diseases across individuals *within a population* and variability in incidence of diseases *across populations*. A high-risk (clinical) approach seeks to modify factors (e.g., behaviors) that put *individuals* at relative risk within a population. A population-based approach is ecological; it seeks to modify environmental factors that cause differences in disease incidence across *populations*. Rose contended that if a population approach is taken, "there is no known biological reason why every population should not be as healthy as the best" (Rose 1992, p. 1). Environmental change is now the central approach to reducing incidence of chronic disease, based largely on experience with tobacco control.

This approach uses policies implemented through all government departments, not just health, to create healthy living conditions, including environments that support nonsmoking, physical activity, and healthy eating. One way to advance this approach is to subject all government policies to health impact assessments (Collins and Koplan 2009; Puska and Stahl 2010). The Canadian Partnership Against Cancer regularly updates its online Prevention Policy Directory to allow research, practice, and policy experts to identify and examine chronic disease prevention policies being implemented within federal, provincial, and territorial jurisdictions in Canada and is considering expanding this to encompass municipal level policies.[1]

Environmental change is driving success in tobacco control. The WHO Framework Convention on Tobacco Control focuses on environmental interventions (e.g., policies related to tobacco packaging and warning labels, smoke-free spaces, tax policy). Such policies create environments that simultaneously (1) support cessation, (2) discourage tobacco use among both new users (to lower prevalence) and current users (to reduce dosage, thus mitigating risk and harm), and (3) minimize exposure to environmental tobacco smoke. Healthy public policy is vital beyond tobacco control. The World Cancer Research Fund and the American Institute for Cancer Research (2009) distilled evidence for 48 policy recommendations designed to substantially reduce cancer risk in populations based on widespread improvement in dietary patterns and physical activity levels, reduced obesity rates, and increased rates of breast feeding.

What type of direct evidence supports use of environmental interventions? It is occasionally feasible to test environmental interventions using randomized trials. For instance, Ludwig et al. (2011) randomized 1,788 women living in public housing in impoverished neighborhoods to receive housing vouchers redeemable only in low-poverty neighborhoods, along with counseling on moving. This intervention led to a small but potentially important reduction in the prevalence of extreme obesity and diabetes more than a decade after the intervention was introduced.

But such randomized trials are rarely feasible. Researchers typically lack the requisite policy levers, large budgets (e.g., for major social marketing campaigns), or influence to effect environmental intervention. Moreover, it is difficult to induce jurisdictions to participate in randomized policy studies.

Thus, with environmental interventions, the major "experiments" are done typically not by researchers, but by "social actors" (Cameron 2009). The role of research is to study innovative interventions as they are implemented, so as to identify what works, for whom, in what context, at what cost. The studies demonstrating improved population health in response to programs in Finland, California, and Toronto described earlier all involved nonrandomized assessments of policy-driven social change. This approach reflects Donald Campbell's (1991) notion of creating a "methodology for an experimenting society" to enable systematic learning from social innovation. In this realm, Green's (2006) adage that "if we want more evidence-based practice, we need more practice-based evidence" is very apt.

There have been many calls for going beyond randomized designs in studying the impact of policies, programs (individually and in combination), and systems designed to reduce disease incidence (Cameron et al. 2007; De Leeuw 2009; Hawe and Potvin 2009; Smith and Petticrew 2010). This has major implications for public health science and practice and links between the two.

---

[1] http://www.cancerview.ca/portal/server.pt/community/prevention_policies/464/prevention_policies_directory

The deepest implication is that the usual notion that intervention research studies precede and inform practice does not always apply with environmental intervention. Scientists may actually impede progress by opposing untested interventions rather than engaging as evaluators of social interventions. This was the experience of Dalip Bal, who headed the groundbreaking California Tobacco Control Program: "Bal is frustrated by colleagues who wait for high-level evidence before acting…. 'Most scientists will say you need a randomized controlled trial level of proof to do a community intervention. That's horse feathers. We tried twenty-five things—twelve worked and we renewed those. Empirical trial and error is the oldest scientific device and we used it to distinction…. Where there is no science you have to go and be venturesome—you can't use the paucity of science as an excuse to do nothing… all the scientists came in behind us and analyzed what we did'" (Sweet and Moynihan 2007).

A second implication is that in the absence of direct evidence of what works, it is critical to enable scientists and practitioners to jointly design innovative population level interventions. Much is known about principles of behavior change (Bandura 1986; Hill and Dixon 2010). Scientists can collaborate with policy and program leaders to discern how to incorporate these principles in intervention design. For instance, Fong and his colleagues (Strahan et al. 2002) distilled principles that could be applied to design of tobacco warning labels and worked with Canadian Cancer Society staff to ensure regulators were able to apply these in determining the design of what were then world precedent-setting Canadian graphic warning labels.

A third implication is that the scientific enterprise must work in concert with the public policy agenda, as research is "grafted on" to policy experiments. Traditional scientific funding mechanisms and practices may need to be augmented with new funding approaches, especially given the evidence of profound misalignment between the evidence generated and the evidence needed (Millward et al. 2003). Special funding programs are evolving (e.g., the Population Health Intervention Research Initiative for Canada, coordinated by the Canadian Institutes of Health Research).

Examples of high-impact research pertinent to the WHO NCD initiative are emerging. For instance, Geoffrey Fong and colleagues mounted the International Tobacco Control Policy Evaluation Project, to deliberately generate evidence required to guide 174 countries implementing the WHO Framework Convention for Tobacco Control (FCTC). They follow cohorts of smokers in over 20 countries in all regions of the world to examine the impact of all policies, as they are implemented, using rigorous methods, built into a sophisticated quasi-experimental study (Fong et al. 2006). Findings are disseminated through FCTC mechanisms and via customized reports and direct consultations with individual countries. Use of research methods (and perhaps infrastructures) developed through such studies may accelerate the broader global NCD prevention effort. A second example is the Canadian Partnership Against Cancer's Coalitions Linking Action and Science for Prevention that enable researchers to work with policy and program leaders in coalitions across jurisdictions within Canada (Manafo et al. 2011).

A fourth implication is that care is required to guide appropriate systematic reviews and syntheses. If RCT evidence is required for strong endorsement of interventions, environmental interventions with the greatest potential to reduce disease incidence may not be supported since they are not generally amenable to study using an RCT. New approaches are emerging which balance rigor with the potential to achieve reduced disease incidence (Swinburn et al. 2005).

In short, interventions at the level of countries, states/provinces/territories, and communities have been shown to reduce disease incidence and disease burden within populations. But there is an urgent need for more evidence about what specific policies, and combinations of policies, will have the greatest effect in improving population health in widely diverse and ever changing contexts. New paradigms and infrastructures are required to support deliberate, efficient, ongoing generation and use of evidence to develop and continually improve policies that reduce disease incidence.

The scope of research required to reduce disease incidence must be broadened. For instance, studies are needed to address the role of corporations in creating environments that either undermine (Bakan 2004; Bakan 2011; Hammond et al. 2006) or enhance (Porter and Kramer 2011) health. The current emphasis on addressing risk factors must expand to include social determinants of health (Evans et al. 1994; Marmot and Wilkinson 2006; Laatikainen et al. 2005; Wilkinson and Pickett 2009) and understanding long-term health impacts of multiple social policies (McLeod et al. 2012; Siddiqi and Hertzman 2007). Evidence of prenatal influences on epigenetics and disease outcomes (Gluckman et al. 2008), possibility including cancer (Eriksson et al. 2010), may build public support for prevention policies, just as evidence of injurious effects of environmental tobacco smoke accelerated societal support for tobacco control.

Links between environmental change and other strategies, described above, can facilitate progress. For instance, in tobacco control, smokers were offered clinical and public health cessation services as restrictive smoking policies were introduced. This synergy facilitated widespread cessation, and provision of cessation services helped create public support for restrictive policies. Moreover, health care providers and organizations that represent them can be powerful advocates for social policy (Collishaw 2011). Clinicians may be more likely to become advocates if they realize that most smokers who quit do so not in response to clinical intervention, but "on their own" with stimulus and support from public policies (Chapman 2011).

1.3 The Need for an Implementation Strategy and Mechanisms

Implementation strategies and mechanisms are required to drive progress within and across jurisdictions. The WHO FCTC provides a model for building coherent efforts and for promoting learning across countries. The WHO NCD initiative has the potential to replicate or build on these international structures.

But the real action is at the level of nations, states/provinces/territories, and communities, where requisite jurisdiction authority and resources are vested. Progress will be accelerated if there is coordination of plans and mutually supportive actions across jurisdictional levels and across sectors (government, NGO, research) within countries.

Models have been created for integrating functions that span jurisdictional levels and sectors to advance cancer control, including primary prevention (Advisory Committee on Cancer Control 1994; Hiatt and Rimer 2003; Kerner et al. 2005). Schematic representations of such integrative models are evolving and being used to help organizations work together coherently to form a cancer/disease prevention "system." Figure 1.2 draws attention to the need for organizations to work together to produce and integrate evidence from traditional pertinent research, evaluation, and surveillance methods.

Interorganizational strategy development and execution is critical to create capacity as implied by Fig. 1.2. Disjointed activities are unlikely to optimize progress. Coherent planning and action is so vital to success that in the foreseeable future, failure of institutions to work in concert to advance their prevention missions may come to be seen by taxpayers and donors as organizational malpractice.

Evidence must guide not only interventions but also the development of the implementation capacity. Although concepts are emerging for facilitating collaboration across organizations (Westley et al. 2006), there is still much to learn. Developmental evaluation (Patton 2010) may enable organizational leaders and researchers working together pragmatically to continually plan, test, and refine new ways of enabling organizations to work together to optimize their individual and collective impact.

Leading organizations are already building interagency support. Specifically, key organizations are building capacity to synthesize and promote use of relevant evidence in decision making. For instance, the Guide to Community Preventive Services, overseen by the Task Force on Community Preventive Services, was established by the US Department of Health and Human Services (DHHS) to develop evidence-informed guidance on which community-based health promotion and disease prevention interventions work and which do not work. The Centers for Disease Control and Prevention provides the Task Force with technical and administrative support (Truman et al. 2000).

To support cancer control, the US National Cancer Institute launched Cancer Control P.L.A.N.E.T. (Plan, Link, Act, Network with Evidence-based Tools) in 2003 to help public health practitioners in the USA find surveillance and intervention research evidence needed to plan, implement, and evaluate their cancer prevention and control programs (Kerner et al. 2005). In 2008, the PLANET website model was adopted and adapted by the Canadian Partnership Against Cancer (the Partnership). The Partnership added additional evidence links to the Canadian PLANET website (e.g., to the Cochrane Collaboration library and the Best Practices Portal of the Public Health Agency of Canada). Appendix Table A.1.1 provides a detailed listing of evidence-based resources for health promotion interventions in general and diet/nutrition, physical activity, sun safety, and tobacco control intervention approaches in particular.

There is an emerging research agenda designed to enable organizations promote evidence to inform action to improve their practices (Lavis et al. 2008a, b, c). This sort of research has potential to improve links between evidence and action and illustrates how research may inform improved interorganizational collaboration.

1.4 Conclusion

There is evidence that population-based initiatives can reduce the incidence and burden of cancer and other chronic diseases. Progress will be accelerated if a strategic approach is taken to investing in and linking interventions delivered by health care providers, high-reach, low-cost programs (e.g., using print, web, and social media platforms), and environmental change through policy. There is a need to develop mechanisms and infrastructures to enable research, policy, and practice communities to work together in organized ways to accelerate progress by deliberately and efficiently generating and using evidence to advance progress in rapidly changing societies around the world.

1.5 Appendix

Table A.1.1 Selected evidence-based health promotion and risk factor prevention web resource links

Subject	Source	Type of review	URL
Consumer health promotion and education	Cochrane Library	Systematic reviews	http://www.thecochranelibrary.com/details/browseReviews/577975/Enabling-consumers-to-know-about-their-health--treatment.html
Diet and nutrition	Research-Tested Intervention Programs (RTIPS)	Individual research project summary evaluations and materials	http://rtips.cancer.gov/rtips/program-Search.do
Health communication and social marketing	Guide to community preventive services	Systematic reviews	http://www.thecommunityguide.org/healthcommunication/campaigns.html
Health intervention programs	Best practices portal	Intervention program descriptions	http://cbpp-pcpe.phac-aspc.gc.ca/intervention/search-eng.html
Obesity prevention in community settings	Guide to community preventive services	Systematic reviews	http://www.thecommunityguide.org/obesity/communitysettings.html
Promoting physical activity: campaigns and informational approaches	Guide to community preventive services	Systematic reviews	http://www.thecommunityguide.org/pa/campaigns/index.html
Promoting physical activity: behavioral and social approaches	Guide to community preventive services	Systematic reviews	http://www.thecommunityguide.org/pa/behavioral-social/index.html
Promoting physical activity: environmental and policy approaches	Guide to community preventive services	Systematic reviews	http://www.thecommunityguide.org/pa/environmental-policy/index.html
Community-wide interventions for increasing physical activity	Cochrane collaboration	Systematic review	http://www.thecochranelibrary.com/details/browseReviews/1052077/Increasing-physical-activity.html
Physical activity	Research-Tested Intervention Programs (RTIPS)	Individual research project summary evaluations and materials	http://rtips.cancer.gov/rtips/program-Search.do
Preventing skin cancer: education and policy	Guide to community preventive services	Systematic reviews	http://www.thecommunityguide.org/cancer/skin/education-policy/index.html

Community-wide sun safety interventions	Guide to community preventive services	Systematic reviews	http://www.thecommunityguide.org/cancer/skin/community-wide/index.html
Sun safety	Research-Tested Intervention Programs (RTIPS)	Individual research project summary evaluations and materials	http://rtips.cancer.gov/rtips/program-Search.do
Reducing tobacco use initiation	Guide to community preventive services	Systematic reviews	http://www.thecommunityguide.org/tobacco/initiation/index.html
Increasing tobacco use cessation	Guide to community preventive services	Systematic reviews	http://www.thecommunityguide.org/tobacco/cessation/index.html
Reducing exposure to environmental tobacco smoke	Guide to community preventive services	Systematic reviews	http://www.thecommunityguide.org/tobacco/environmental/index.html
Restricting minors' access to tobacco products	Guide to community preventive services	Systematic reviews	http://www.thecommunityguide.org/tobacco/restrictingaccess/index.html
Decreasing tobacco use among workers	Guide to community preventive services	Systematic reviews	http://www.thecommunityguide.org/tobacco/worksite/index.html
Preventing tobacco use in young people	Cochrane Library	Systematic reviews	http://www.thecochranelibrary.com/details/browseReviews/579463/Preventing-tobacco-use-in-young-people.html
Psychological approaches to reducing tobacco use	Cochrane Library	Systematic reviews	http://www.thecochranelibrary.com/details/browseReviews/579465/Psychological-approaches.html
Reducing tobacco use in specific groups	Cochrane Library	Systematic reviews	http://www.thecochranelibrary.com/details/browseReviews/578671/Interventions-in-specific-groups.html
Reducing tobacco use in specific settings	Cochrane Library	Systematic reviews	http://www.thecochranelibrary.com/details/browseReviews/579467/Interventions-in-specific-settings.html

(continued)

Table A.1.1 (continued)

Subject	Source	Type of review	URL
Reducing tobacco use with mass media approaches	Cochrane Library	Systematic review	http://www.thecochranelibrary.com/details/browseReviews/578691/Mass-media-programmes.html
Tobacco use and government policies	Cochrane Library	Systematic reviews	http://www.thecochranelibrary.com/details/browseReviews/578675/Effects-of-government-policy-on-tobacco-use.html
Tobacco control	Research-Tested Intervention Programs (RTIPS)	Individual research project summary evaluations and materials	http://rtips.cancer.gov/rtips/programSearch.do
Worksite health promotion	Guide to community preventive services	Systematic reviews	http://www.thecommunityguide.org/worksite/index.html

References

Abrams DB, Orleans CT, Niaura RS, Goldstein MG, Prochaska JO, Velicer W. Integrating individual and public health perspectives for treatment of tobacco dependence under managed health care: A combined stepped-care and matching model. *Annuals of Behavioral Medicine* 1996; 18:290-304.

Advisory Committee on Cancer Control, National Cancer Institute of Canada. Bridging research to action: A framework and decision-making process for cancer control. *CMAJ* 1994; 151:1141-1146.

Bakan J. *The corporation: The pathological pursuit of profit and power.* New York: Free Press, 2004.

Bakan J. *Childhood under siege: How big business targets children.* New York: Free Press, 2011.

Bandura A. *Social foundations of thought and action.* Englewood Cliffs, NJ: Prentice-Hall, 1986.

Barnoya J, Glantz SA. (2004). Association of the California tobacco control program with declines in lung cancer incidence. *Cancer Causes Control* 2004; 15:689-695.

Cameron R, Manske S, Brown K, Jolin M, Murnaghan D, Lovato C. Integrating public health policy, practice, evaluation, surveillance, and research: The school health action planning and evaluation system. *Am J Publ Hlth* 2007; 97:648.

Cameron R. *Beyond dissemination and implementation research: Integrating evidence and action.* Invited Plenary Address, 2nd Annual NIH Conference on the Science of Dissemination and Implementation: Building Research Capacity to Bridge the Gap from Science to Service, Bethesda, MD, 2009.

Campbell DT. Methods for the experimenting society. *American Journal of Evaluation* 1991; 12:223-260.

Campbell H.S, Ossip-Klein D, Bailey L, Saul J. Minimal dataset for quitlines: A best practice. *Tobacco Control* 2007; 16:16-20.

Chapman S. Tar wars over smoking cessation. *Br Med J* 2011; 342: d5008.

Collins J, Koplan J P. Health impact assessment: A step toward health in all policies. *JAMA* 2009; 302:315-317.

Collishaw N. *Beyond smoking cessation services: More doctors needed as tobacco control advocates.* Presented at Physicians for a Smoke-free Canada, September, 2011.

De Leeuw E. Evidence for healthy cities: Reflections on practice, method and theory. *Health Promotion International* 2009; 24(S1): i19-i36.

Eriksson JG, Thornburg K L, Osmond C, Kajantie E, Barker DJP. The prenatal origins of lung cancer. I. The fetus. *American Journal of Human Biology* 2010; 22:508-511.

Evans RG, Barer ML, Marmor TR. (Eds.). Why are some people healthy and others not? *The Determinants of Health of Populations.* New York: Aldine de Gruyter, 1994.

Fong GT, Cummings KM, Shopland DR. Building the evidence base for effective tobacco control policies: The international tobacco control policy evaluation project (the ITC project). *Tobacco Control* 2006; 15(Suppl III): iii1-iii2.

Free C, Whittaker R, Knight R, Abramsky T, Rodgers A, Roberts IG. Txt2stop: a pilot randomised controlled trial of mobile phone-based smoking cessation support. *Tobacco Control* 2009; 18:88-91.

Glasgow RE, Vogt TM, Boles SM. Evaluating the public health impact of health promotion interventions: The RE-AIM framework. *Am J Pub Hlth* 1999; 89:1322-1327.

Gluckman PD, Hanson MA, Phil D, Cooper C, Thornburg KL. Effect of in utero and early-life conditions on adult health and disease. *New Engl J Med* 2008; 359:61-73.

Green LW. (2006). Public health asks of systems science: To advance our evidence-based practice, can you help us get more practice-based evidence? *Am J Pub Hlth* 2006; 96:406-409.

Green LW, Orleans T, Ottoson J, Cameron R, Pierce J, Bettinghaus E. (2006). Inferring strategies for disseminating physical activity policies, programs and practices from the successes of tobacco control. *Am J Prev Med* 2006; 31(4S):S66-S81.

Greenwald P, Cullen JW, Weed D. Introduction: Cancer prevention and control. *Seminars in Oncology* 1990; 17:383–390.
Hammond D, Collishaw N, Callard C. Tobacco industry research on smoking behaviour and product design. *Lancet* 2006; 367:781-87.
Hawe P, Potvin L. What is population health intervention research? *Can J Publ Hlth* 2009; 100: I8-I13.
Hiatt RA, Rimer BK. A new strategy for cancer control. *Cancer Epidemiol Biomarkers Prev* 2003; 12:705-712.
Hill D, Dixon H. Achieving behavioural changes in individuals and populations. In J. M. Elwood & S. B. Sutcliffe (Eds.), *Cancer control.* Oxford: Oxford University Press, 2010, pp 43-62.
Hogg W, Dahrouge S, Russell G, Tuna M, Geneau R, Muldoon L et al. Health promotion activity in primary care: Performance of models and associated factors. *Open Medicine* 2009; 3:165-173.
Kerner JF, Guirguis-Blake J, Hennessy KD, Brounstein PJ, Vinson C, Schwartz RH et al. Translating research into improved outcomes in comprehensive cancer control. *Cancer Causes and Control* 2005; 16(Suppl. 1): 27-40.
Laatikainen T, Critchley J, Vartiainen E, Salomaa V, Ketonen M, Capewall S. Explaining the decline in coronary heart disease mortality in Finland between 1982 and 1997. *Am J Epidemiol* 2005;162:764-773.
Lavis JN, Moynihan R, Oxman AD, Paulsen EJ. Evidence-informed health policy 4 - case descriptions of organizations that support the use of research evidence. *Implementation Science* 2008a; 3(56).
Lavis JN, Moynihan R, Oxman AD, Paulsen EJ. Evidence-informed health policy 1 - synthesis of findings from a multi-method study of organizations that support the use of research evidence. *Implementation Science* 2008b; 3(53).
Lavis JN, Moynihan R, Oxman AD, Paulsen EJ. Evidence-informed health policy 3 - interviews with the directors of organizations that support the use of research evidence. *Implementation Science* 2008c; 3(55).
Ludwig J, Sanbonmatsu L, Gennetian L, Adam E, Duncan GJ, Katz LF et al. Neighborhoods, obesity, and diabetes - a randomized social experiment. *New Engl J Med* 2011; 365:1509-1519.
Manafo E, Petermann L, Lobb R, Keen D, Kerner J. Research, practice, and policy partnerships in pan-Canadian coalitions for cancer and chronic disease prevention. *Journal of Public Health Management Practice* 2011; 17: E1–E11.
Manske SR, Miller S, Moyer C, Phaneuf MR, Cameron R. Best practice in group-based smoking cessation: Results of a literature review applying effectiveness, plausibility and practicality criteria. *American Journal of Health Promotion* 2004; 18: 409-423.
Marmot MG, Wilkinson RD. editors. *Social determinants of health.* Oxford, England: Oxford University Press, 2006.
McDonald PW. Population-based recruitment for quit smoking programs: An analytic review of communication variables. *Preventive Medicine* 1999; 28:545-557.
McLeod CB, Hall PA, Siddiqi A, Hertzman C. How society shapes the health gradient: Work-related health inequalities in a comparative perspective. *Annual Reviews of Public Health* 2012; 33:59-73.
Millward LM, Kelly MP, Nutbeam D. *Public health intervention research - the evidence.* Health Development Agency, London, 2003.
Naiman A, Glazier RH, Moineddin R. (2010). Association of anti-smoking legislation with rates of hospital admission for cardiovascular and respiratory conditions. *CMAJ* 2010; 182: 761-767.
Patton MQ. *Developmental evaluation: Applying complexity concepts to enhance innovation and use.* New York: Guilford Press, 2010.
Peckham S, Hann A, Boyce T. Health promotion and ill-health prevention: The role of general practice. *Quality in Primary Care* 2011; 19:317-323.
Porter ME, Kramer MR. Creating shared value. *Harvard Business Review* 2011; January-February (Reprint R1101C), 1-17.

Potvin L, Jones CM. Twenty-five years after the Ottawa charter: The critical role of health promotion for public health. *Can J Publ Hlth* 2011;102:244-248.

Puska P. Successful prevention of non-communicable diseases: 25 year experience with North Karelia project in Finland. *Public Health Medicine* 2002; 4:5-7.

Puska P, Stahl T. Health in all policies – the Finnish initiative: Background, principles, and current issues. *Annual Review of Public Health* 2010; 31:315-328.

Rose G. *Strategies of prevention: The individual and the population.* Oxford University Press: Oxford, England, 1992.

Ross L, Nisbett RE. *The person and the situation: Perspectives of social psychology.* New York: McGraw-Hill, 1991.

Shahab L, McEwen A. Online support for smoking cessation: A systematic review of the literature. *Addiction* 2009; 104:1792-1804.

Siddiqi A, Hertzman C. Towards an epidemiological understanding of the effects of long-term institutional changes on population health: A case study of Canada versus the USA. *Social Science & Medicine* 2007; 64:589-603.

Smith RD, Petticrew M. Public health evaluation in the twenty-first century: Time to see the wood as well as the trees. *Journal of Public Health* 2010; 32: 2-7.

Smoke-Free Ontario – Scientific Advisory Committee. *Evidence to guide action: Comprehensive tobacco control in Ontario.* Toronto, ON: Ontario Agency for Health Protection and Promotion, 2010.

Spoth R. Translating family-focused prevention science into effective practice: Towards a translational impact paradigm. *Current Directions in Psychological Science* 2008; 17:415-421.

Stead LF, Perera R, Lancaster T. A systematic review of interventions for smokers who contact quitlines. *Tobacco Control* 2007; 16(Suppl 1): i3-i8.

Strahan EJ, White K, Fong G, Fabrigar LR, Zanna MP, Cameron R. Enhancing the effectiveness of tobacco package warning labels: A social psychological perspective. *Tobacco Control* 2002; 11:183-190.

Sweet M, Moynihan R. Improving population health: The uses of systematic reviews. *Milbank Memorial Fund* Centers for Disease Control and Prevention, New York, NY, 2007; 1:73.

Swinburn B, Gill T, Kumanyika S. Obesity prevention: a proposed framework for translating evidence into action. *The International Association for the Study of Obesity--Obesity Reviews* 2005; 6:23-33.

The World Bank Human Development Network. *The growing danger of non-communicable diseases: Acting now to reverse course.* Conference Edition, 2011; pp. 1-14.

Truman BI, Smith-Akin CK, Hinman AR, Gebbie KM, Brownson R, Novick LF et al. Developing the guide to community preventive services - overview and rationale. *Am J Prev Med* 2000; 18(1S):18-26.

Westley F, Zimmerman B, Patton MQ. *Getting to maybe: How the world is changed.* Random House: Toronto, 2006.

Wilkinson R, Pickett K. *The spirit level: Why more equal societies almost always do better.* London: Allen Lane, 2009.

Willett WC, Koplan JP, Nugent R, Dusenbury C, Puska P, Gaziano TA. Prevention of chronic disease by means of diet and lifestyle changes. In D. T. Jamison, et al. (Eds.), *Disease control priorities in developing countries* (2nd edition). Washington (DC): World Bank, 2006.

World Cancer Research Fund / American Institute for Cancer Research. *Policy and action for cancer prevention. Food, nutrition, and physical activity: A global perspective.* Washington, DC: American Institute for Cancer Research, 2009.

World Health Organization / Health and Welfare Canada / Canadian Public Health Association. *The Ottawa charter for health promotion.* Ottawa: World Health Organization, 1986.

Yarnall KSH, Pollak KI, Ostbye T, Krause KM, Michener JL. Primary care: Is there enough time for prevention? *Am J Publ Hlth* 2003; 93:635-641.

Chapter 2
Preventing Cancer by Ending Tobacco Use

Neil Collishaw and Cynthia Callard

2.1 Introduction

Widely accepted epidemiological evidence about the health hazards of smoking was first published in the early 1950s (Doll and Hill 1950; Wynder and Graham 1950). By the early 1960s, the causal link between smoking and lung cancer and several other diseases had been definitively established and was documented in reports of the British Royal College of Physicians and Surgeons (Royal College of Physicians of London, Committee on Smoking and Atmospheric Pollution 1962) and the United States Surgeon General (United States Public Health Service 1964). As time went on, more and more diseases were found to be linked to smoking and passive smoking. By 2004, the United States Surgeon General had identified over 50 diseases and conditions caused or possibly caused by tobacco smoke (Surgeon General 2004). Over a dozen of these are cancers. It has recently been estimated that 19.4 % of all new cases of cancer in the United Kingdom are attributable to tobacco smoke (Parkin 2011). Similar results could be expected for countries at a similar mature stage of the tobacco epidemic (Lopez et al. 1994). Cancers caused by smoking occur disproportionately at sites with the poorest prognosis, such as lung, oesophagus and pancreas (American Cancer Society 2011). As a result, cancer caused by smoking or passive smoking accounts for a higher proportion of cancer deaths than other cancer cases — one-quarter to one-third of all cancer mortality (Cancer Research UK 2011; Canadian Cancer Society 2003).

Throughout the whole of the latter half of the twentieth century, many people believed that the link between smoking and disease was "not proven" (Oreskes and Conway 2010). However, because of a series of court settlements in the United States that required the release of previously secret tobacco industry documents,

N. Collishaw (✉) • C. Callard
Physicians for a Smoke-Free Canada, 1226 A Wellington Street,
Ottawa, ON K1Y 3A1, Canada
e-mail: ncollishaw@smoke-free.ca

A.B. Miller (ed.), *Epidemiologic Studies in Cancer Prevention and Screening*, Statistics for Biology and Health 79, DOI 10.1007/978-1-4614-5586-8_2,

scholars now have access to an extraordinary cache of information in over 13 million previously secret documents. Scholarly analyses of these documents have revealed that the "not proven" sentiment prevailed because the tobacco industry deliberately created it and maintained it over decades, even in the face of definitive scientific information to the contrary (Brandt 2007, 2012; Oreskes and Conway 2010; Michaels 2008). In an extensive trial initiated by the United States Department of Justice, tobacco companies were found guilty of racketeering and conspiracy under the US Racketeer Influenced and Corrupt Organizations Act. Their misdemeanours are documented in the judgement against them (Kessler 2006).

2.2 Progress in Tobacco Control to Date

Most of the tobacco control measures implemented to date seek to discourage tobacco use by smokers and potential smokers; they can be characterized as demand reduction measures. Other measures can be imagined that would seek to alter the current structure of the tobacco industry in ways favourable to public health protection. These can be thought of as supply control measures. One example would be an upper limit on the number of cigarettes permitted to be sold. Another example would be government-imposed conditions and restrictions under which tobacco companies may be permitted to earn profits. To date, governments have mainly eschewed use of supply control measures in constructing their tobacco control policies.

Partly because of the tobacco industry's campaign to manufacture doubt and uncertainty where none existed, governments were slow to act to control the tobacco epidemic. Among the countries that pioneered tobacco control measures were Norway, Finland and Singapore, which implemented tobacco advertising bans and other control measures in the 1970s. Canada, Australia and New Zealand followed with advertising bans, requirements for warnings on packages and other control measures in the late 1980s and early 1990s.

The 1990s also saw the first steps towards development of the Framework Convention on Tobacco Control (FCTC), a global tobacco control treaty. It came into force in 2005 and boasted 174 Parties by the end of 2011. The treaty codifies in international law the elements of the comprehensive tobacco control programmes that were already in force in a few countries. Most elements of the FCTC are demand reduction measures. They encourage or require Parties to adopt a series of tobacco control measures that include:

- Higher tobacco taxes to discourage consumption
- Bans on smoking in public places and workplaces
- Reporting of toxic substances in tobacco
- Large health warnings on packages (preferably with pictures)
- Extensive restrictions or bans on tobacco advertising
- Health education, health promotion
- Smoking cessation services

- Controls on smuggling
- Bans on sales to minors
- Promotion of alternative livelihoods for displaced tobacco workers
- Facilitation of legal liability action against tobacco companies

Other measures include guarding against the interference of the tobacco industry in the setting of public health policy, encouragement for general strengthening of tobacco control and provisions for further research, monitoring, reporting and cooperation. The existence of the FCTC and its rapid ratification by a large number of countries may have helped quicken the pace of adoption of tobacco control measures around the world. However, the FCTC is far from being fully implemented. Despite recent progress, only 6 % of the global population lives in countries that have comprehensive advertising bans and 15 % live in countries with large, graphic health warnings on cigarette packages (World Health Organization 2011). Even with the FCTC in force, the tobacco industry is continuing its longstanding practice of opposing national tobacco control measures. For example, Philip Morris has launched a challenge of Australia's new law requiring plain packaging. Philip Morris contends that the new law is a violation of a bilateral investment treaty between Australia and Hong Kong, a claim rejected by the Australian government legal team (Australian Government, Attorney General's Department 2011). Many FCTC-compliant laws have recently been contested in national courts. In some cases, the tobacco industry has succeeded in having tobacco control laws weakened or overturned. In all cases, litigation or the threat of litigation can slow or weaken the adoption of national tobacco control measures (Corporate Accountability International 2005). Tobacco companies also can and do challenge tobacco control laws in international tribunals. Currently, aspects of national tobacco control laws of FCTC Parties Norway, Australia and Uruguay are being challenged in international tribunals by the tobacco companies (Webster 2011).

2.3 Structural Impediments Will Slow Further Progress

By law, tobacco corporations are compelled to make profits. Under current corporate law, profit-making is a legal requirement that imposes an obligation on tobacco company management to seek to minimize the impact of public health measures to reduce smoking. In the 1980s, Player's cigarettes were advertised in Canada by means of the advertisement shown on the left of Fig. 2.1. In 1988, cigarette advertising was banned with certain limited exceptions for sponsorship advertising. When that law (The Tobacco Products Control Act*)* was invalidated in 1995, it was replaced by the Tobacco Act in 1997, which also banned tobacco advertising, also with certain limited exceptions for sponsorship advertising. Even after this second law was passed, Imperial Tobacco Company of Canada managed to skate through the regulations and find a way to continue advertising Player's cigarettes, using practically the same imagery as they had been using a decade earlier, while remaining technically within the law. The post-advertising ban example is shown in the

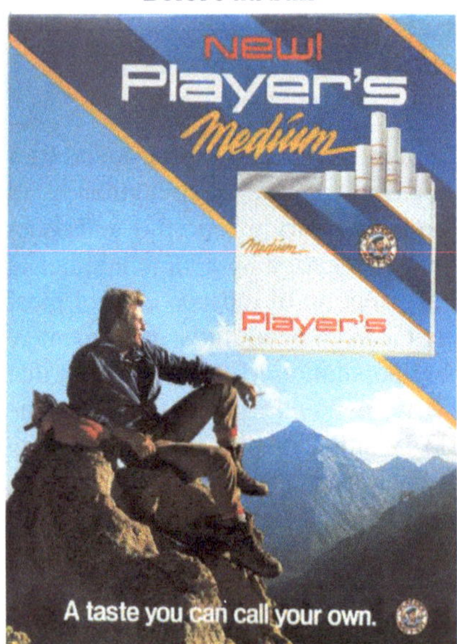

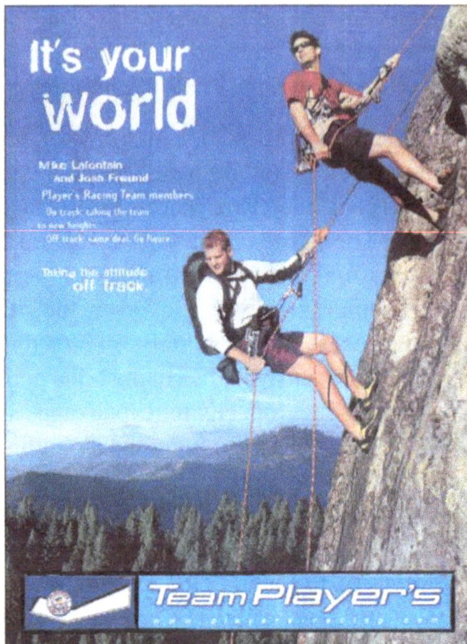

Fig. 2.1 Canadian advertisements for Player's cigarettes in the 1980s (*left panel*) and in 1998, two advertising bans later (*right panel*)

right-hand panel of Fig. 2.1. That legal loophole was closed and all tobacco sponsorship advertising has disappeared from Canadian media. Nevertheless, Imperial Tobacco was able to stretch out tobacco advertising, using their preferred imagery, for more than a decade after tobacco advertising had supposedly been prohibited.

State tobacco monopolies, even if they do not make profits for shareholders, are nevertheless required to maximize financial return to the state. There too, making money is given higher priority under law than protecting health. Tobacco companies do not adopt tobacco control measures; they adapt to them. It can be expected that in the future, unless their fiduciary obligations are fundamentally altered, tobacco companies will continue to oppose, weaken and mitigate tobacco control measures, particularly if they may threaten profit-making (Callard et al. 2005a).

2.4 More and Better Demand Reduction Measures Will Be Needed

The FCTC has proven itself an excellent tool for improving tobacco control around the world. In spite of the slow rate of progress of FCTC implementation and tobacco industry countermeasures, more and more countries are implementing effective tobacco control measures. As mentioned earlier, the FCTC mainly mandates demand reduction measures. Even if it were fully implemented in all countries, there is scope and justification for more tobacco demand reduction measures. There is a specific provision in the FCTC for Parties to implement stronger tobacco control measures than those required by the FCTC. Some of these additional demand reduction measures could include:

- Large warnings on packages, occupying 80–100 % of the largest surfaces of the package
- Plain and standardized packaging (currently being implemented in Australia)
- Retail display bans (currently in force in Canada, Iceland, Thailand and a few other countries)
- Bans on promotional allowances to wholesalers and retailers

Despite tobacco industry countermeasure, there has been progress in curbing the tobacco epidemic. For example, smoking prevalence declined from 50 % of adults in Canada in the mid-1960s to just 20 % in 2010 (Physicians for a Smoke-Free Canada 2011). In addition, at least two jurisdictions have proposed ambitious near-term targets for tobacco control, based largely on an expanded set of demand reduction measures. California has proposed targets of 10 % adult smoking prevalence and 8 % smoking prevalence for high-school-aged youth to be achieved by the end of 2014 (California Department of Public Health 2011). Australia has set a target of adult daily smoking prevalence of 10 % or less by 2018 (Australian Government 2011). Based on their success to date, both jurisdictions are on track to achieve these targets. However, while progress is being made in some countries in tobacco control, tobacco companies are expanding markets in others, particularly in Asia. The net result has been that global consumption of cigarettes remains high. It was estimated to be about six trillion cigarettes in 2011 (Euromonitor International 2011).

Even if all FCTC measures were implemented, as well as additional demand reduction measures, the combination of the powerful addictiveness of tobacco and the structural imperative that requires tobacco companies to oppose and weaken all public health measures that may threaten profits mean that we cannot expect to appreciably quicken the pace of progress against the global tobacco epidemic, unless something changes and changes radically.

2.5 A Paradigm Shift: Some Options for Supply Control Measures

More progress could be made if supply control measure were added to our current armamentarium of demand control measures for tobacco control. Supply control measures would change the ways that tobacco companies do business, to bring them more nearly in line with public health objectives. Governments have been reluctant to consider supply control measures, and their use has been discouraged by the World Bank (World Bank 1999). Nevertheless, some observers have proposed more comprehensive tobacco control measures that would include both demand and supply control measures. A few governments are also considering expanding tobacco control to include supply control measures.

2.5.1 *Proposals to Make Finland and New Zealand Tobacco-Free Nations*

Ending tobacco use has been set as a national goal by the governments of Finland and New Zealand. In the case of Finland, the 2010 Tobacco Act states that the government aims to "put an end to the use of tobacco products in Finland" (Ministry of Social Affairs and Health of Finland 2010). An official document of the New Zealand government (but not a statute) states, "the Government agrees with a longer term goal of reducing smoking prevalence and tobacco availability to minimal levels, thereby making New Zealand essentially a smoke-free nation by 2025". The same document also states, "The Government agrees to investigate further options for measures to reduce tobacco supply" (New Zealand Government 2010). Both of these governments have set bold objectives to make their countries tobacco-free. The New Zealand government did state that is would be considering a variety of policy proposals, including tobacco supply reduction proposals. However, neither the government of Finland nor the government of New Zealand has yet specified precisely how their ambitious goals might be accomplished. Others, however, have provided suggestions that these and other governments could consider.

2.5.2 *The Sinking Lid (New Zealand)*

A group of New Zealand researchers (Thomson et al. 2010) has proposed that a comprehensive set of demand control measures be combined with gradually more restrictive supply control measures, such as a 10 % per year reduction in manufacturing and import quotas for tobacco products (the sinking lid), until importation and sale of tobacco ceased or reached an acceptable low level (e.g. under 1 % prevalence). The researchers have proposed that the ever-declining tobacco supply quota be sold at auction to tobacco manufacturers. Increasing scarcity of quota would drive up its price, which would, in turn, drive up the price of cigarettes, further reducing prevalence. The authors acknowledge that such a system might work best, at least initially, in a geographically isolated country with no domestic tobacco manufacturing industry, such as New Zealand.

2.5.3 *The Tobacco Supply Agency (Australia)*

An Australian researcher (Borland 2003) has proposed that a monopsonistic agency be set up as the sole buyer and distributor of domestic and imported tobacco products. Through selective buying and regulation, such an agency could require manufacturers to supply more harm-reduced products and phase out the most harmful products. The new Tobacco Control Agency could also eliminate advertising, require plain packaging and large health warnings and otherwise restrict or even eliminate altogether communication by tobacco manufacturers with consumers. While the practicality of this proposal has been questioned (Liberman 2006), Borland has replied, "I think we should confront the fox of the tobacco industry rather than Liberman's approach of fixing holes in the fence of regulation" (Borland 2006). No nation has yet adopted the regulated market model.

2.5.4 Performance-Based Targets and Reversing Incentives (United States)

Stephen Sugarman, a Professor of Law at the University of California at Berkeley, has examined how performance-based regulation might be applied to health-threatening consumer products including cigarettes, alcohol, guns, junk food and motor vehicles (Sugarman 2009). Sugarman suggests that the ultimate performance-based measure for tobacco control would be reduced tobacco-caused disease and death, but its achievement would take too long to be a practical standard in a revised regulatory system. Instead, he proposes using reliable data on smoking rates as a satisfactory performance standard around which new tobacco control regulations could be built. Sugarman suggests that there be substantial financial penalties proposed if specified smoking prevalence reduction targets were not met. Sugarman expresses a preference for a penalty-only scheme as likely the most politically attractive. However, he also outlines a reward and penalty option that could be used, should the latter prove to be the more politically attractive. Under this scheme, firms would continue to be penalized for failing to meet targets. The added feature is that they would receive generous financial bonuses for surpassing their targets.

2.5.5 Performance-Based Targets and Reversing Incentives (Canada)

A Canadian team (Callard et al. 2005a, b) has proposed that, as an ideal outcome, control of the tobacco supply should be transferred to a non-profit agency with a public health purpose to phase out tobacco. Various ways of achieving this transfer and various structures for the operation of such a non-profit agency were proposed.

Later, it was recognized that "the world is not yet ready for wholesale replacement of institutions and structures by new ones" (Physicians for a Smoke-Free Canada 2010). They went on to describe a new system of performance-based regulation that would require existing tobacco companies to meet public health goals of year-over-year reductions in tobacco use. However, some significant change would have to happen for the tobacco industry to actually want to achieve significant public health purposes.

Large-scale performance-based regulation cannot be contemplated for the tobacco industry unless motivation for them to work in favour of public health can be created. It was proposed that the profit-making incentives be reversed. Some judicious combination of rewards and penalties could be constructed that would penalize companies with profit-negating penalties if targeted reductions in smoking prevalence were not met and reward them with profits if prevalence reduction targets were surpassed. This model (Physicians for a Smoke-Free Canada 2010) is similar to one proposed by Sugarman (2009). In this way, tobacco corporations could continue to fulfil their fiduciary responsibilities to make profits for their shareholders, but now they would be striving to accomplish tobacco prevalence reductions, a public health goal.

2.6 Discussion and Conclusions

The tobacco industry would almost certainly oppose any of the schemes outlined here. They would especially oppose supply control measures that they would see a direct attack on the way they do business. In the case of proposals for reversing incentives, one would not want to embark on such schemes unless there was also a willingness to transfer tobacco supply from profit-making enterprises to a non-profit agency with public health purpose, should the tobacco industry prove intransigent in their opposition to a new system of making profits through reversed incentives and performance-based regulation.

It has been suggested that there is a sound business case for purchasing the tobacco industry and transferring it to non-profit agencies with a public health purpose (Callard 2010; Collishaw 2011; Callard and Collishaw 2012). The sound business case applies both at the national and global levels. Using performance-based regulations and reversed incentives, a scheme to phase out tobacco over a couple of decades has the advantage that it could be done within existing structures and tobacco companies could still earn profits for their shareholders, with the important difference that profitability would be achieved by selling fewer cigarettes, not more. This route to profits would nevertheless necessarily end in 20–30 years when tobacco consumption reached near-zero levels. Two to three decades would be plenty of time for tobacco corporations to redeploy their capital into other profit-making pursuits. Like other future scenarios for tobacco control, no discernable steps are being taken towards implementation of performance-based regulation of tobacco.

There are early indications that governments in Finland and New Zealand wish to devise schemes to make their countries tobacco-free. Their wishes, however, have not yet been translated into concrete actions. Encouragingly, schemes proposed by researchers in New Zealand, Australia, the United States and Canada supply some ideas that could eventually be translated into government policy.

All proposals reviewed here recognize the fundamental conflict between the fiduciary obligation of tobacco companies to make money for their shareholders and the public health objective of reducing tobacco use to near-zero levels. Still other proposals not reviewed here also make the observation that the tobacco industry is a roadblock to the achievement of tobacco control and propose various solutions, all of which would alter the current structure or profit-making potential of the tobacco industry in some way (Glantz 1993; Liberman 2003; Enzi 2007; Hall and West 2008; Gerace 1999; Sugarman 2009; Gilmore et al. 2010; Khoo et al. 2010; Malone 2010; Rand Europe 2010; Tobacco Strategy Advisory Group 2010). A variety of options for restructuring to achieve public health goals have been proposed. While the structures proposed differ, they all seek to resolve or at least mitigate the fundamental conflict between the tobacco industry's goal of maximizing tobacco sales and the public health goal of phasing out tobacco. All these schemes share another characteristic—not one has been implemented. Moreover, apart from the official statements by Finland and New Zealand, there is little indication that even first steps along the road to planned supply and demand reduction of tobacco leading to its phase-out or near phase-out in a prescribed period of time are even being contemplated anywhere in the world. The only exception is the Himalayan Kingdom of Bhutan, which has banned the sale, but not the use, of tobacco products (Ugen 2003).

What would such first steps be? Before a solution can be implemented, there would first have to be widespread recognition that a problem exists. In open democratic societies, for a change that would be felt by millions of people, at least a very substantial minority would have to perceive that there was a problem and want something to be done about it. We are still a very long way from that situation. When asked who is responsible for the problem of uptake of smoking by youth, only 7 % of Canadians cite the tobacco industry (Canadian Tobacco Use Monitoring Survey 2010). Much larger proportions cited friends and peers (41 %), parents (22 %) and young people themselves (16 %). Few recognize that an oft-repeated objective of Imperial Tobacco Company of Canada was "to support the continued social acceptability of smoking" (Imperial Tobacco Limited 1988). Imperial Tobacco succeeded and continues to succeed in this objective. It is likely that they succeed by frequent, subtle and indirect influences on the friends, peers, parents and young people popularly believed to be responsible for the uptake of smoking by youth.

Greater awareness of the role of the tobacco industry in sustaining the tobacco epidemic is needed. The Health Officers Council of British Columbia (2011) has recognized this need, not only with respect to tobacco but also about alcohol and illicit drugs. They have recommended "that a national commission of inquiry be established to recommend ways of increasing emphasis on public health oriented approaches to alcohol, tobacco, currently illegal, prescription and other psychoactive substances". They would call on such a commission "to make recommendations for coherent and comprehensive public health oriented psychoactive substances related policies and programs". Such a commission of inquiry would raise public awareness of the control of tobacco and other psychoactive substances and could well be a very good initial step towards fostering greater public understanding of the need for a sound public health approach to the control of tobacco and other psychoactive substances.

References

American Cancer Society. *Cancer Facts and Figures*; 2011

Australian Government. *National Tobacco Campaign;* 2011. From http://www.quitnow.gov.au/internet/quitnow/publishing.nsf/Content/ntc-2009-2013-lp

Australian Government, Attorney-General's Department. *Investor-State Arbitration - Tobacco Plain Packaging*; 2011. From http://ag.gov.au/www/agd/agd.nsf/page/8F5B65DEBCAED226CA25796D006B4857

Borland R. A strategy for controlling the marketing of tobacco products: A regulated market model. *Tobacco Control* 2003; 12:374–382.

Borland R. Why not seek clever regulation? A reply to Liberman. *Tobacco Control* 2006; 15:339–340.

Brandt AM. Inventing conflicts of interest: A history of tobacco industry tactics. *Am J Pub Hlth* 2012; 102:63–71.

Brandt AM. *The Cigarette Century: The rise, fall and deadly persistence of the product that defined America.* 2007. New York: Basic Books.

California Department of Public Health. *Tobacco Education and Research Oversight Committee (TEROC).* Retrieved 2011 29-December from Saving Lives, Saving Money: Towards a Tobacco-Free California 2012-2014 - Mission, Vision, Goal, Principles, Objectives and Strategies (DRAFT): http://www.cdph.ca.gov/services/boards/teroc/Documents/Draft%20Master%20Plan%202012%20Principles%20Objectives%20and%20Strategies.pdf

Callard C. Follow the money: How the billions of dollars that flow from smokers in poor nations to companies in rich nations greatly exceed funding for global tobacco control and what might be done about it. *Tobacco Control* 2010; 19:285–290.

Callard C, Collishaw N. Exploring vector space: Overcoming resistance to direct control of the tobacco industry. *Tobacco Control* 2012; (in press).

Callard C, Thompson D, Collishaw N. *Curing the Addiction to Profits: A supply-side approach to phasing out tobacco.* 2005a; Ottawa, Canada: Canadian Centre for Policy Alternatives.

Callard C, Thompson D, Collishaw N. Transforming the tobacco market: why the supply of cigarettes should be transferred from for-profit corporations to non-profit enterprises with a public health mandate. *Tobacco Control* 2005b; 14:278–283.

Canadian Cancer Society. *From 21,000 cancer deaths could be prevented if people had quit smoking sooner.* 2003; http://www.cancer.ca/Canada-wide/About%20us/Media%20centre/CW-Media%20releases/CW-2003/21%20000%20cancer%20deaths%20could%20be%20prevented%20if%20people%20had%20quit%20smoking%20sooner.aspx?sc_lang=en. Retrieved 2011 28-December.

Canadian Tobacco Use Monitoring Survey. *Unpublished tabulations prepared by Physicians for a Smoke-Free Canada* 2010.

Cancer Research UK. *Smoking and Cancer.* Retrieved 2011 28-December from http://info.cancerresearchuk.org/healthyliving/smokingandtobacco/

Collishaw N. *European Conference on Tobacco or Health* 2011. From Phasing out tobacco: http://ectoh.org/documents/Neil%20Collishaw%202011%20Phasing%20out%20tobacco-7%20-%20v11.pdf

Corporate Accountability International. *Big Tobacco's Attempts to Derail the Global Tobacco Treaty: Cases from Battleground Countries* 2005.

Doll R, Hill A B. Smoking and carcinoma of the lung: preliminary report. *BMJ* 1950; ii (4682): 739–48.

Enzi M. *Bill S.1834. 110th Congress, First Session* 2007.

Euromonitor International. *Passport - Legislation: The Tobacco Control Noose Tightens.* 2011.

Gerace T. The toxic tobacco law: "appropriate remedial action". *J Publ Hlth Policy* 1999; 20: 394–407.

Gilmore AB, Branston JR, Sweanor D. The case for OFSMOKE: how tobacco price regulation is needed to promote the health of markets, government revenue and the public. *Tobacco Control* 2010; 19: 423–430.

Glantz SA. Removing the incentive to sell kids tobacco: a proposal. *JAMA* 1993; 269: 793–794.

Hall W, West R. Thinking about the unthinkable: a de facto prohibition on smoked tobacco products. *Addiction* 2008; 103: 873–874.

Imperial Tobacco Limited. *1988 Overview. Exhibit Number AG-51* (Vols. 77, page 15335). Montreal Court of Appeal, Case Numbers 500-09-001296-912 and 500-090001297-910. 1991. Joint Record, 1988.

Kessler G. *United States of America v. Philip Morris USA et al., Civil Action No. 99-2496 (GK). Amended Final Opinion.* 2006. Retrieved 2010 йил 01-June from http://www.justice.gov/civil/cases/tobacco2/amended%20opinion.pdf

Khoo D, Koong HN, Berrick A J. Phaisng out tobacco: proposal to deny access to tobacco for those born from 2000. *Tobacco Control* 2010; 19: 355–360.

Liberman J. The future of tobacco regulation: a response to a proposal for fundamental institutional change. *Tobacco Control* 2006; 15:333–338.

Liberman J. Where to for tobacco regulation: time for new approaches? *Drug and Alcohol Review* 2003; 22: 461–469.

Lopez A, Collishaw N, Piha T. A descriptive model of the cigarette epidemic in developed countries. *Tobacco Control* 1994; 3:242–247.

Malone RA. Imagining thngs otherwise: new endgame ideas for tobacco control. *Tobacco Control* 2010; 19:349–350.

Michaels D. *Doubt is their product: How industry's assault on science threatens your health.* 2008. New York: Oxford University Press.

Ministry of Social Affairs and Health of Finland. *The aim of the Tobacco Act is to put an end to smoking in Finland [Finnish government media release].* 2010. Retrieved 2011 21-December from http://www.stm.fi/tiedotteet/tiedot/view/1522179#en

New Zealand Government. *Government response to the Report of the Maori Affairs Committee on its Inquiry into the tobacco industry in Aotearoa and the consequences of tobacco use for Maori (Final Response).* 2010. Retrieved 2011 21-December from http://www.parliament.nz/NR/rdonlyres/3AAA09C2-AD68-4253-85AE-BCE90128C1A0/188520/DBHOH_PAP_21175_GovernmentFinalResponsetoReportoft.pdf

Oreskes N, Conway EM. *Merchants of Doubt: How a handful of scientists obscured the truth on issues ranging from tobacco smoke to global warming.* 2010. New York: Bloomsbury Press.

Parkin D. Tobacco-attributable cancer burden in the UK in 2010. *Br J Cancer* 2011;105: S6–S13.

Physicians for a Smoke-Free Canada. *Smoking in Canada.* 2011. From http://www.smoke-free.ca/factsheets/pdf/prevalence.pdf

Physicians for a Smoke-Free Canada. *Future options for tobacco control: Performance-based regulation of tobacco.* 2010.

Rand Europe. *Assessing the impacts from revising the Tobacco Products Directive: Study to support a DG SANCO impact assessment. Final Report.* 2010.

Royal College of Physicians of London, Committee on Smoking and Atmospheric Pollution. *A report of the Royal College of Physicians of London on smoking in relation to cancer of the lung and other diseases.* 1962. Toronto: McClelland and Stewart.

Sugarman SD. Performance-based regulation: Enterprise responsibility for reducing death, injury and disease caused by consumer products. (D. U. Press, Ed.) *Journal of Health Politics, Policy and Law* 2009; 34: 1035–1077.

Surgeon General. *The health consequences of smoking: a report of the Surgeon General.* 2004. Atlanta: Department of Health and Human Services, Centers for Disease Control and Prevention, National Center for Chronic Disease Prevention and Health Promotion, Office of Smoking and Health.

The Health Officers Council of British Columbia. *Public Health Perspectives for Regulating Psychoactive Substances: What we can do about alcohol, tobacco and other drugs.* 2011.

Thomson G, Wilson N, Blakely T, Edwards R. Ending appreciable tobacco use in a nation: using a sinking lid on supply. *Tobacco Control* 2010; 19: 431–435.

Tobacco Strategy Advisory Group. *Building on our gains, taking action now: Ontario's Tobacco Control Strategy for 2011–2016.* Ontario Ministry of Health Promotion and Sport, Toronto, 2010. From http://www.mhp.gov.on.ca/en/smoke-free/TSAG%20Report.pdf

Ugen S. Bhutan: the world's most advanced tobacco control nation? *Tobacco Control* 2003; 12:431–433.

United States Public Health Service. *Smoking and Health. Report of the Advisory Committee to the Surgeon General of the Public Health Service.* 1964. Centre for Disease Control.

Webster PC. Tobacco control measures under industry assault. *CMAJ* 2011; 183: E1233–E1234.

World Bank. *Curbing the Epidemic: Governments and the Economics of Tobacco Control.* Washington, 1999.

World Health Organization. *WHO Report on the Global Tobacco Epidemic.* Geneva, 2011.

Wynder EL, Graham EA. Tobacco smoking as a possible etiologic factor in bronchiogenic carcinoma; a study of 684 proved cases. *JAMA* 1950; 143: 329–336.

Chapter 3
Prevention of Occupationally Induced Cancer

Aaron Blair, Karin Hohenadel, Paul Demers, Loraine Marrett, and Kurt Straif

3.1 Occupational Causes of Cancer

Observations on workers provided some of the earliest information on the causes of cancer and other diseases. Ramazzini, in the 1700s, described many occupational diseases in *De Morbis Artificum Diatriba* (Bisetti 2006), and Percival Pott (1775) linked scrotal cancer in chimney sweeps to the nature of their work and exposure to soot providing the first identification of a chemical carcinogen. Expansion of the effort to identify occupational causes of cancer in the twentieth century through laboratory and epidemiologic investigations greatly increased our understanding of hazards in the workplace. Siemiatycki et al. (2004), in evaluation of the results of the International Agency for Research on Cancer (IARC) Monograph Program for the Evaluation of Carcinogenic Risks to Humans, found 31 % (28 of 89) of group 1 carcinogens were largely identified and characterized from the occupational arena, as were 42 % of the substances classified in group 2A (probably carcinogenic to humans) and group 2B (possibly carcinogenic to humans). Although the rate of identification of new workplace carcinogens may have diminished in recent decades (Blair et al. 2011), findings from studies of the workplace still play an important role

A. Blair (✉)
Occupational and Environmental Epidemiology Branch, Division of Cancer Epidemiology and Genetics, National Cancer Institute, Executive Plaza South, Room 8008, Bethesda, MD, USA
e-mail: blaira@mail.nih.gov

K. Hohenadel • P. Demers
Occupational Cancer Research Centre, Cancer Care Ontario, Toronto, ON, Canada

L. Marrett
Prevention and Cancer Control, Cancer Care Ontario, Toronto, ON, Canada

K. Straif
Section of IARC Monographs, International Agency for Research on Cancer, Lyon, France

A.B. Miller (ed.), *Epidemiologic Studies in Cancer Prevention and Screening*, Statistics for Biology and Health 79, DOI 10.1007/978-1-4614-5586-8_3,

in the identification of new human carcinogens, and the list of suspected occupational exposures that need further evaluation continues to grow (Straif 2008).

Given the large number of occupational exposures (and workplace conditions, such as shift work) implicated in the development of cancer, a number of efforts have been taken to estimate the proportion of cancer that might be due to occupational factors. Although there has been considerable debate regarding the utility and accuracy of such efforts (Saracci and Vineis 2011), estimates of the fraction of all cancers attributed to occupational exposures have generally been around 5 % (Straif 2008). This overall estimate, however, does not fully describe the impact of occupational exposures for several reasons. First, the contribution of occupational carcinogens to the overall burden of cancer should also be viewed in relation to the relative contributions from other categories of established cancer risk factors. The estimated fraction of cancers related to occupational exposures is similar to that for most other groups of risk factors, and only the estimated contributions from diet and tobacco are considerably larger (Doll and Peto 1981). Second, there is considerable variation in the reliability of the estimates of burden from the various categories of carcinogenic factors. For example, the estimated contribution from diet is probably more speculative than that for occupation. Third, there is considerable variation in the occupational contribution by type of cancer. The lung is the most frequent target organ for established occupational carcinogens (about one-third of the IARC class 1 occupational carcinogens affect the lungs) (Tomatis et al. 1997), and approximately twenty percent of this cancer in men may have an occupational origin (Nurminen and Karjalainen 2001; Rushton et al. 2010; Steenland et al. 2003; Straif et al. 2009). This is important because of the general lack of effective treatment and high mortality rate for lung cancer. Fourth, the cancer burden from occupational exposures is largely borne by blue-collar workers. Occupational exposures for these workers are typically not under their control, and the attributable fraction for cancer among these workers is considerably larger than the overall population value. This was well expressed by Doll and Peto (1981) when they noted that "Occupational cancer, moreover, tends to be concentrated among relatively small groups of people among whom the risk of developing the disease may be quite large, and such risks can usually be reduced or even eliminated, once they have been identified. The detection of occupational hazards should therefore have a higher priority in any program of cancer prevention than their proportional importance might suggest."

Although a considerable number of occupational exposures have been established as human carcinogens, our understanding of workplace hazards is far from complete. Many important workplace substances have not been fully evaluated and new exposures enter the workplace each year. Even for established workplace carcinogens, studies continue to provide new and valuable information on cancer risk in relation to low levels of exposure, individual susceptibility, and links with new cancer sites. Recent IARC deliberations for Monograph Volume 100 expanded the number of cancers linked to many established or suspected occupational carcinogens. Among the 87 agents listed as human carcinogens before Volume 100, for 25 substances there was sufficient evidence to add additional cancer sites as related to the exposure, and for 11 exposures there was limited evidence for additional sites

(Cogliano et al. 2011). For example, working groups concluded that there was sufficient evidence to link cancers of the larynx and of the ovary with asbestos exposure, in addition to long-established links with lung cancer and mesothelioma (Straif et al. 2009). The identification of new cancer sites associated with previously labeled carcinogenic substances can sometimes significantly increase the number of cancers associated with certain occupational exposures, as occurred with designation of leukemia as a cancer caused by formaldehyde, in addition to the previous link with cancer of the nasopharynx, a very rare tumor (Cogliano et al. 2011).

It is clear that occupationally induced cancers are an important contributor to the overall cancer burden and that they remain a public health concern. A recent survey of individuals from the scientific, medical, industry, and worker communities underscored this concern and identified occupational exposures and topics that they considered priority issues for future research (Hohenadel et al. 2011a).

3.2 Societal Efforts to Control Occupational Exposures

Because of the number of workplace factors that are known or suspected human carcinogens, efforts have been undertaken by the public and private sectors to eliminate or control exposure and reduce cancer risk. Control of occupational risk factors can be accomplished by a number of approaches, including eliminating the use of the hazardous material entirely, use of closed production technology, changing production methods, use of protective devices to limit risk by reducing exposures, and changing work practices or schedules, such as might be necessary to mitigate the effects of night shift work (Cherrie 2009).

Classification systems for carcinogens (e.g., IARC (Cogliano et al. 2011)) are an essential component of the effort to control hazardous workplace exposures. Information from these classification systems are used for regulation, hazardous product labeling, and material safety data sheets. Establishment of occupational exposure limits is also used to control exposure to carcinogens. Regulatory agencies in many countries perform such standard-setting activities. Some nongovernmental organizations are also involved. Organizations involved in recommending exposure limits, such as the American Conference of Governmental Industrial Hygienists and the European Union's Standing Committee on Occupational Exposures, generally use a large margin of safety for carcinogens as well as a carcinogen notation. However, other guideline-setting organizations such as the German MAK Committee will not set exposure limits for carcinogens without a known threshold for effect, and some regulating bodies have requirements to reduce exposure to as low as reasonably achievable (often referred to as ALARA). Perhaps surprisingly, relatively few carcinogens have been banned outright (e.g., asbestos in many countries). Other workplace carcinogens, such as benzidine and bis(chloromethyl)ether, have been banned in several countries or have had the scope of their usage reduced and strictly regulated. Some jurisdictions have passed toxic-use reduction legislation to encourage, or require, companies to reduce the use of hazardous substances through substitution with less toxic substances or through changes in industrial processes or work practices.

The underlying goal of all these activities is to eliminate or lower exposures and reduce cancer risk. These efforts have been successful in reducing exposure. Symanski and colleagues (1998a) assembled information from 119 published papers and other data resources to evaluate changes in occupational exposures over time. They found exposure levels decreased over time in 78 % of the studies and increased in 22 %. The decrease in exposure levels ranged from 4 % to 14 % per year, with a median annual decline of 8 % (Symanski et al. 1998b). Exposures declined more rapidly in manufacturing than mining, for aerosols than vapors, for studies including biological-based monitoring than those with only airborne monitoring, and for exposures measured after 1972 than those obtained earlier.

In the United Kingdom, Creely et al. (2006), using data from the National Exposure Database (NEDB), found that workplace exposures decreased between the early 1980s and early 2000s for dust and fumes in the rubber industry, toluene in the paint industry, respirable dust and respirable quartz in quarries, and wood dust in several industries. Thus, although there is evidence that efforts to reduce many exposures in industry have been successful over the past few decades, Cherrie et al. (2007) also found that the average exposure for 12 of 19 substances evaluated from the NEDB still exceeded the British occupational exposure limits, indicating that work is not complete and that additional intervention efforts are needed.

It is also important to recognize that exposure to workplace carcinogens remains quite common, especially in some industrial sectors. For example, shift work involving circadian disruption, classified as probably carcinogenic to humans based on limited evidence for increased risk of breast cancer (Cogliano et al. 2011), impacts approximately 20 % of the working populations in industrialized countries. Two other very common nonchemical exposures are occupational sun exposure and environmental tobacco (secondhand) smoke. The latter has diminished dramatically in many countries due to the introduction of regulations banning smoking in public places and workplaces, but occupational sun exposure remains common. The estimate from CAREX Canada is that approximately 10 % of the workforce has outdoor jobs. Other common exposures include diesel engine exhaust, polycyclic aromatic hydrocarbons, crystalline silica, benzene, and wood dust (http:\\www.carexcanada.ca). Millions of workers remain exposed to established or suspected carcinogens based on the recent efforts by the WHO to estimate the global burden of occupational disease (Driscoll et al. 2005).

Despite the number of occupational exposures labeled as definite or possible human carcinogens and the sizable effort in recent times to eliminate exposures or control their levels, there are few studies that specifically evaluate the effectiveness of these intervention efforts in reducing cancer rates in the workplace (Stayner et al. 1996; Tomatis et al. 1997). The conduct of such studies is challenging. The most direct approach would be through epidemiologic studies designed to compare cancer risks before and after exposure modification. These, however, are rare. Mirabelli (2009) found only five epidemiologic studies that assessed changes in cancer risk after efforts to control occupational exposure to asbestos or benzene. A recent effort focusing on asbestos found nine such studies among the voluminous literature on asbestos (Hohenadel et al. 2011b), and the primary purpose of most of these reports was actually hazard identification.

There are probably a number of reasons for this paucity of studies on the effectiveness of exposure control on disease prevention. First, control of exposure may itself be seen as the end point of the disease prevention effort. After all, causality has been established and actions to restrict exposure to an acceptable level have been designed and undertaken. Thus, it might appear that the most important activity is to monitor exposure to make sure target exposure limits are not exceeded. Exposure monitoring, including biomonitoring to assess all exposure routes and susceptible populations, is probably easier than monitoring an anticipated reduction in disease occurrence in relation to exposure control. Second, the assumption that removing or reducing exposure will result in a decrease in disease is not only rational but backed up by empirical evidence on some carcinogens. There is a wealth of information on changes in cancer risk following reduction or cessation of tobacco smoking (IARC 2007). Thus, one might conclude that direct evidence is not required for every carcinogen. The change in cancer risk following cessation of smoking, however, varies somewhat by cancer site, and it might not be unreasonable to expect such differences could also occur for various occupations, which have a much greater diversity of exposure–cancer combinations than with tobacco. Empiric information on such differences, should they occur, would provide important evidence regarding the effectiveness of standard setting. Exposure-response patterns used in the evaluation and characterization of occupational hazards for cancer can also be used to predict changes in disease occurrence that might be expected from reduction in exposure. Armstrong and Darnton (2011) found that the shape of the exposure-response relationship and the distribution of exposure were important in the prediction of the reduction in occupational disease associated with exposure control. Third, for most occupational carcinogens, the time period from achieving critical exposure until development of cancer symptoms or diagnosis is typically long and may span decades. Thus, the time required before changes in cancer rates could be observed following exposure reduction might be equally long. However, lung cancer, which typically has a long latency following smoking initiation, shows a reduction in risk after cessation of smoking compared to continuing smokers in just a few years (IARC 2007). Fourth, the design of epidemiologic studies to compare cancer rates after exposure changes is challenging for several reasons. Direct comparison in a single workplace is difficult because many of the workers employed when the exposure modification took place will have already experienced earlier and heavier exposures. This contamination complicates isolating the cancer risks from the lower exposure levels after intervention from earlier, higher levels. Use of workers first employed after the exposure control would avoid the "contamination" problem, but this would most likely result in age at exposure and other differences between workers employed before and after the change that would complicate comparisons between the two groups. Selecting a "comparison" facility where exposure modification has not occurred would be another option, but this may introduce other problems and it would certainly increase the cost of the study. Finally, there may be no obvious source of funding for studies of an "established" workplace carcinogen. Funding for epidemiologic studies is largely devoted to hazard identification or characterization. Establishment of an exposure standard is probably a disincentive for funding for further study, rather than an advantage.

Registries of exposed workers and occupational cancers (Anttila et al. 1996; Bruske-Hohlfeld et al. 1997; McCormack et al. 2012; Straif and Silverstein 1997; Scarselli et al. 2010a, 2010b) are resources that may be used to assess prevention and protection measures. Compensation for occupational diseases is a type of surveillance that can provide an indication of changes in the cancer burden from occupational exposures following exposure elimination or reduction. However, this approach heavily depends on the legal context and is probably most effective for cancers that are overwhelmingly tied to a specific occupational exposure, such as mesothelioma. There are not many such sentinel cancers. This approach would not work well for lung cancer from asbestos exposure because cancer of the lung is often associated with other occupational carcinogens and many nonoccupational factors. A study of compensation and cancer registry databases in Ontario found that only 35 % of Ontarians diagnosed with mesothelioma between 1980 and 2002 filed for worker's compensation (Payne and Pichora 2009). Although an estimated 1 to10 lung cancers occur from asbestos exposure for every mesothelioma (Albin et al. 1999), the Ontario study found that only one-half as many lung cancers as mesotheliomas were awarded compensation in relation to asbestos exposure (Pichora and Payne 2007).

3.3 Evidence for Reduction in Cancer from Control of Workplace Exposure

Despite the challenges in evaluating the effectiveness of workplace prevention efforts, there are a few examples in the literature that demonstrate changes in cancer occurrence are associated with reductions in exposure. An early effort compared the incidence of bladder cancer in a cohort of benzidine manufacturing workers before and after exposure-reduction efforts (Meigs et al. 1986). The risk of bladder cancer risk was considerably greater among men first employed during the earliest years of the plant operation and before preventive measures were undertaken than among those employed later, even after rates were adjusted for duration of follow-up. Rates of nasal cancer were high during the early part of the twentieth century when respirable dust control in the wood furniture industry was lacking. Hayes et al. (1986) found that nasal cancer rates were considerably lower among workers in the Netherlands first entering the industry after 1940 than those entering earlier. In fact, no nasal cancers were found among those entering after 1941 when controls on wood dust exposure were introduced. Lung cancer among chloromethyl ether workers was dramatically lower among those exposed more recently than those employed in the industry earlier when exposures were higher (Swerdlow 1990). Follow-up, however, among the more recent workers may not have been sufficiently long to allow for the full impact of the exposure on disease occurrence, particularly because lower exposures may result in longer latencies. The risk of nasal cancer among nickel refinery workers in Norway was considerably lower among those entering the industry around 1960s than among those entering in the 1930s, when exposures were higher (Magnus et al. 1982). The risk of angiosarcoma of the liver decreased dramatically from those first employed in vinyl chloride industry in the 1940s to those first employed in the 1960s, consistent with a reduction of exposure (Boffetta et al. 2003). Risk of lung cancer decreased with time since last exposure to arsenic among smelter workers, which is a type of exposure control (Lubin et al. 2008).

In a recent effort to examine the effectiveness of asbestos-related interventions, a systematic review of the published literature was conducted to identify studies that evaluated changes in occurrence of lung cancer, mesothelioma, or overall malignancy with changes in exposure (Hohenadel et al. 2011b). The review examined 744 papers cited in the IARC Monographs on asbestos (volumes 7, 14 and 100C) and 350 articles found on PubMed since the last monograph (from March 2009 to December 2010). From these 1,094 epidemiological papers, nine provided information on changes in cancer risk subsequent to attempts at control of asbestos exposure. Decreases in risk of lung cancer, mesothelioma, and/or overall malignancy were evaluated in all studies and some studies additionally included information on other cancer sites. Exposure interventions included efforts to reduce asbestos dust exposure by application of closed-drum mixing and introducing wet processes, production discontinuation and factory closures, and total governmental bans. Although a number of decreases in cancer rates were observed in these studies, results were complex and few overall discernible patterns emerged across studies. It did appear that decreases in risk tended to occur for lung cancer sooner than for mesothelioma; that for studies providing information on risk by timing of exposure or change in exposure, relative risks started to decline 10–15 years after exposure control for both lung cancer and mesothelioma; and that in some cases, the decline in risk appeared to begin prior to the actual exposure intervention.

These findings underscore the challenges in evaluating patterns of relative risk following occupational exposure interventions. First, few studies were conducted specifically to measure the effectiveness of interventions on reducing cancer risk. Second, the interventions described, the cancers evaluated, and the length of the follow-up periods varied substantially for the different studies. This made it largely impossible to create summary variables or to perform meta-analyses, across studies to assess overall changes in disease patterns. Third, the approach to handling potential confounders, such as tobacco smoking, varied among the studies, and often the numbers of cases were small (particularly for mesothelioma). Still, this review provides evidence that interventions on asbestos exposure have been effective in decreasing cancer risk, and it highlights the need for studies on interventions in the future to more fully characterize these efforts for established occupational carcinogens.

In some situations, it is possible to look at the impact of an intervention on cancer risks at a population level. Because most mesotheliomas are caused by workplace exposure to asbestos, it is a good target for ecologic-/geographic-based efforts to assess the impact of exposure-based regulations on disease rates over time. Use of asbestos in many industrialized countries peaked in the 1970s, providing an opportunity to track subsequent changes in mesothelioma rates in the population. Assuming a 30–40-year lag, reflecting the latency of this disease, rates should be peaking now or in the next decade for the earliest interventions. Sweden, which passed regulations to restrict exposure to asbestos in the mid-1970s, saw a stabilization of the incidence rate of pleural mesothelioma in the 1990s (Hemminki and Hussain 2008). In Canada, where regulation was initiated somewhat later, the incidence of mesothelioma has continued to rise (Marrett et al. 2008; Kirkham et al. 2011). In Great Britain, the peak for mesothelioma is projected for 2015 with a rapid decline thereafter (Hodgson et al. 2005; Tan et al. 2010).

3.4 Future Needs

A number of past and present occupational exposures have been identified as known or suspect carcinogens. Societal efforts to control many of these exposures and to reduce cancer risks have been implemented, particularly in developed countries. Intervention efforts may not be as extensive in developing countries and where enforcement of legal standards – if they exist – may be lacking all together. Although research efforts devoted to the identification of occupational hazards and major investments in exposure control activities are commonplace, relatively little attention or resources has been devoted to assessing the success of these efforts. Although information on prevention is sometimes obtained in studies focusing on evaluation of occupational hazards, resources for these studies may be diminishing also.

Some information on prevention of cancer from exposure control can be gleaned from currently available data resources, but a more thorough assessment would allow a more complete documentation of the benefits of these actions. The literature on established occupational carcinogens should be carefully surveyed to extract information that may be buried in papers that have an etiologic orientation, as was found for asbestos (Hohenadel et al. 2011b). Changes in cancer rate over time and by geographic area can continue to be used to evaluate changes for cancers that are sentinels for an occupational exposure, such as mesothelioma and angiosarcoma of the liver. Unfortunately this approach cannot be used for most occupational exposure–cancer associations because few exposures result in such sentinel cancers.

Some information on disease rates following changes in exposure can probably be retrieved from unpublished data in completed studies. Cohort studies in industry often span time periods that include significant exposure modification, and these could perhaps be used to relate reduction in exposure to changes in disease rates. Case-control studies might also be used for this purpose, although occupational exposure assessment is often not sufficient for the task.

Studies specifically designed to evaluate changes in cancer risks following exposure intervention are desirable. They are needed to provide information on various aspects of the exposure control process, including the success of different exposure control approaches; the consistency across different age, gender, and exposure subgroups; multiple changes of exposure limits; and possible effect modification by lifestyle and other occupational exposures. Documented information on successful interventions on occupational carcinogens at low and moderate levels, as well as at high levels, would provide additional incentives for occupational cancer control.

References

Albin M, Magnani C, Krstev S, Rapiti E, and Shefer I. Asbestos and cancer: An overview of current trends in Europe. *Environ Health Perspect* 1999; 107(Suppl 2): 289–298.

Anttila A, Heikkila P, Nykyri E, Kauppinen T, Pukkala E, Hernberg S, Hemminiki K. Risk of nervous system cancer among workers exposed to lead. *J Occup Environ Med* 1996; 38:131–136.

Armstrong BG, Darnton A. Estimating reduction in occupational disease burden following reduction in exposure. *Occup Environ Med* 2011; 65:592–596.

Bisetti AA. Bernardino Ramazzini and occupational lung medicine. *Ann NY Acad Sci* 2006; 534:1029–1037.

Blair A, Marrett L, Beane Freeman L. Occupational cancer in developed countries. *Environmental Health* 2011; 10: (Suppl 1) 59.

Boffetta P, Matisane L, Mundt KA, Dell LD. Meta-analysis of studies of occupational exposure to vinyl chloride in relation to cancer mortality. *Scand J Work Environ Health* 2003; 29: 220–229.

Bruske-Hohlfeld I, Mohner M, Wichmann HE. Predicted number of lung cancer cases in Germany among former uranium miners of the Wismut. *Health Physics* 1997; 72:3–9.

Cherrie JW. Reducing occupational exposure to chemical carcinogens. *Occup Med* 2009; 59:96–100.

Cherrie JW, Van Tongeren M, Semple S. Exposure to occupational carcinogens in Great Britain. *Ann Occup Hyg* 2007; 51:653–664.

Cogliano VJ, Baan R, Straif K, Grosse Y, Lauby-Secretan B, Ghissassi FE et al. Preventable exposures associated with human cancers. *J Natl Cancer Inst* 2011; 103:1827–1839.

Creely KS, Van Tongeren M, While D, Soutar AJ, Tickner J, Agostini M et al. *Trends in inhalation exposure; mid 1980s till present.* HSE report RR460. 2006; Sudbury, UK: HSE books, Available at http://www.hse.gov.uk/research/rrhtm/rr460.htm.

Driscoll T, Nelson DI, Steenland K, Leigh J, Concha-Barrientos M, Fingerhut M, Pruss-Ostun A. The global burden of disease due to occupational carcinogens. *Am J Ind Med* 2005; 48: 419–431.

Doll R, Peto R. The causes of cancer: quantitative estimates of avoidable risks of cancer in the United States today. *J Natl Cancer Inst* 1981; 66:1191–1308.

Hayes RB, Gerin M, Raatgever JW, de Bruyin A. Wood-related occupations, wood dust exposure and sinonasal cancer. *Am J Epidemiol* 1986; 124:569–577.

Hemminki K, Hussain S. Mesothelioma incidence has leveled off in Sweden. *Int J Cancer* 2008; 122:1200–1201.

Hodgson JT, McElvenny DM, Darnton AJ, Price MJ, Peto J. The expected burden of mesothelioma mortality in Great Britain from 2002 to 2050. *Br J Cancer* 2005; 92:587–593.

Hohenadel K, Pichora E, Marrett L, Bukvic D, Brown J, Harris SA, et al. Priority issues in occupational cancer research: Ontario stakeholder perspectives. *Chronic Disease Injuries Canada* 2011a; 31:147–151.

Hohenadel K, Straif K, Demers PA, Blair A. The effectiveness of asbestos-related interventions in reducing rates of lung cancer and mesothelioma: a systematic review. *Occupational and Environmental Medicine* 2011b; 68 (Suppl 1) A71 doi:10.1136/oemed-2011-100382.229.

IARC. *Tobacco Control: Reversal of Risk after Quitting Smoking*. IARC Handbooks on Cancer Prevention. 2007; Volume 11. Lyon, France.

Kirkham TL, Koelhoorn MW, McLeod CH, Demers PA. Surveillance of mesothelioma and workers' compensation in British Columbia, Canada. *Occup Environ Med* 2011; 66:30–35.

Lubin JH, Moore LE, Fraumeni JF Jr, Cantor KP. Respiratory cancer and inhaled inorganic arsenic in copper smelters workers: A linear relationship with cumulative exposure that increases with concentration. *Environ Health Perspect* 2008; 116:1661–1665.

Magnus K, Andersen A, Hogetveit AC. Cancer of respiratory organs among workers at a nickel refinery in Norway. *Int J Cancer* 1982; 30:681–685.

Marrett LD, Ellison LF, Dryer D. Canadian cancer statistics at a glance: mesothelioma. *CMAJ* 2008; 178:677–678

McCormack V, Peto J, Byrnes G, Straif K, Boffetta P. Estimating the asbestos-related lung cancer burden from mesothelioma mortality. *Br J Cancer* 2012 Jan 10 doi:10.1038/bjc2011.563. [Epub ahead of print].

Meigs JW, Marrett LD, Ulrich FU, Flannery JT. Bladder tumor incidence among workers exposed to benzidine: a thirty-year follow-up. *J Natl Cancer Inst* 1986; 76:1–8.

Mirabelli D. Evidence of effectiveness and prevention of occupational cancer. *Epidemiologia & Prevenzione* 2009; 33:74–78.

Nurminen M, Karjalainen A. Epidemiologic estimate of the proportion of fatalities related to occupational factors in Finland. *Scandinavian Journal of Work Environment Health* 2001; 27:161–213.

Payne JL, Pichora E. Filing for workers' compensation among Ontario cases of mesothelioma. *Can Respirat J* 2009; 16:148–152.

Pichora EC, Payne JI. Trends and characteristics of compensated occupational cancer in Ontario, Canada, 1937–2003. *Am J Ind Med* 2007; 50:980–991.

Pott P. *Chirurgical Observations Relative to the Cataracts, the Polypus of the Nose, the Cancer of the Scrotum, the Different Kinds of Ruptures and Mortifications of the Toes and Feet.* 1775; London, T.J. Carnegy.

Rushton L, Bagga S, Brown T, Cherrie J, Holmes P, Fortunato L et al. Occupational and cancer in Britain. *Brit J Cancer* 2010; 102:1428–1437.

Saracci R, Vineis P. Environment and cancer: the legacy of Lorenzo Tomatis. *Environmental Health* 2011; 10: (Suppl 1) 51.

Scarselli A, DiMarzio D, Marinaccio A, Iavicoli S. The register of exposed workers to carcinogens: legislative framework and data analysis. *Med Del Lavoro* 2010a; 101:9–18.

Scarselli A, Massari S, Binazzi A, DiMarzio D, Scano P, Marinaccio A, Iavicoli S. Italian National Registry of Occupational Cancers: data system and findings. *J Occup Environ Med* 2010b; 52:346–353.

Siemiatycki J, Richardson L, Straif K, Lateille B, Lakhani R, Campbell S. et al. Listing occupational carcinogens. *Environ Health Perspect* 2004; 112:1447–1459.

Stayner L, Kuempel E, Rice F, Prince M, Althouse R. Approaches for assessing the efficacy of occupational health and safety standards. *Am J Ind Med* 1996; 29:353–357.

Steenland K, Burnett C, Lalich N, Ward E, Hurrell J. Dying for work: The magnitude of US mortality from selected causes of death associated with occupation. *Am J Ind Med* 2003; 43, 461–482.

Straif K. The burden of occupational cancer. Occup Environ Med 2008; 65:787–788.

Straif K, Benbrahim-Tallaa L, Baan R, Grosse Y, Secretan B, El Ghissassi F et al. A review of human carcinogens—Part C: metals, arsenic, dusts, and fibres. *Lancet Oncology* 2009; 10:453–454.

Straif K, Silverstein M. Comparison of U.S. Occupational Safety and Health Administration Standards and Germn Berufsgenossenschaften guidelines for Preventive Occupational Health Examinations. *Am J Ind Med* 1997; 31:373–380.

Swerdlow AJ. Effectiveness of primary prevention of occupational exposures on cancer risk. In: Hakama M, Beral V, Cullen JW, Parkin DM (eds). *Evaluating effectiveness of primary prevention of cancer*. IARC Scientific Publication 1990; No. 103, Lyon France, pp 23–56.

Symanski E, Kupper LI, Rappaport SM. Comprehensive evaluation of long term trends in occupational exposure: part 1. Description of the database. *Occup Environ Med* 1998a; 55:300–309.

Symanski E, Kupper LI, Rappaport SM. Comprehensive evaluation of long term trends in occupational exposure: part 2. Predictive models for declining exposures. *Occup Environ Med* 1998b; 55:310–316.

Tan E, Warren N, Darnton AJ, Hodgson JT. Projection of mesothelioma mortality in Britain using Bayesian methods. *Br J Cancer* 2010; 103:430–436.

Tomatis L, Huff J, Hertz-Picciotto I, Sandler DP, Bucher J, Boffetta P et al. Avoided and avoidable risks of cancer. *Carcinogenesis* 1997; 18:97–105.

Chapter 4
Human Papillomavirus Vaccination for the Prevention of Cervical and Other Related Cancers

F. Xavier Bosch

4.1 Establishment of the Causality Link Between HPV Infections and Cancer

4.1.1 Etiology

The etiology of cervical cancer has been significantly linked to persistent infection with up to 15 strains of human papillomavirus (HPV). The association is consistent worldwide, and causality has been generally accepted based on molecular epidemiological studies, including prevalence surveys, case–control studies, cohort studies using cervical intraepithelial neoplasia (CIN) of grade 2/3 as surrogate endpoints, and screening studies. More recently, HPV vaccination trials have consistently concluded that vaccination against HPV types 16 and 18 could virtually eliminate the occurrence of HPV 16-/18-related CIN 2/3 if given to individuals not carrying the infection at the time of vaccination, thus providing the ultimate proof of causality in human populations.

An International Agency for Research on Cancer (IARC) Monograph Working Group concluded that there was sufficient evidence in humans for the carcinogenicity of HPV types 16, 18, 31, 33, 35, 39, 45, 51, 52, 56, 58, and 59 in the cervix (IARC 2007). HPV types 26, 66, 68 73, and 82 were found to be associated with cervical cancer in some case–control studies, but the prevalence was very low in case series. For some rare types (HPV types 26, 53, 68, 73, and 82), the odds ratios (OR) observed are of similar magnitude to that of HPV 66 but, given the low prevalence

F.X. Bosch (✉)
Head, Cancer Epidemiology Research Program (CERP),
Catalan Institute of Oncology (Institut Català d'Oncologia - ICO)
& Bellvitge Biomedical Research Institute (IDIBELL),
Avda. Gran Via 199-203 08907 L'Hospitalet de Llobregat
(Barcelona), Barcelona, Spain,
e-mail: admincerp@iconcologia.net

A.B. Miller (ed.), *Epidemiologic Studies in Cancer Prevention and Screening*, Statistics for Biology and Health 79, DOI 10.1007/978-1-4614-5586-8_4,

observed in cases, these types were temporarily classified as "probably" carcinogenic or, for HPV 66, as "limited evidence"(Bouvard et al. 2009). The consensus to date is that HPV is the central and necessary cause of cervical cancer and that at least fifteen HPV types are capable of inducing an invasive cancer.

4.1.2 HPV DNA Type Distribution in Cervical Cancer and Rationale for HPV 16 and 18 Vaccines

The distribution of HPV types in cervical cancer has been published in a pooled analysis of about 3,000 cases from the IARC program (Munoz et al. 2004) and in a meta-analysis of about 14,000 cases (Smith et al. 2007). The eight most common HPV types detected in both series, in descending order of frequency, were HPV types 16, 18, 45, 31, 33, 52, 58, and 35, and these are responsible for about 90% of all cervical cancers worldwide. Two of the types – HPVs 16 and 18 – are consistently found associated with at least 70% of the cases on several worldwide estimates (Bosch et al. 1995; de Sanjose et al. 2010; Munoz et al. 2004), and these were identified as the two types included in the first generation of virus-like particle (VLP) HPV vaccines. The results have been recently confirmed in two landmark studies, one in the US population (Wheeler et al. 2009) and a large international survey, including specimens from close to 40 countries and slightly over 10,000 cervical cancer cases (de Sanjose et al. 2010).

These two studies are critical because they used unified criteria for the fieldwork, centralized laboratory protocols both for pathology and for HPV testing and typing, and unified statistical treatment of the data, particularly on the causality attribution to any given HPV type when multiple infections were detected in a specimen. These two studies largely overcome the limitations inherent to meta-analyses and other forms of literature summaries. The HPV type distributions in cancer are geographically consistent in identifying HPV 16 and 18 followed by 45, 31, and 33 as the leading HPV types with moderate variability in the third and subsequent types (e.g., in the cases from Asia – particularly from Japan – where HPV types 58, 33, and 52 were relatively common). These distributions are sensitive to the technologies employed for HPV testing and typing as well as to the methods used to attribute causality when there are multiple HPV types in a given specimen. Of interest is the finding that cervical adenocarcinoma is a subtype of cervical cancer related almost solely to three HPV types (16, 18, and 45), with a tenfold gap in prevalence between the third most common type and any other type (de Sanjose et al. 2010).

4.1.3 The Role of HPV in Genital Cancers Other than Cervical

The available clinical and epidemiological studies indicate that cancers of the vagina and of the anus resemble cancer of the cervix with respect to the role of HPV. In both cases, HPV DNA is detected in the majority of tumors and particularly of their precursor lesions. In recent reviews, between 64% and 91% of vaginal cancer cases and 82% and 100% of vaginal intraepithelial neoplasia of grade 3 (VAIN 3) lesions are HPV DNA positive. In anal cancers in both genders, HPV DNA is detected in 88–94%. An estimated 40–50% of cancers of the vulva have also been associated with HPV as have some 40% of the penile carcinomas. The evidence available for some of these sites is not as comprehensive as for cervical cancer, although causality has been generally recognized (Forman 2012; IARC 2007).

In all HPV-positive anogenital cancers, HPV 16 is the most common HPV type detected, followed by HPV types 18, 31, and 33. The combined contribution of HPV 16 and 18 has been estimated in a range of 88–93%, significantly higher that the relative contribution to cervical cancer (de Vuyst et al. 2009; Miralles-Guri et al. 2009).

4.1.4 The Role of HPV in Head and Neck Cancers

HPV DNA can be consistently identified in a significant fraction of cancers of the oropharynx (i.e., in the 40–50% range) and in smaller proportions of the specimens of the remaining cancer of the oral cavity and the larynx (5–15%) (Gillison 2012; Gillison et al. 2000).

Cancers of the head and neck and particularly of the oropharynx are becoming of increasing interest since time trends suggest that incidence is on the rise; it strikes young individuals of both genders, is unrelated to alcohol or tobacco consumption, and linked to patterns of sexual behavior involving multiple partners and oral sex (D'Souza et al. 2007; Heck et al. 2010; Rintala et al. 2006). For these cancers, no screening opportunities have been previously identified. In estimates and projections of the cancer incidence in the USA, it has been estimated that numerically these cancers are likely to become more frequent than cervical cancer (Chaturvedi et al. 2011). Similar trends have been observed in the Nordic countries (Nasman et al. 2009). However, the natural history of oral HPV infections and the additional risk factors of neoplastic transformation as well as the characterization of the preneoplastic lesions that could be amenable to screening are largely unknown.

Of interest is the observation that HPV-related head and neck cancers are of increased sensitivity to treatments with chemotherapy and radiotherapy as compared to the HPV unrelated cases, usually linked to alcohol and tobacco consumption. HPV testing is increasingly adopted as part of the routine diagnostic workup of these cancers and is a useful guide to clinical management (Ragin and Taioli 2007).

4.2 Phase III Vaccination Trials: Synthesis of the Critical Results

There are currently two HPV vaccines identified as Gardasil® (Merck & Co., Inc., Whitehouse Station, NJ, USA) and Cervarix® (GlaxoSmithKline Biologicals, Rixensart, Belgium). Gardasil targets two oncogenic HPV types (16 and 18) and two nononcogenic HPV types (6 and 11) responsible for genital warts and respiratory papillomatosis. Cervarix targets two oncogenic HPV types (HPV 16 and 18) and is formulated with a novel adjuvant ASO4 included to boost the immune response. The essential results of the phase III clinical trials have been already provided, and these two vaccines are currently licensed in over 120 countries. Most developed countries have introduced HPV vaccines into routine vaccination programs with specific recommendations, and more than one hundred million doses have already been distributed in 2011.

Phase III results for both vaccines are available for women in the 15–26 age range (Table 4.1). Trials have examined vaccine efficacy (VE) in several cohorts of HPV-unexposed and HPV-exposed women and in several age ranges. For simplicity, results in Table 4.1 are presented in qualitative format and reflect VE in the most appropriate study cohort. In addition, several ancillary protocols have been completed or are under way including bridging studies in the 9–15 years of age for both girls and boys and in the 26–45 years of age women. More limited information is also available of the VE in adult men and in special populations (immunosuppressed transplant patients, HIV-infected populations, infants, and others).

These two vaccines have shown to date a very high efficacy against the predefined endpoint lesions (HPV 16- or 18-related CIN 2 or superior [CIN 2+]), adequate safety and tolerability profiles, high immunogenicity, duration of protection so far of 7–8 years, and strong indications of ability to induce immune memory. Some degree of cross protection against CIN 2+ related to other HPV types (HPV 31 for both vaccines and HPV 33 and 45 for Cervarix) has been documented. Therefore, the global estimates of the protection against cervical cancer of the currently available vaccines in properly vaccinated populations range from strictly 70% of the cervical cancer cases attributed to HPV 16 and 18 to a range of 75–80% adding non-vaccine HPV-type cross protection. The latter however still requires some additional evaluation in terms of quantification of the vaccine efficacy estimates and on the potential duration of the protective effect of the types not included in the vaccine. None of the vaccines has shown therapeutic activity. Finally, it is important to note that these estimates show little geographic variation; thus, these vaccines should be considered of global validity.

The limitations of current vaccines are known and include the lack of therapeutic effect, the limited impact of the cross protection effect, and, as a consequence of the two, the requirement to continue some form of screening programs among vaccinated women. Finally, the cost of the production technology is high translating into the high cost of the vaccine at least in the early years after introduction in developed countries (Centers for disease control and prevention. 2009; European center for disease prevention and control 2008; Markowitz et al. 2007; Schiller et al. 2008).

In addition to the pivotal phase III trials, additional research has generated critical information to guide the use of the HPV vaccines. Among the most relevant results, trials that have examined vaccine efficacy among women up to the age of 45 have shown that even though the antibody titers generated by vaccination are lower, protection against persistent infection and CIN 2+ lesions is high (Castellsague

Table 4.1 Phase III trials of HPV vaccine in 2012: synthesis of the most important features and results (Adapted from Bosch et al. (2008) and Schiller et al. (2008))

	End point	Gardasil®	Cervarix®	Comments
Key features	*Viral types included*	6, 11, 16, 18	16, 18	Introduced since 2006
	Target	Protection from cancer (CIN 2+) & genital warts	Protection from cancer (CIN 2+)	CIN 2+ as surrogate of cervical cancer for phase III trials
	Adjuvant	Aluminum salts	Aluminum salts + AS 04[a]	AS 04 is a non specific stimulant of the immune response
	Safety	Safe	Safe	In controlled trials & post introduction surveillance
	Tolerance	Acceptable	Acceptable	Compliance with a three dose regime is very high
Immunology results	*Immune response (Antibodies)*	High Ab levels to HPV 16 for 7–8 years.	High Ab levels to HPV 16 & 18 for 7–8 years	Sero-conversion in all vaccinated women with both vaccines
		Decline of the Ab levels to HPV 18 at 5+ years	Correlation of Ab titers in serum and vaginal secretions	Ab titers to Cervarix® higher than to Gardasil® at 24 months in a comparative trial
	Duration of clinical protection	7–8 years	7–8 years	Duration of studies in 2009/10. Models predict long term duration (20+)
	Bridging studies	9–15 boys and girls; 26–45	9–15; 26–45	Support clinical indications of vaccination, ages 9 and above
	Immunologic memory	Booster effect following a fourth dose at year 5	Booster effect following a fourth dose	Induction of B cells to Cervarix® superior to Gardasil® at 24 months in a trial
Efficacy results	*CIN 2+ (HPV 16/18)*	Proven	Proven	Protection 95–100%
	CIN 3+ (HPV 16/18)	Proven	Proven	Protection close to 100%. *Estimated prevention from cervical cancer 70 + %*
	VIN/VAIN (HPV 16/18)	Proven	Reported	Protection 95–100%

(continued)

Table 4.1 (continued)

	End point	Gardasil®	Cervarix®	Comments
	Genital warts in women (HPV 6/11)	Proven	Viral types not included in the vaccine	Strong suggestion of herd immunity on male genital warts following massive vaccination of women (>70% to age 26) in Australia
	Genital warts in men (HPV 6/11)	Proven	Viral types not included in the vaccine	
	Anal cancer	Reported	Probable	Analogy with cervical cancer
Other results and clinical impact	Cross protection CIN 2+	Proven HPV 31	Proven HPV 31, suggestive HPV 33, 45 and 51	Likely impact on cervical cancer: Increase by 6–12% (76–82%)
	CIN 2+ independent of HPV type	43%	70%	Estimated in HPV naive cohorts at study entry
	CIN 3+ independent of HPV type	43%	93%	
	Treatments reduction	23%	26%	Independent of viral type
	Therapeutic effect	None	None	No impact on prevalent infections
	Penile cancer	Probable	Probable	Analogy with genital warts in males
	Oral Y pharyngeal cancer	Probable	Probable	Analogy with cervical cancer
	Juvenile papillomatosis laryngeal	Probable	No	Plausible following massive reduction of HPV 6 y 11 in women of reproductive age

CIN cervical intraepithelial neoplasia
Gardasil® (Merck & Co., Inc., Whitehouse Station, NJ USA)
Cervarix® (GlaxoSmithKline Biologicals, Rixensart, Belgium)

et al. 2011). This observation prompts the suggestion of expanding the use of HPV vaccines beyond the currently recommended age groups.

Although protection against other cancer sites was not the primary objective of the phase III trials, vaccinated women showed a remarkable reduction of the incidence of preneoplastic lesions of the vulva (VIN 2/3), the vagina (VAIN 2/3), and in some trials of the preneoplastic lesions of the anal canal (AIN 2/3). Trials of the Gardasil vaccine have shown very high efficacy in the protection against genital warts in both males and females (Schiller 2012; Schiller et al. 2008).

The vaccine efficacy observed in preventing genital warts in vaccinated men and the herd immunity observed among male populations coexisting with a highly vaccinated female population in Australia allow the speculation that vaccination will also protect vaccinated males against the HPV-related fraction of penile carcinomas. It is unlikely that a specific trial would ever evaluate specifically the preventive potential of HPV vaccines against such a rare disease. However, the observation deserves long-term monitoring of trends in penile cancer incidence in populations that introduce male vaccination or that achieve very high vaccination rates among women.

There is little information on the preventive potential against the HPV-related cancers of the oropharynx or on the reduction of respiratory papillomatosis of the newborn and infants following generalized introduction of the vaccine Gardasil that includes VLPs of HPV 6 and 11 as antigens.

4.3 HPV Vaccine Introduction and Early Population-Based Results

HPV vaccines were first used in 2006 and gained rapid support among international and national licensing offices and advisory boards. General recommendations gave priority (and in many instances allocated state-supported vaccination costs) to young girls/adolescents prior to the average ages at onset of sexual activity. Catch-up vaccination of sexually active women is more variable across countries. Licensing has been generally granted to ages 45 based on a limited number of trials showing safety, immunogenicity, and efficacy against persistent HPV infection and CIN 2+ lesions.

In countries with centralized programs and state-supported vaccine costs, coverage of the target populations (adolescents and young girls) is very high, and in a few settings, early evaluations of the clinical impact have already been shown. For example, in Australia an enlarged vaccination program offered for 2 years free vaccination to women up to the age of 26. The program was well coordinated among all stakeholders, and coverage reached a significant 65–70% of the target population, girls 12–14, and some 50% coverage of the catch-up older population, women 15–26. In the program Gardasil was the only vaccine used. Early results were provided in an ecological type of study reporting on the relative contribution of genital warts to the series of clinical cases attended in a STD clinic in Melbourne (the average number of annual patients at the clinic was reported as close to 53,000 per year of which some 5,000 attended because of genital warts). In this noncontrolled clinical observation, 3 years after vaccine introduction a significant reduction in the diagnosis of genital warts has been recorded, and some indication of herd immunity is being documented. The latter is observed by a significant reduction in the number of episodes of genital warts among heterosexual males (largely non-vaccinated) in the same clinics where the reduction among females was documented. In the same analyses, genital warts in male homosexuals during the interval remained constant as was the level of all other STDs (Fairley et al. 2009). The analyses strongly suggest that the reduction in incidence of genital warts in males was a consequence of the high vaccination coverage of the female population in the same age range. A significant reduction of the cases of CIN 1+ and CIN 2+ in these populations has been also recorded within the first 4 years of the vaccination program (Brotherton et al. 2011).

Very high coverage rates with Cervarix have also been achieved in the United Kingdom among the target populations aged 12–13 and the catch-up population of up to 18 years of age. A significant advantage in coverage has been generally observed in areas where vaccination is offered in the context of school-based programs. Similar observations have been reported within countries (i.e., the different autonomous regions in Spain) by comparing subpopulations served by school-based programs with populations served by health center-based programs. Even with an equivalently centralized subsidy of the vaccine costs (the cost of the vaccination program has to be regionally supported), compliance is far better if controlled school-based programs are implemented.

A number of other examples have been reported from developing areas of the world where HPV vaccination has been introduced as part of controlled demonstration programs. One of such programs was led by the Program for Appropriate Technology in Health (PATH) and explored strategies of vaccine introduction in four areas in Peru, Vietnam, India, and Uganda. These projects have concluded among others that vaccine acceptance by the population is satisfactory, that a strategy of using school-based vaccination programs in urban areas is highly appropriate but combined programs of school and outreach visits are necessary in areas where the population is dispersed and school attendance is likely to be insufficient. Moreover, strategies based on campaigns in Uganda (Child Days Plus) unveiled the complexity of targeting girls based on age rather than on school grade. The former, particularly if age is restricted to single cohorts, generated a significant time loss and reduced coverage in trying to verify age.

In other populations of the developing world such as Bhutan or Panama where HPV vaccine was offered free of charge, vaccination coverage has been very satisfactory (Markowitz 2012).

4.4 Issues in Vaccine Use and Introduction

Early indications following phase III trials were strongly driven by the priority of preventing cervical cancer. At this stage, however, advances in the understanding of the spectrum of cancers related to HPV, the results of additional vaccination trials, and the evolution of vaccine costs strongly indicate that some of the original preventive indications are unnecessarily self-limited.

4.4.1 Single-Gender Vaccination

HPV was first recognized as a cause of cervical neoplasia, and all subsequent preventive efforts were oriented toward cervical cancer, the second most frequent cancer in women worldwide. However, research has identified the same HPV types, notably HPV 16, as the cause of a fraction of almost all genital tract cancers in men and women and more recently, of a significant fraction of cancers of the oral cavity and oropharynx. Furthermore, HPV vaccine trials in males have shown the potential of HPV vaccines to prevent genital warts (if Gardasil is used) and anal preinvasive lesions (AIN 2/3).

Previous experiences with other vaccines (i.e., rubella) showed that in certain cultural environments, female-only vaccination prompted rumors and negative attitudes toward vaccination on the grounds of unjustified side effects or more extravagant proposals such as the existence of international plots to sterilize young women or other. As a result, interruption or irregular coverage of all vaccines occurred, and subsequent outbreaks of previously controlled infections such as polio virus occurred and spread to areas where the disease was already considered under control. Gender-neutral vaccination and incorporation of the HPV vaccines into the expanded program of immunization (EPI) would bypass the problem and facilitate coverage (Kane 2012).

Major arguments in favor of male vaccination are the following: (1) the expected impact on herd immunity in populations where vaccination coverage among women is low (somehow arbitrarily defined as below 70%); (2) the impact of reducing genital warts in men, especially men who have sex with men (MSM), if Gardasil is used; (3) the impact on HPV-related cancers in males; and (4) avoidance of concerns in the population on the importance and motivation for HPV vaccination, potentially triggered by the promotion of single-gender vaccination.

Some of the deterrents of the male vaccination proposal at this stage are the following: (1) the late acquisition of the evidence of the burden of HPV-related conditions in men as compared to the early focus on cervical cancer, (2) the limited evidence on the impact of HPV vaccines in men, and (3) the high price of the vaccines leading to concerns that male immunization is not cost-effective.

In this rapidly evolving field, vaccination trials among males have been satisfactorily conducted and licensing by regulatory agencies has already occurred in the USA and other countries. However, formal introduction into routine vaccination public programs has not yet been proposed. Some male populations at high risk of HPV infections and HPV-related cancers (i.e., MSM) are potential target groups for first introduction of male HPV vaccination (Advisory Committee on Immunization Practices 2011; Palefsky et al. 2011).

4.4.2 Target Age Groups for Vaccination

The introduction of HPV vaccines into the routine immunization programs of peri-adolescent girls in most developed countries is a major first step of preventive oncology (Global Advisory Committee on Vaccine Safety 2009). However, the target ages for vaccination offer a canopy of national alternatives with limited scientific rationale. While all regulatory offices recognize the priority to vaccinate girls before sexual behavior starts (in the range of 9–14 years of age), in Europe alone, the upper limit for vaccine recommendations range from single cohorts below the age of 14 in Spain and Norway to age 18 in the UK or Belgium, to age 23 in France and to age 26 in some regions in Italy and in Greece. More interestingly, the vaccination program in Australia, with an estimated national vaccination coverage of 50% in women up to the age of 26 with Gardasil, achieved an almost disappearance of genital warts and a significant reduction of CIN 2+ lesions in the 4-year interval following the introduction of the vaccination program.

Vaccination trials in women up to the age of 45 (Castellsague et al. 2011) have also shown that vaccine efficacy is high among women that are HPV DNA negative at study entry. It is known that HPV exposure can occur at any age group as long as the person is sexually active. Therefore, vaccination can offer some degree of prophylactic benefit at any age group, and the major deterrent to a generalized vaccination program with a difficult-to-determine upper age limit is vaccine cost. The discussion becomes particularly relevant when considering the reduction of the frequency of screening events required for vaccinated women and additional cost benefit analyses will have to be conducted accordingly.

4.4.3 Predicted Impact of Vaccinating Sexually Active Adult Women

Phase III HPV vaccination trials have provided efficacy estimates in different cohorts, mimicking potential users in the population at large. The preventive value of HPV vaccines is better expressed in women that are naïve to the relevant HPV types at study entry, and VE decayed rapidly when vaccinated cohorts were evaluated irrespective of the HPV status at study entry and with case counting starting on the day after the first dose is delivered (usually described as intention-to-treat [ITT] or total vaccinated cohort [TVC] type of analyses). Based upon these observations in the early reports of the trials (interim analyses and analyses within the first 2/3 years of follow-up), VE and vaccination of adult sexually active women was considered of little interest. However, with the observation of larger number of individuals for longer periods of follow-up, VE estimates for the ITT/TVC cohorts significantly increased in both vaccine trials (Garland et al. 2007; Herrero et al. 2011). This is explained because the CIN 2+ cases that are attributable to prevalent HPV infections or low-grade lesions at study entry tend to occur in the first years of follow-up and equally so in both the vaccinated and the control groups. However, as time elapses, cases related to *de novo* HPV infections are observed, and VE estimates increase significantly. Therefore, the potential for prevention of programs that target the general population at large irrespective of their HPV status at vaccination still needs to be assessed. Cost benefit analyses and related screening protocols will also have to pay attention to this observation.

4.4.4 Cost of the Vaccines

The price of the vaccines when first introduced was significantly higher than any other widely used infant vaccines and similar to the initial prices of hepatitis B vaccines. Cost benefit analyses based on prices above 100€ per dose in the private markets and similar in the public markets strongly limited the rapid introduction of the vaccine into developing countries and severely reduced vaccine indications in developed countries by restricting the target populations to one single age cohort in several of them. As expected, major efforts have been invested in lowering the price of vaccines including massive negotiations for procurement, tiered prices for emerging economies, and very low prices for GAVI-eligible countries. Other opportunities for price reduction in the future will probably come from ongoing studies evaluating alternative options such as two-dose regimes or different forms of packaging and delivering systems.

With rapidly decreasing prices, the economic limitations that modulated the age ranges covered by the public system in developed countries may change and move toward wider vaccination indications such as the one adopted by the Australian Government. These considerations are likely to be particularly important in emerging economies and other regions in the world (i.e., eastern European countries, Turkey, Mexico, etc.) that are now at the planning phases of their national policies for cervical cancer prevention (Andrus et al. 2008).

4.4.5 Alternative Uses of HPV Vaccines

Ongoing trials and demonstration programs are now evaluating two-dose vaccination regimes instead of three, using either of the available vaccines. Initial results in the

Costa Rica trial (Herrero et al. 2011) looked at women who received one or two doses of Cervarix instead of a standard 3-dose regimen. In this trial, even one dose showed high antibody titers, not inferior to the titers in people receiving the conventional three-dose schedule. Assessment of the efficacy and duration of protection with one or two doses requires further validation in formal comparative trials that are currently underway in India, Canada, and elsewhere.

Alternative schedules using longer intervals between the doses are other alternatives that are being tested in Mexico, Vietnam, and in Quebec, Canada, using schedules at 0, 6, and 60 months (Kreimer et al. 2011; Neuzil et al. 2011). The protocol should be able to assess the efficacy of two doses as well as the convenience and impact of a booster dose 5 years after initiation of the vaccination scheme. Short-term results from the program in Mexico suggest that two doses at 0 and 6 months induce higher antibody titers than the conventional 0 and 1 or 2 months. No efficacy results are so far available from these studies.

One of the programs with Cervarix is examining the validity of administering the vaccine to infants aged 4 months with a view to incorporate them into the EPI schedules. Further studies in 0–1-year-olds and coadministration formulations with the other EPI vaccines would represent a major advantage in terms of achieving high coverage and vaccination of males as well as females. However, to date no major programs are under way to examine these options.

4.5 Prospects for Second-Generation Vaccines and Impact on Preventive Strategies

Research is actively ongoing on the preparation of so-called second-generation vaccines that would overcome some of the limitations of current vaccines.

The first objective of the second-generation HPV vaccines will be to address the spectrum of HPV types by increasing the number of antigens. Trials of a nonavalent HPV (including HPV 6, 11, 16, 18, 45, 31, 33, 52, 58) vaccine targeting protection against the HPV types that cause 90% of cervical cancer as well as genital warts are currently in advanced phase III trials, and results are awaited in 2012.

A similar end result could be achieved (i.e., VE >90%) by Cervarix if the reported impact on CIN 3+ lesions irrespective of HPV type (93.2%VE) is shown to persist over time.

Other alternatives to increase the valency of HPV vaccines are exploring L2-based constructs and cheaper high-throughput production systems. These vaccines are currently in the early days and entering phase I trials (Jagu et al. 2009).

Figure 4.1 (adapted from Bosch 2009) shows a speculative diagram on plausible protocols for cervical cancer prevention with broad-spectrum vaccines in developing and developed countries. Details of several of the steps of the proposal will require additional clinical research for verification and recommendation.

According to the scheme, HPV vaccination of women could be proposed as broad as feasible in terms of age groups while retaining the emphasis on young pre-

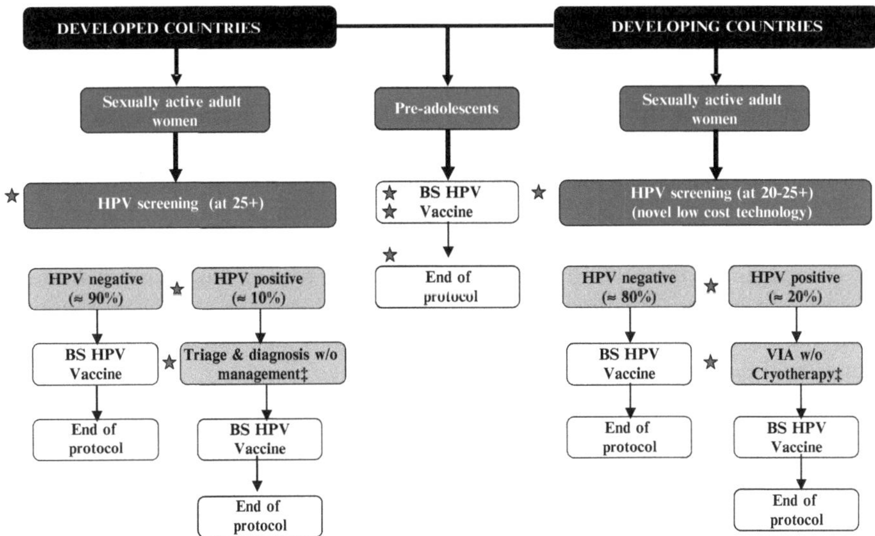

Fig. 4.1 Cervical cancer prevention strategies using broad-spectrum HPV vaccines. *BS* broad spectrum, *HPV* human papillomavirus, *VIA* visual inspection with acetic acid. = Details of such protocols would require additional clinical research; = Vaccination event (Adapted from (Bosch 2009))

sexual initiation girls who would not need further screening. Needless to say, some safety evaluations of the proposal would be necessary in focused clinical trials early in the process.

Vaccinated sexually active young women (i.e., before the ages of 25/30 but years after sexual initiation) could be offered a single-event HPV screening when reaching the age of 25 or 30. The screen would identify the group of women that were already HPV positive before vaccination and remained persistently infected who would then be followed.

Women at ages 30–45+could be offered broad-spectrum HPV vaccines at the time that a single HPV screen is offered. In the screening event, women found HPV negative (80–90% of the target population) will complete the HPV BS vaccination program with no further screening requirements over their lifetime. For women that turned out to be HPV positive, diagnostic and follow-up procedures (colposcopy/biopsy/surgery) could be activated in parallel with completion of the vaccination scheme. Following treatment of the CIN 2+ cases identified, HPV screening could be further used once/twice in their lifetime as a proof of cure and a safety net.

Whatever the final format of the protocols, broad-spectrum vaccines have the potential to (1) alleviate the health services demand of the repeated screening protocols currently in use, (2) influence the cost benefit analyses in favor of generalized vaccination, and (3) trigger a significant reduction in cervical cancer mortality over a medium term, well before the long-term benefits of the generalized adolescent HPV vaccination are clearly visible.

Developing countries would follow a similar protocol, while using an adapted HPV testing system (i.e., the careHPV™ Test, Qiagen Gaithersburg, Inc., MD, USA) and triage protocol for women testing HPV positive (Blumenthal et al. 2005; Sankaranarayanan et al. 2005). The HPV DNA test adapted for use in developing populations achieved significant features of simplicity (average lab technicians can be trained to use them), technical demands (do not require electricity or running water), and output (sampling and testing can be achieved in significant numbers over one shift period) thus allowing for strategies of testing and treating within the duration of the preventive event.

In brief, the use of BS HPV vaccines should significantly reduce or terminate the requirement for continuous screening among vaccinated adolescents and dramatically simplify the strategy for cervical cancer prevention in sexually active adult women in both developed and developing countries. They will help closing the equity gap in cervical cancer prevention between developed and developing populations.

4.6 Screening Implications of Generalized HPV Vaccination

4.6.1 Developed Populations

It has been repeatedly shown that under the best technical conditions, using the Pap smear as the primary screening test, paired with colposcopy and biopsy as the diagnostic tools, the achievable reduction in cervical cancer incidence and mortality is in the range of 50–80% in countries with centrally organized efforts. In countries with opportunistic screening, the impact in cervical cancer reductions is generally lower. Likewise, it could be speculated that the reduction in cervical cancer incidence would be in the 80–85 + % range using HPV tests as the primary screening option with some additional triage test (cytology, HPV typing, p16 + Ki 67 stains) to guide management. Even in well-screened populations in Sweden or within a private insurance plan in California, some cervical cancer cases occur, and these are attributed to either lack of participation to the screening program (56–64% of the cases), false-negative results of the Pap smear (32–24% of the cases), or lack of follow-up of women found at high risk in the cytology results (13–11% of the cases) (Andrae et al. 2008; Leyden et al. 2005). These seem to be nowadays the population limits of Pap smear-based screening programs.

Developed countries have now the opportunity to benefit from HPV-related technologies by implementing strategic combinations of population-based HPV vaccination with a second-generation screening technology program for the prevention of cervical cancer. Vaccinated populations will experience a dramatic reduction in the incidence of CIN 2+ due to HPV 16 and 18 (over 60% of the CIN 2+ cases), and consequently the validity of the Pap smear as primary screening test will suffer.

A reduction by half of the underlying prevalence of the conditions of interest (CIN 2+) will imply a significant loss in predictive value (Franco et al. 2006, 2009). Populations such as the Australian or the British that are currently vaccinating women that will soon enter the recommended screening age groups are appropriate scenarios to test at a large scale the validity of HPV-based tests as primary screening tools and will serve as guidance for future planning in other countries.

Additional public health and clinical research will help define the details of the most effective and cost-effective combinations of mass vaccination and second-generation screening and triage protocols. However, it can now be speculated that in defined developed populations with good preventive care services and adequate attention to immigrant populations, cervical cancer can be drastically reduced to achieve the level of disease elimination within a reasonable time frame.

4.6.2 Developing Populations

With few exceptions, developing populations have irregularly benefited from the conventional Pap smear-based screening strategy, and numerous reviews have documented the reasons for the failure. Many of these are structural and social, thus requiring significant improvement of the public health services to achieve the results described for developed populations. This being the case, cervical cancer remains the third leading cancer in women worldwide and the number one or second cancer in women in 82% of the 127 developing nations. Moreover, because in these countries cervical cancer strikes at young ages and significantly so among young women (i.e., <45 years of age), cervical cancer is a major component of the number of years of life lost to cancer.

In recent years, low-technology tests for secondary prevention of cervical cancer in developing countries have been proposed and evaluated, such as direct visual inspection of the cervix with acetic acid (VIA). The validity of the test is limited, requires careful training and supervision of the observers, and has generated inconsistent results in different settings. These methods are usually included in "see and treat" or "screen and treat" programs in order to minimize attrition in the follow-up of screened women. However, the number of false positives and overtreatments is considerable, and its use has not been generally endorsed (Cuzick et al. 2008).

In contrast to the limited success of Pap smear-based screening programs, developing countries have achieved outstanding results in vaccinating the infant and pediatric age groups. Vaccination in the expanded program of immunization (EPI) is very high in virtually all developing populations, thanks to a great extent to international organizations and donors such as the World Health Organization (WHO), GAVI (formerly The Global Alliance for Vaccines and Immunisation), the United Nations Children's Fund (UNICEF), the Bill & Melinda Gates Foundation, and others. Eradication of small pox was archived, and elimination or significant control of polio, measles, and other infectious diseases has been successful in most developing nations. Therefore, vaccination against HPV seems a relevant option as well as a realistic one to address cervical cancer prevention. Like in developed countries, adult sexually active women in extensive populations in developing countries could benefit from the already available novel form of HPV DNA screening test, technologically adapted to be used in low development level scenarios (Andrus et al. 2008; Qiao et al. 2008; Sankaranarayanan et al. 2008, 2009; World Health Organization 2009).

4.7 Opportunities for Research and Progress

Academic research has made tremendous advancements in providing the understanding of the causes of cervical cancer and generating the technology to prevent it both at the primary and secondary levels. Anticipated developments in the years to come can be summarized as follows:

4.7.1 Etiology

Completion of studies linking and quantifying the impact of HPV infections in the etiology of anogenital cancer and cancer of the head and neck.

4.7.2 Screening

Screening programs in the public system are likely to gradually adopt HPV tests as the primary screening tool. The related clinical protocols will require additional studies to define the management of HPV+women with normal cytology. HPV DNA testing technologies adapted to developing countries (i.e., careHPV Test) will be gradually tested and introduced in developing countries.

4.7.3 HPV Vaccines

Research on novel HPV vaccines to be developed will continue both in the direction of increasing the valence of the vaccines and/or by including therapeutic components in the vaccine products.

4.7.4 Adoption of HPV Vaccines

Continued developments in vaccine development should evolve in parallel to (and learn from) the implementation experiences. Efforts to introduce HPV vaccines in all countries should be strongly encouraged, and it would be unjustified to delay it on the grounds of the promise of better vaccines on the horizon.

4.7.5 Integrated Cervical Cancer Control

Logistical research and modeling studies will help define the most adequate strategies to address comprehensive cancer prevention strategies in extensive areas and populations where no preventive options are available nowadays.

4.7.6 Disease Awareness and Medical Education

These will aim at (1) increasing the low level of awareness on the impact of cervical cancer worldwide and particularly in developing countries, (2) addressing issues of cervical cancer as a single-gender disease and the stigma of being linked to a sexually transmitted infection (STI), and (3) counteracting the negative publicity on vaccines and HPV vaccination in the media.

4.7.7 Social Consensus on Cervical Cancer Prevention

Political efforts are now needed toward introducing the concepts of cervical cancer elimination and eradication and help reaching the stage at which the public health community at large embarks on the required worldwide effort.

4.8 Conclusion

Technologies to dramatically reduce the impact of cervical and other HPV-related cancers are now available. HPV vaccines and HPV-based screening tests might represent the technical requirements to begin closing the equity gap in cervical cancer prevention between developed and developing countries.

4.8.1 Notes

The author would like to express sincere thanks to Cris Rajo and Ion Espuña in the preparation of the manuscript.

The study has been partially supported by Spanish public grants from the Instituto de Salud Carlos III (grants FIS PI030240, FIS PI061246, RCESP C03/09, RTICESP C03/10, RTIC RD06/0020/0095 and CIBERESP), from the Agència de Gestió d'Ajuts Universitaris i de Recerca (AGAUR 2005SGR 00695 and 2009SGR126), from the Marató de TV3 Foundation (051530), and from GlaxoSmithKline Biologicals, Sanofi Pasteur MSD & Merck & Co, Inc., who had no role in the preparation of this manuscript.

4.8.2 Conflict of Interest Disclosure

FXB has received travel and consultancy fees from MSD, GSK, Qiagen, and SPMSD. Through the Catalan Institute of Oncology, he has administered research and educational grants from GSK, MSD, and SPMSD.

References

Advisory Committee on Immunization Practices. Recommendations on the use of quadrivalent human papillomavirus vaccine in males. *MMWR Morb Mortal Wkly Rep* 2011; 60:1705–1708.

Andrae B, Kemetli L, Sparen P, Silfverdal L, Strander B, Ryd W et al. Screening-preventable cervical cancer risks: evidence from a nationwide audit in Sweden. *J Natl Cancer Inst* 2008; 100:622–629.

Andrus J K, Sherris J, Fitzsimmons JW, Kane MA, Aguado MT. Introduction of human papillomavirus vaccines into developing countries - international strategies for funding and procurement. *Vaccine* 2008; 26: Suppl 10 K87–K92.

Blumenthal PD, Lauterbach M, Sellors JW, Sankaranarayanan R. Training for cervical cancer prevention programs in low-resource settings: focus on visual inspection with acetic acid and cryotherapy. *Int J Gynaecol Obstet* 2005; 89: Suppl 2 S30–S37

Bosch FX. Broad-spectrum human papillomavirus vaccines: new horizons but one step at a time. *J Natl Cancer Inst* 2009; 101:771–773.

Bosch FX, Manos MM, Munoz N, Sherman M, Jansen AM, Peto J et al. Prevalence of human papillomavirus in cervical cancer: a worldwide perspective. International biological study on cervical cancer (IBSCC) Study Group. *J Natl Cancer Inst* 1995; 87:796–802.

Bosch F, de Sanjosé S, Castellsagué X. Evaluating the potential benefits of universal worldwide human papillomavirus vaccination. *Therapy* 2008; 5:305–312.

Bouvard V, Baan R, Straif K, Grosse Y, Secretan B, El Ghissassi F et al. A review of human carcinogens--Part B: biological agents. *Lancet Oncol* 2009; 10:321–322.

Brotherton JM, Fridman M, May CL, Chappell G, Saville AM, Gertig DM. Early effect of the HPV vaccination programme on cervical abnormalities in Victoria, Australia: an ecological study. *Lancet* 2011; 377:2085–2092.

Castellsague X, Munoz N, Pitisuttithum P, Ferris D, Monsonego J, Ault K et al. End-of-study safety, immunogenicity, and efficacy of quadrivalent HPV (types 6, 11, 16, 18) recombinant vaccine in adult women 24–45 years of age. *Br J Cancer* 2011; 105:28–37.

Centers for Disease Control and Prevention. *Reports of health concerns following HPV vaccination*. Centers for Disease Control and Prevention. 2009

Chaturvedi AK, Engels EA, Pfeiffer RM, Hernandez BY, Xiao W, Kim E et al. Human papillomavirus and rising oropharyngeal cancer incidence in the United States. *J Clin Oncol* 2011; 29:4294–4301.

Cuzick J, Arbyn M, Sankaranarayanan R, Tsu V, Ronco G, Mayrand MH et al. Overview of human papillomavirus-based and other novel options for cervical cancer screening in developed and developing countries. *Vaccine* 2008; 26: Suppl 10 K29–K41.

de Sanjose S, Quint WG, Alemany L, Geraets DT, Klaustermeier JE, Lloveras B et al. Human papillomavirus genotype attribution in invasive cervical cancer: a retrospective cross-sectional worldwide study. *Lancet Oncol* 2010; 11:1048–1056.

De Vuyst H, Clifford GM, Nascimento MC, Madeleine MM, Franceschi S. Prevalence and type distribution of human papillomavirus in carcinoma and intraepithelial neoplasia of the vulva, vagina and anus: a meta-analysis. *Int J Cancer* 2009; 124:1626–1636.

D'Souza G, Fakhry C, Sugar EA, Seaberg EC, Weber K, Minkoff HL et al. Six-month natural history of oral versus cervical human papillomavirus infection. *Int J Cancer* 2007; 121:143–150.

European Center for Disease Prevention and Control (ECDC). Guidance for the introduction of HPV vaccines European countries. htttp://edcdeuropa.eu/pdf/HPV_report.pdf. 2008

Fairley CK, Hocking JS, Gurrin LC, Chen MY, Donovan B, Bradshaw CS. Rapid decline in presentations of genital warts after the implementation of a national quadrivalent human papillomavirus vaccination programme for young women. *Sex Transm Infect* 2009; 85:499–502.

Forman D. Burden of HPV infections & related disease. *Vaccine* 2012. In the Press

Franco EL, Cuzick J, Hildesheim A, de Sanjose S. Chapter 20: Issues in planning cervical cancer screening in the era of HPV vaccination. *Vaccine* 2006; 24: Suppl 3S3/171–S3/177.

Franco EL, Mahmud SM, Tota J, Ferenczy A, Coutlee F. The expected impact of HPV vaccination on the accuracy of cervical cancer screening: the need for a paradigm change. *Arch Med Res* 2009; 40:478–485.

Garland SM, Hernandez-Avila M, Wheeler CM, Perez G, Harper DM, Leodolter S et al. Quadrivalent vaccine against human papillomavirus to prevent anogenital diseases. *N Engl J Med* 2007; 356:1928–1943.

Gillison, ML. HPV and diseases of the upper airway: head and neck cancer and respiratory papillomatosis. *Vaccine* 2012. In the Press

Gillison ML, Koch WM, Capone RB, Spafford M, Westra WH, Wu L et al. Evidence for a causal association between human papillomavirus and a subset of head and neck cancers. *J Natl Cancer Inst* 2000; 92:709–720.

Global Advisory Committee on Vaccine Safety, 17–18 December 2008. *Wkly Epidemiol Rec* 2009: 84:37–40.

Heck JE, Berthiller J, Vaccarella S, Winn DM, Smith EM, Shan'gina O et al. Sexual behaviours and the risk of head and neck cancers: a pooled analysis in the International Head and Neck Cancer Epidemiology (INHANCE) consortium. *Int J Epidemiol* 2010; 39:166–181.

Herrero R, Wacholder S, Rodriguez AC, Solomon D, Gonzalez P, Kreimer R et al. Prevention of Persistent Human Papillomavirus Infection by an HPV16/18 Vaccine: A Community-Based Randomized Clinical Trial in Guanacaste, Costa Rica. *Cancer Discovery* 2011; 1:408–419.

IARC. IARC monograph series vol 90. *Human Papillomaviruses* Lyon: International Agency for Research on Cancer. 2007.

Jagu S, Karanam B, Gambhira R, Chivukula SV, Chaganti RJ, Lowy DR et al. Concatenated multitype L2 fusion proteins as candidate prophylactic pan-human papillomavirus vaccines. *J Natl Cancer Inst* 2009; 101:782–792.

Kane M. Implementation of HPV Immunization in the Developing World. *Vaccine* 2012; In the Press

Kreimer AR, Rodriguez AC, Hildesheim A, Herrero R, Porras C, Schiffman M et al. Proof-of-principle evaluation of the efficacy of fewer than three doses of a bivalent HPV16/18 vaccine. *J Natl Cancer Inst* 2011; 103:1444–1451.

Leyden WA, Manos MM, Geiger AM, Weinmann S, Mouchawar J, Bischoff K et al. Cervical cancer in women with comprehensive health care access: attributable factors in the screening process. *J Natl Cancer Inst* 2005; 97:675–683.

Markowitz L E. HPV Vaccine Introduction - The First Five Years. *Vaccine* 2012; In the Press

Markowitz LE, Dunne EF, Saraiya M, Lawson HW, Chesson H, Unger ER. Quadrivalent Human Papillomavirus Vaccine: Recommendations of the Advisory Committee on Immunization Practices (ACIP). *MMWR Recomm Rep* 2007; 56(RR-2):1–24.

Miralles-Guri C, Bruni L, Cubilla AL, Castellsague X, Bosch FX, de Sanjose S. Human papillomavirus prevalence and type distribution in penile carcinoma. *J Clin Pathol* 2009; 62:870–878.

Munoz N, Bosch FX, Castellsague X, Diaz M, de Sanjose S, Hammouda D et al. Against which human papillomavirus types shall we vaccinate and screen? The international perspective. *Int J Cancer* 2004; 111:278–285.

Nasman A, Attner P, Hammarstedt L, Du J, Eriksson M, Giraud G et al. Incidence of human papillomavirus (HPV) positive tonsillar carcinoma in Stockholm, Sweden: an epidemic of viral-induced carcinoma? *Int J Cancer* 2009; 125:362–366.

Neuzil KM, Canh d G, Thiem VD, Janmohamed A, Huong VM, Tang Y et al. Immunogenicity and reactogenicity of alternative schedules of HPV vaccine in Vietnam: a cluster randomized non-inferiority trial. *JAMA* 2011; 305:1424–1431.

Palefsky JM, Giuliano AR, Goldstone S, Moreira ED, Jr, Aranda C, Jessen H et al. HPV vaccine against anal HPV infection and anal intraepithelial neoplasia. *N Engl J Med* 2011; 365:1576–1585.

Qiao YL, Sellors JW, Eder PS, Bao YP, Lim JM, Zhao FH et al. A new HPV-DNA test for cervical-cancer screening in developing regions: a cross-sectional study of clinical accuracy in rural China. *Lancet Oncol* 2008; 9:929–936.

Ragin CC, Taioli E. Survival of squamous cell carcinoma of the head and neck in relation to human papillomavirus infection: review and meta-analysis. *Int J Cancer* 2007; 121:1813–1820.

Rintala M, Grenman S, Puranen M, Syrjanen S. Natural history of oral papillomavirus infections in spouses: a prospective Finnish HPV Family Study. *J Clin Virol* 2006; 35:89–94.

Sankaranarayanan R, Bhatla N, Gravitt PE, Basu P, Esmy PO, Ashrafunnessa KS et al. Human papillomavirus infection and cervical cancer prevention in India, Bangladesh, Sri Lanka and Nepal. *Vaccine* 2008; 26: Suppl 12 M43–M52.

Sankaranarayanan R, Gaffikin L, Jacob M, Sellors J, Robles S. A critical assessment of screening methods for cervical neoplasia. *Int J Gynaecol Obstet* 2005; 89: Suppl 2 S4–S12.

Sankaranarayanan R, Nene BM, Shastri SS, Jayant K, Muwonge R, Budukh AM et al. HPV screening for cervical cancer in rural India. *N Engl J Med* 2009; 360:1385–1394.

Schiller JT. A review of Clinical Trials of Human Papillomavirus Prophylactic vaccines. *Vaccine* 2012; 30 Suppl 5:123–138.

Schiller JT, Castellsague X, Villa LL, Hildesheim A. An update of prophylactic human papillomavirus L1 virus-like particle vaccine clinical trial results. *Vaccine* 2008; 26: Suppl 10 K53–K61.

Smith JS, Lindsay L, Hoots B, Keys J, Franceschi S, Winer R et al. Human papillomavirus type distribution in invasive cervical cancer and high-grade cervical lesions: a meta-analysis update. *Int J Cancer* 2007; 121:621–632.

Wheeler CM, Hunt WC, Joste NE, Key CR, Quint WG, Castle PE. Human papillomavirus genotype distributions: implications for vaccination and cancer screening in the United States. *J Natl Cancer Inst* 2009; 101:475–487.

World Health Organization. Meeting of the Immunization Strategic Advisory Group of Experts November 2008 – conclusions and recommendations. *Weekly Epidemiological Record* 2009; 84:1–16.

Chapter 5
Prevention of Cancers Due to Infection

Hideo Tanaka

5.1 Hepatitis B Virus and Hepatocellular Carcinoma

5.1.1 Virus Transmission

HBV is classified into at least 10 genotypes (A to J) and several subtypes based on sequence divergence of the entire HBV genomic sequence of >8 % for genotypes and 4–8 % for subtypes (Cao 2009; McMahon 2009; Kurbanov et al. 2010). Genotype A is prevalent in sub-Saharan Africa, Northern Europe, and Western Africa. Genotype B is found in Japan (B1) (Orito et al. 2001), Taiwan, China, Indonesia, Vietnam, Philippines, (B2-5), Alaska, Northern Canada, and Greenland (B6). Genotype C (subtypes C1-5) mainly exists in East and Southeast Asia. Genotype D with subtypes D1-D5 is prevalent in Africa, the Mediterranean region, and India. Genotype E is endemic in West Africa. Genotype F (subtypes F1-4) is found in Central and South America. Genotype G has been reported in France, Germany, and the United Status.

The modes of transmission leading to the development of chronic HBV carriers are likely different among HBV genotypes. In East Asian countries, where genotype B and C are the dominant genotypes, perinatal or vertical transmission plays an important role in spreading HBV and subsequent chronicity. The likelihood of transmission resulting in chronic infection from an HBeAg-positive mother or HBeAg-negative but HBsAg-positive mother before the introduction of HBV vaccination was reported to be in the range of 70–90 % and 6–21 % in Taiwan, respectively (Beasley et al. 1977; Tsai et al. 1984; Ko et al. 1986). In adults, the

H. Tanaka (✉)
Division of Epidemiology and Prevention, Aichi Cancer Center Research Institute, Osaka, Japan
e-mail: hitanaka@aichi-cc.jp

A.B. Miller (ed.), *Epidemiologic Studies in Cancer Prevention and Screening*, Statistics for Biology and Health 79, DOI 10.1007/978-1-4614-5586-8_5,

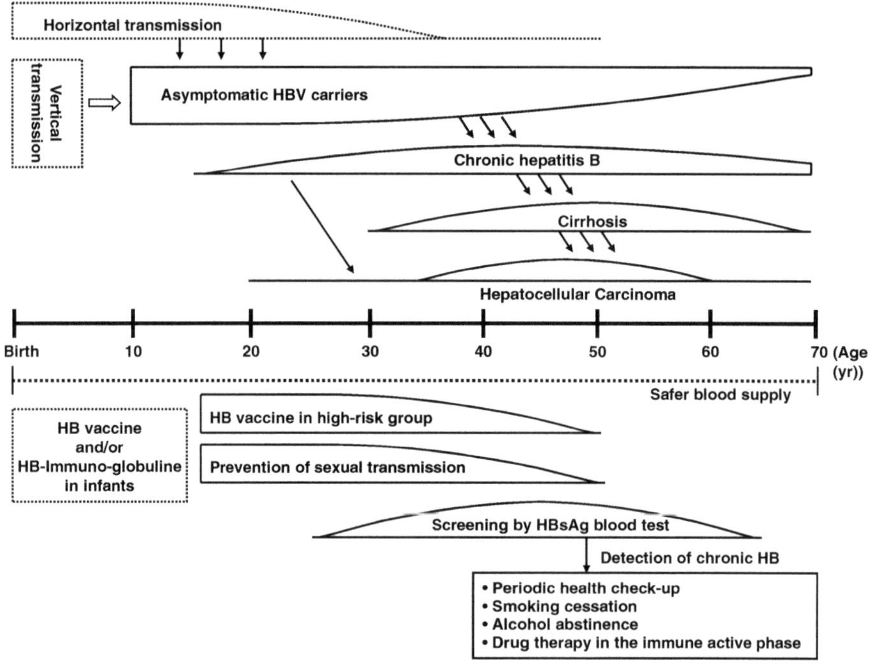

Fig. 5.1 Natural history of HBV infection and prevention of HBV-related HCC

major routes of transmission are sexual intercourse and needles. The remaining genotypes are frequently found in areas where horizontal transmission is the main mode of transmission. Since spreading of transmission in an area is considered to be positively correlated with accumulated duration of carrier state among the population, the likelihood of chronicity after transmission is important to consider when developing strategies of HBV eradication. The likelihood of developing persistent HBV infection after acute hepatitis B was reported to be higher in patients with genotype A (23 %) than in those with genotype B (11 %) or C (7 %) in Japan (Suzuki et al. 2005). A nationwide survey conducted in Japan reported that the prevalence of HBV genotype A in chronic hepatitis B patients increased from 1.7 % in 2000 to 3.5 % in 2006 (Matsuura et al. 2009). A recent genome-wide association study of chronic hepatitis B showed that genetic variation in the *HLA-DQ* genes was strongly associated with the risk of persistent HBV infection (Mbarek et al. 2011). This study indicates the importance of host genetic factors in the clearance of HBV.

5.1.2 Natural History of Chronic Hepatitis B

In the natural history of chronic HBV infection (Fig. 5.1), seroconversion of HBeAg and seroclearance of HBsAg are important events with an estimated annual incidence of 12 % and 2 %, respectively (Chen et al. 2002; Hsu et al. 2002; Kao et al. 2004; Liu et al. 2010). Earlier HBeAg seroconversion to an HBeAb-positive state is usually involved in a favorable clinical outcome, whereas late or absent HBeAg seroconversion after multiple hepatitis flares is likely to accelerate the progression of chronic hepatitis to cirrhosis.

A cohort study conducted in Taiwan with a mean follow-up of 52 months indicated that genotype C infection had a significantly lower rate of spontaneous HBeAg seroconversion than genotype B (27 % vs. 47 %) (Kao et al. 2004). Clinical observations reported from Hong Kong and Japan showed that chronic hepatitis B (CHB) patients with genotype C were more prone to develop advanced fibrosis, cirrhosis, and HCC than genotype B patients (Sumi et al. 2003; Yuen et al. 2004). A community-based prospective cohort study conducted in Taiwan showed that HBV carriers with genotype C had 2.35 times significantly higher risk of developing HCC than HBV carriers with genotype B (Yang et al. 2008). A recent genome-wide association study of chronic HBV carriers with HCC and without HCC demonstrated that one intronic single-nucleotide polymorphism in 1p36.22 was highly associated with HBV-related HCC (Zhang et al. 2010). This finding indicates the importance of host genetic factors as well as virus genetic factors in disease progression in chronic HBV carriers. In the clinical setting, it is important to predict HCC risk in CHB patients using available clinical markers as well as patients' demographic factors. Yuen et al. (Yuen et al. 2009) followed 820 CHB patients and determined that male gender (rate ratio (RR) 2.98), increasing age (RR 1.07), and higher HBV DNA level (RR 7.31) were independent risk factors for the development of HCC. Using these factors with the optimal cut-off point, they showed the prediction of the 5- and 10-year risks for the development of HCC with sensitivity of >84 % and specificity of >76 % (Yuen et al. 2009).

Several environmental factors that are considered to be associated with disease progression and the development of HCC in HBV carriers have been established. Dietary aflatoxins were classified as established carcinogens of HCC (IARC 1993) in some areas of developing countries, where HBV infection is endemic. Heavy drinking is a well-known risk factor for developing HCC (IARC 1988) and is possibly a liver carcinogen mainly by accelerating liver inflammation which is causally involved in the development of cirrhosis (Adami et al. 1992; Tsukuma et al. 1993). In 2004, IARC reported that there is sufficient evidence for the association between tobacco smoking and liver cancer, mainly, HCC (IARC 2004). Coinfection of human immunodeficiency virus (HIV) and HBV is relatively prevalent in sub-Saharan Africa, and it is increasing in Southeast Asia. One cohort study conducted in the Han Chinese population (Yang et al. 2011) indicated that HIV infection has a significant impact on the natural progression of HBV infection not only in HBV carriers who were horizontally infected but also in those who usually have perinatal HBV infection. Coinfection with HBV and HCV is rare worldwide, and assessment of their interaction for HCC risk was inconsistent. A recent published meta-analysis that included 59 studies that assessed the association between HBV/HCV monoinfection and coinfection for HCC risk demonstrated that the risk of coinfection is not significantly greater than that of HBV/HVC monoinfection (Cho et al. 2011).

This finding may be reasonable from current biological knowledge that superinfection of one virus tends to inhibit infection of the other virus among coinfected cases (Sheen et al. 1992; Chu et al. 1998).

5.1.3 *Effectiveness of HBV Vaccine*

Several clinical trials reported the efficacy of HB vaccine in preventing HBsAg-positive chronic status occurring through perinatal HBV infection (Beasley et al. 1983; Tsai et al. 1984; Lo et al. 1985a; Lo et al. 1985b). In Taiwan, a nationwide HB vaccination program for preventing vertical HBV transmission was introduced in 1984, and consistent effectiveness in reducing the prevalence of HBV infection among children and adolescents was revealed by comparing the prevalence before and after the program was launched (Chen et al. 1996; Hsu et al. 1999; Ni et al. 2001). Likewise, in other previously endemic areas, Gambia (Whittle et al. 1995) and Malaysia (Ng et al. 2005), vaccination was proven to be very successful in reducing the rate of HBV infection. Consequently, a decreasing trend in the incidence of HBV-related HCC in the program-received generation was expected. Chang et al. (Chang et al. 1997) reported that the average annual incidence (per 100,000 children) of HCC in children 6–14 years of age declined from 0.70 in 1981–1986, to 0.57 in 1986–1990, to 0.36 in 1990–1994 ($P<0.01$). This important finding demonstrated that a nationwide universal vaccination program protected children not only from becoming chronic HBV carriers but also from developing HCC in a HBV-prevalent population.

In Taiwan, since it was reported that HB immunity as defined by anti-HBs seropositivity decreased to 50 % in 15 years after universal HBV vaccination (Lu et al. 2009), the necessity and age at which a boost would be administered among anti-HBs-negative adolescents were discussed. However, an HB vaccine that has lost protective (10 < mIV/mL) anti-HBs antibody usually shows a rapid anamnestic response when boosted (Zanetti et al. 2005). This probably means that immunological memory for HBsAg can outlast antibody detection, providing long-term protection against HBV infection and the development of the carrier state (West and Calandra 1996). Therefore, at least for immunocompetent individuals, booster doses of HB vaccine do not seem to be necessary to ensure long-term protection (Banatvala and Van Damme 2003).

Among HBV low-endemic countries, the United Kingdom, Scandinavian countries, and Japan have adopted a vaccination program targeted to well-defined risk groups. In Japan, a nationwide prevention program utilizing passive-active immunoprophylaxis for infants born to HBsAg-positive mothers was introduced in 1986 (Koyama et al. 2003). This program was expected to reduce the prevalence of chronic HBV infection and prevent the occurrence of HBV-related HCC among the program-acquired generations. To evaluate this effect, we reviewed the annual reports from a nationwide survey of childhood solid tumors (aged 0–14 years) during 1981–2008 (Tajiri et al. 2011). The incidence of HBV-HCC rapidly declined from 2001 when all of the program-acquired generation become 15 years old and over, whereas the incidence of hepatoblastoma was almost stable during the same period (Tajiri et al. 2011). This finding indicates that this high-risk approach introduced in Japan has reduced the occurrence of HBV-related HCC in childhood.

5.1.4 *Treatment of Chronic Hepatitis B*

There has been cumulative evidence that early treatment and viral suppression in patients with CHB greatly reduce the risk of progression to cirrhosis, HCC, and eventual death (Fattovich et al. 2008; Chang et al. 2010). Treatment is more effective during the immune-active phase of the disease when rates of progressive fibrosis are increased. There are two possible treatment approaches including stimulating the immune system through pegylated interferon or suppressing viral load through nucleotide analogs. Since CHB patients often remain asymptomatic and therefore are undiagnosed before progression to severe liver disease, a screening program by a HBsAg blood test in targeted populations should be considered.

5.2 Hepatitis C Virus and Hepatocellular Carcinoma

5.2.1 *Viral Transmission*

HCV was first identified in 1988 as a RNA virus in the Flaviviridae family (Choo et al. 1989) and is now classified into 6 major genotypes (Simmonds et al. 1993; Bukh et al. 1994; Robertson et al. 1998). Recent molecular clock analysis of the sequences of HCV isolates indicated that HCV-1b penetrated Japan and Europe in the 1920s and 1940s, respectively; the HCV-4a population showed exponential growth in South Africa in the 1950s; HCV endemics were dated in the 1960s for both in the United States (HCV-1a) and former Soviet Union (HCV-3a) and HCV-6a in the late 1970s in Hong Kong (Tanaka et al. 2006a). The initial spread time of HCV is considered to be associated with the time trend in the incidence of HCC with considerable time lag in each area (Tanaka et al. 2006a).

HCV is mainly transmitted by the parenteral route. Direct percutaneous exposure, that is, the sharing of contaminated needles or syringes among drug abusers and blood transfusion on blood products from infectious donors (prior to screening) is the most efficient route of transmission. A recent systematic review estimated that the prevalence of anti-HCV among injection drug users (IDUs) in 25 countries ranged from 60 % to 80 % and that about 10.0 million IDUs worldwide might be anti-HCV positive (Nelson et al. 2011). The probability of spontaneous viral clearance in these HCV-parenterally exposed groups is estimated to be 30 %–50 % on the basis of HCV RNA-negative rates among anti-HCV-positive individuals in HCV-endemic regions (Tanaka et al. 1994). This means that about 50 %–70 % of those infected with HCV through parenteral exposure will develop a chronic persistent infection. Sexual transmission occurs inefficiently, but is attributed to transmission in the United States because of the large number of individuals at risk (Alter 1997). Perinatal transmission of HCV is less common than perinatal transmission of HBV and HIV. A study from Japan demonstrated that the probability of HCV transmission from mother to infant is 6 % among babies born to mothers with anti-HCV and 10 % among babies born to mothers with HCV RNA (Ohto et al. 1994). The rate of spontaneous viral clearance among children with vertically acquired infection observed in the United States was 9 % (Abdel-Hady et al. 2011).

5.2.2 *Factors Associated with the Development of HCC*

Many cohort studies and cross-sectional studies of asymptomatic HCV carriers indicated that 50 %–80 % of persons with chronic HCV infection progress to chronic hepatitis. Since most HCV-associated HCC occurs in the presence of cirrhosis, HCV infection may lead to HCC through the indirect mechanism of immune-mediated damage and subsequent liver cell turnover, although the HCV core protein has been shown to exhibit oncogenic properties (Moriya et al. 1998; Anzola 2004). In population-based cohort studies, assuming that most of the HCV carriers are asymptomatic, the rate ratio of the effect of HCV chronic infection on the development of HCC ranged from 21.5 to 35.8 (Osella et al. 2000; Hara et al. 2001; Sun et al. 2003; Ishiguro et al. 2011), whereas the rate ratio among voluntary blood donors was 126 (95 % CI 79–202) (Tanaka et al. 2004). Most of the HCV-related HCC cases occur after age 60. A well-designed retrospective cohort study indicated that the age of patients is more significant than the duration of HCV infection for HCC development among patients with posttransfusion HCV (Hamada et al. 2002). This result is convincing with the finding that the rate of progression of fibrosis was proportional to patient age at the time of HCV infection, and patient age was the main factor associated with progression to fibrosis (Anzola 2004).

Although heavy alcohol drinking has been recognized as a risk factor for primary liver cancer, most of the epidemiologic studies showing a positive association did not limit the study subjects to individuals with chronic HCV infection. However, a systematic review of epidemiologic evidence reported in Japan, where HCV-related HCC is etiologically dominant, concluded that there is convincing evidence that alcohol drinking increases the risk of primary cancer (Tanaka et al. 2008a). This finding strongly indicates that heavy alcohol drinking increases the risk of HCC among individuals with chronic HCV infection. A similar notion is plausible in the association of cigarette smoking with the risk of HCV-related HCC, which was supported through the finding that cigarette smoking probably increases the risk of primary liver cancer in a systematic review of epidemiologic studies conducted in the Japanese population (Tanaka et al. 2006b).

There have been several epidemiologic data to indicate that obesity is associated with an increased risk of liver cancer. Ohki et al. (2008) conducted a cohort study enrolling 1,431 patients with chronic hepatitis C and reported that being overweight ($25 < BMI \leq 30$) and obesity ($BMI > 30$) were shown to be an independent risk factor with a hazard ratio of 1.86 and 3.10, respectively, as compared with underweight patients ($BMI \leq 18.5$). Coinfection with HIV appears to increase the risk of progression of HCV-induced liver disease due to insufficient immune control of HCV chronicity and subsequent risk of HCC (Graham et al. 2001; Thomas 2002). There have been several epidemiological studies that showed an inverse association of coffee drinking with the risk of primary liver cancer. To confirm the association, a meta-analysis of coffee consumption and risk of liver cancer was performed using data from 4 cohort studies (4 from Japan) and 5 case-control studies (2 from Italy, 2 from Japan, 1 from Greece) (Larsson and Wolk 2007). They found that consumption of coffee may reduce the risk of liver cancer; the summary relative risk of coffee consumption per 2 cups/day increment among the subjects with a history of liver diseases was 0.56 (95 % CI 0.35–0.91). As the source populations mostly consisted of patients with HCV-related HCC, this finding suggests that coffee intake may reduce the risk of HCC among individuals with chronic HCV infection.

5.2.3 *Prevention of HCV-Related HCC*

At present, as there is no vaccine to prevent HCV infection, interrupting parenteral transmission is very important. Testing of blood donations for anti-HCV and additionally HCV RNA has led to substantial decrease in the number of posttransfusion hepatitis C cases in many developed countries. The use of disposable needles and syringes in health-care settings is important to reduce HCV infection in the general population. The effectiveness of these measures was demonstrated in the Japanese population in that the spread of HCV essentially ended by the early 1990s at the latest, as evidenced by the recent very low incidence of HCV infection among repeat donors (Sasaki et al. 1996; Tanaka et al. 1998). We have also shown that the termination of HCV spread has led to a decrease in the incidence of HCV-related HCC by the early 2000s at the latest on the population level (Tanaka et al. 2008b). In the United States, Europe, Australia, New Zealand, and southern China, however, the most important mode of HCV transmission is now by IDU (Dore et al. 2003; Garten et al. 2005; Farrell 2007). Avoiding sharing of needles and blood-contaminated syringes is thought to be important in preventing HCV transmission by IDU and is also effective in preventing concomitant HIV infection. On the other hand, attempts to prevent IDU by educational measures and public awareness campaigns have not been conspicuously successful (Madden and Cavalieri 2007) (Fig. 5.2).

There has been strong evidence that the incidence of HCC among patients with chronic HCV infection can be reduced by antiviral therapy, achieving a sustained

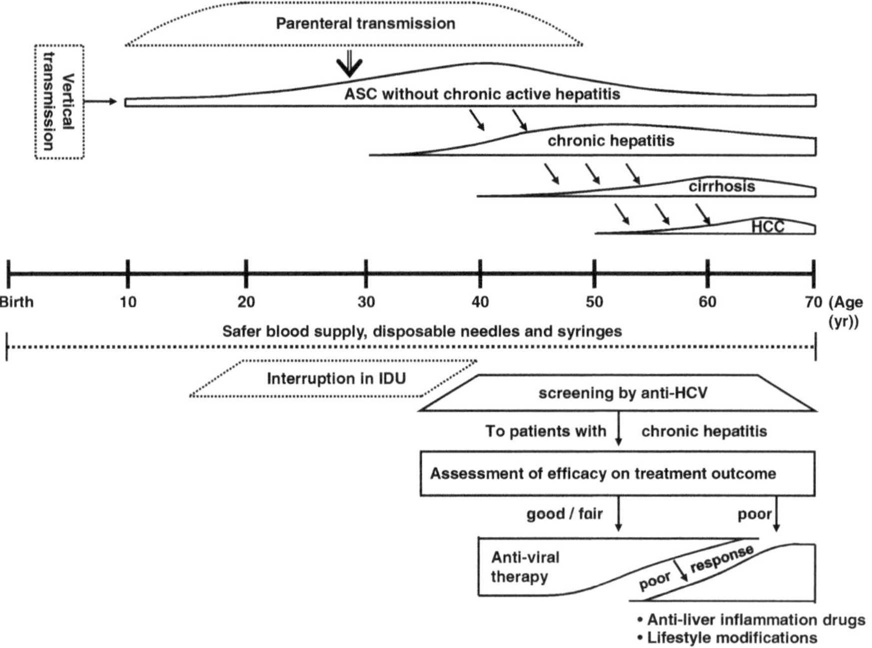

Fig. 5.2 Natural history of chronic HCV infection and prevention of HCV-related HCC

viral response (SVR) that is nearly equivalent to viral eradication. SVR has been particularly likely by treatment with interferon in combination with ribavirin (Ueno et al. 2009). However, this treatment is effective in less than 50 % of the patients with a high viral load of genotype 1 (Mangia et al. 2005). Viral factors, including the serum quantity of HCV RNA and HCV genotype, and host factors of gender, BMI, the presence of steatosis and liver fibrosis, and genetic variations near the *IL28* gene on chromosome 19 have been reported to be significant predictors of treatment outcome (Tanaka et al. 2009). A recent clinical trial revealed that telaprevir, a new protease inhibitor, in combination with peg-interferon alfa-2b and ribavirin led to a high SVR rate (34–88 %) among difficult-to-treat patients with genotype 1 chronic hepatitis C (Hayashi et al. 2012). As the majority of individuals with chronic hepatitis C are asymptomatic, a community-based anti-HCV screening system in HCV-prevalent populations has been a priority in Japan since 2002 (Tanaka et al. 2008).

Patients with chronic hepatitis C who do not achieve SVR with antiviral therapy and patients who have viral and host factors for a potential poor response to antiviral treatment need other strategies to prevent HCC. It may be possible to treat these patients with ursodeoxycholic acid and/or glycyrrhizin to improve liver inflammation, which was reported to reduce the incidence of HCC among patients with interferon-resistant active chronic hepatitis C (Ikeda et al. 2006). For these patients, lifestyle modification such as avoiding heavy alcohol drinking, smoking, and obesity is likely to be important.

5.3 *H. pylori* Infection and Gastric Cancer

5.3.1 Transmission

About half of the world's population is estimated to be infected with *H. pylori,* a spiral-shaped, gram-negative bacterium. It is usually transmitted during early childhood possibly through oral-oral and oral-fecal routes in humans and colonizes the gastric epithelium. A systematic review on acquisition of *H. pylori* infection indicated that infected mothers, fathers, and siblings are independent risk factors for childhood *H. pylori* infection (Weyermann et al. 2009). Inadequate sanitation practices, low social class, the use of well water instead of municipal water, and male gender were reported to be associated with acquisition and/or remaining of *H. pylori* childhood infection (Queiroz et al. 2012). In developed countries, improvement of sanitation and hygiene has been responsible for a dramatic reduction in transmission during the last few decades and was involved in the clear birth cohort effect on the prevalence of *H. pylori* infection in the general population.

5.3.2 Factors Associated with the Development of Gastric Cancer in Chronically H. pylori-Infected Subjects

H. pylori was acknowledged by a working group of the IARC (1994) as a cause of stomach cancer. It has been causally associated with non-cardia gastric adenocarcinoma and gastric lymphoma, with an estimated attributable fraction of around 75 % for both diseases (Parkin 2006). Non-cardia gastric adenocarcinoma is the consequence of a multistep and multifactorial process. It starts from chronic inflammatory gastritis in the antrum which is induced by persistent *H. pylori* infection that is thought to form the initial lesion. It may progress to multifocal chronic atrophic gastritis, intestinal metaplasia, dysplasia, and finally invasive carcinoma (Correa 1992). However, as only a small proportion of infected subjects developed adenocarcinoma, it raises the question of why it causes cancer in only a minority of those infected.

H. pylori are genetically highly diverse bacteria, and several genes/genotypes have been associated with strain virulence, and consequently disease progression (Basso et al. 2008). Several recent studies showed that virtually all cases of non-cardia adenocarcinoma occur in subjects infected with strains positive for the cytotoxin-associated (CagA) gene, which is present in about 60 % of strains in Western countries (Gonzalez and Agudo 2012). CagA-positive strains translocate the CagA protein into gastric epithelial cells by a type IV secretion system, which seems to play a pivotal role in the development of gastric atrophy (Hamajima et al. 2006). CagA positivity is strongly associated with positivity for the vacuolating cytotoxin (VacA) s1/m1 genotype (Plummer et al. 2007), which is involved in higher degrees of inflammation, with the presence of epithelial damage in the gastric mucosa and progression of precancerous lesion (Gonzalez et al. 2011).

As to host genetic factors, polymorphisms of *IL-1B* and *TNF-A* showed relatively consistent association with risk of *H. pylori* infection, possibly due to inhibition of gastric acid secretion (Hamajima et al. 2006). Polymorphisms of *PNPNII*, *IL-2*, and *IL-13* were reported to be significantly associated with the risk of gastric atrophy (Hamajima et al. 2006). Recently, we investigated the *ABO* genotype and risk of *H. pylori* infection, atrophic gastritis, and gastric cancer in 703 cancer patients and 1,465 non-cancer patients (Nakao et al. 2011). The results showed that gastric cancer risk increased with the addition of the *A* allele (P trend <0.001), and decreased with the addition of the B allele (P trend $=0.023$), the odds ratio (OR) of atrophic gastritis was 0.73 (95 % CI 0.53–1.09) for blood type B relative to blood type A, and the OR of *H. pylori* infection was 0.39 (95%CI 0.17–0.87) for *BB* genotype relative to *AA* genotype (Nakao et al. 2011). These findings suggest that the *ABO* gene locus may influence the development of gastric cancer through persistent *H. pylori* infection and subsequent development of atrophic gastritis.

As to lifestyle factors, smoking elevates the risk of gastric cancer (Fujino et al. 2005) as well as the risk of precancerous lesions, intestinal metaplasia, and dysplasia (Kneller et al. 1992; You et al. 2000; Kato et al. 2004), and promotes the grade of atrophic gastritis in *H. pylori*-infected subjects (Nakamura et al. 2002). There are abundant case-control and cohort data on intake of salt or salty foods and risk of stomach cancer (Wang et al. 2009). It was biologically confirmed that a high-salt diet dose-dependently enhanced *H. pylori*-associated gastritis and stomach carcinogenesis in Mongolian gerbils (Kato et al. 2006). Intake of fresh fruits and vegetables was inversely associated with gastric cancer risk (Inoue et al. 1996), possibly attributed to their high concentrations of antioxidant substances.

5.3.3 Prevention of *H. pylori*-Induced Gastric Cancer

Eradication of *H. pylori* to prevent gastric cancer has been widely debated, and a recent meta-analysis of six randomized trials suggested that *H. pylori* eradication therapy reduces gastric cancer risk (RR 0.65, 95%CI 0.43–0.98) (Fuccio et al. 2009). There are several observational and randomized controlled studies that showed that eradication inhibits progression of or even improves gastric mucosal atrophy in patients with atrophic gastritis (Correa et al. 2000; Sung et al. 2000; Ohkusa et al. 2001; Watanabe et al. 2003; Arkkila et al. 2006). Similarly, eradication therapy is assumed to be efficient in inhibiting progression of intestinal metaplasia in randomized controlled trials (Sung et al. 2000; Leung et al. 2004). From this accumulated evidence, a consensus has been reached that *H. pylori* eradication therapy in patients with atrophic gastritis is effective for preventing gastric cancer (Asaka et al. 2010). The Japanese guidelines for the management of *H. pylori* infection recommended that the first-line eradication therapy of *H. pylori* be 1 week of triple therapy using a proton-pump inhibitor combined with two antibiotics, amoxicillin and clarithromycin (Asaka et al. 2010). However, the success rate of eradication from this regimen has recently fallen to 80 % or below because of the increasing incidence of clarithromycin resistance. Therefore, some alternative regimens to improve the success rate are needed (Chuah et al. 2011). When attempting to find appropriate patients for *H. pylori* eradication therapy, a screening method using serum testing of *H. pylori* antibody combined with pepsinogen I and II is possibly useful before the endoscopic examination. Serum pepsinogen testing is clinically useful for the prediction of gastric lesions in *H. pylori*-infected persons (Toyoda et al. 2012).

When we consider primary prevention of *H. pylori*-associated gastric cancer by lifestyle interventions, high-risk approaches targeting *H. pylori*-infected individuals are not very cost-effective because the number of individuals in the target population is quite large and the lifetime risk of developing gastric cancer in the targeted individuals is relatively small. In contrast, nationwide health promotion activities such as tobacco control and changes in dietary habits such as reducing salt intake and increasing fruit and vegetable intakes are likely to be a realistic approach to preventing the development of *H. pylori*-induced gastric cancer. Recently, we performed an age-period-cohort analysis of gastric cancer mortality rates in Japan between 1950 and 2004 and found that a decreasing period effect was observed from 1950, before improvements in detection and treatment of gastric cancer (Tanaka et al. 2012). This decreasing period effect occurred during a period when the Japanese people reduced dietary salt intake and therefore supports the utility of population approaches of lifestyle modification for prevention of *H. pylori*-induced gastric cancer.

5.4 Other Infections That Cause Malignancies

5.4.1 Epstein-Barr Virus (EBV)

EBV establishes a latent infection and lifelong persistence in more than 90 % of the world population. It is transmitted through saliva and initially infects the epithelium of the oropharynx, from which it subsequently spreads into B cells of the lymphoid tissue (Young and Rickinson 2004). EBV has been determined as a carcinogenic agent of Burkitt's lymphoma, nasopharyngeal carcinomas, Hodgkin lymphoma (NHL), and non-Hodgkin lymphoma in immunosuppressed subjects (IARC 1997). Vaccines for preventing primary EBV infection are currently under investigation.

5.4.2 Human T-Cell Leukemia Virus Type I (HTLV-1)

HTLV-1, the first human retrovirus that was identified, has a causal role in acute T-cell leukemia/lymphoma (ATL) (IARC 1996). ATL develops only in HTLV-1-infected persons and ATL cells contain monoclonal integrated HTLV-1 provirus. HTLV-1 carriers are clustered in southern Japan, southern Philippines, northern Iran, West and Central Africa, the Caribbean, and in American Indian populations and Melanesian populations of Australia and the Pacific (Tajima and Takezaki 1999). Viral transmission mostly occurs from mother to child during breast feeding. It was reported that the overall infection rate from carrier mother to her children was 10–30 % in Japan (Tajima and Hinuma 1992). After a latency period that has been shown to last an average of 60 years, approximately 7 % of male and 2 % of female HTLV-1 carriers will develop ATL (Tajima and Kuroishi 1985; Murphy et al. 1989). As viral eradication by an antiviral drug is not realistic, prevention of chronic infection is important. Breast feeding has been shown to reduce the risk of vertical transmission (Takezaki et al. 1997).

5.4.3 *Parasitic Infections*

Chronic infections with the liver flukes, *Opisthorchis viverrini (O. viverrini)* and *Clonorchis sinensis (C. sinensis)*, are both risk factors for cholangiocarcinoma (IARC 1994). *O. viverrini* is endemic in the Mekong River basin in Thailand, Laos, Cambodia, and Vietnam, while *C. sinensis* is endemic in southern and northern China, Southern Taiwan, Southern Korea, and northern Vietnam (Keiser and Utzinger 2005; Hong and Fang 2012). Infection with these liver flukes occurs mainly through ingestion of raw and/or fermented river fishes (Songserm et al. 2012) whose muscles contain metacercariae of the flukes. The most available preventive measure is considered to be community-based intervention changing the cooking (eating) style of these dangerous foods; this has been challenging in the Khon Kaen area, where the incidence of cholangiocarcinoma is the highest in the world (Kamsa-Ard et al. 2011). Praziquantel (PZQ) is an effective agent in eradicating liver flukes from the biliary tree. The results of a recent large-scale trial in China indicated the efficacy of one or two mass-chemotherapy treatments with PZQ in a year targeting the whole population in a *C. sinensis* highly endemic area (Choi et al. 2010). However, as humans cannot acquire a sufficient immune response to protect from reinfection, cointerruption of the routes of transmission is strongly recommended.

Schistosoma haematobium (*S. haematobium*) infection plays a causative role in the development of bladder cancer (Mostafa et al. 1999). The infectious cercariae of this fluke are transmitted through human skin during wading and swimming in rivers and ponds where its snail host lives. Approximately 110 million people in sub-Saharan Africa are infected with *S. haematobium*.

5.4.4 *Human Immunodeficiency Virus Type I (HIV-I) and Human Herpes Virus 8 (HHV-8)*

HIV has been classified as carcinogenic to humans for Kaposi sarcoma and NHL (IARC 1996). Subsequently, increased risks for several other cancers including

Hodgkin disease, anal cancer, cervical cancer, and seminoma in HIV-positive subjects have been reported. HIV, however, is not carcinogenic *per se* and interacts with the risk for many virus-associated cancers which are induced by immunodeficiency. The introduction of highly active antiretroviral therapy for treating HIV-positive adults has led to a decline in the incidence of AIDS-defining cancers in the US AIDS population through 1991–2005, although the incidence of non-AIDS-defining cancers has been increasing by aging (Shiels et al. 2011).

HHV-8, known as Kaposi sarcoma herpes virus, is a casual factor for the development of Kaposi sarcoma and a few rare lymphoproliferative disorders (Du et al. 2007). South America and Africa have relatively high prevalence rates possibly through mother-to-child transmission and inter-sibling transmission, whereas Europe and North America have low prevalence rates where it is mainly transmitted through receptive anal intercourse.

References

Abdel-Hady M, Bunn SK, Sira J, Brown RM, Brundler MA, Davies P, et al. Chronic hepatitis C in children-review of natural history at a National Centre. *J Viral Hepat* 2011; 18:e535–540.

Adami HO, Hsing AW, Mclaughlin JK, Trichopoulos D, Hacker D, Ekbom A, et al. (1992). Alcoholism and liver cirrhosis in the etiology of primary liver cancer. Int J Cancer 51:898–902.

Alter MJ. Epidemiology of hepatitis C. *Hepatology* 1997; 26(Suppl 1): 62S–65S.

Anzola M. Hepatocellular carcinoma: role of hepatitis B and hepatitis C viruses proteins in hepatocarcinogenesis. *J Viral Hepat* 2004; 11:383–393.

Arkkila PE, Seppala K, Farkkila MA, Veijola L, Sipponen P. Helicobacter pylori eradication in the healing of atrophic gastritis: a one-year prospective study. *Scand J Gastroenterol* 2006; 41:782–790.

Asaka M, Kato M, Takahashi S, Fukuda Y, Sugiyama T, Ota H, et al. Guidelines for the management of Helicobacter pylori infection in Japan: 2009 revised edition. *Helicobacter* 2010; 15:1–20.

Banatvala JE, Van Damme P. Hepatitis B vaccine -- do we need boosters? *J Viral Hepat* 2003; 10:1–6.

Basso D, Zambon CF, Letley DP, Stranges A, Marchet A, Rhead JL, et al. Clinical relevance of Helicobacter pylori cagA and vacA gene polymorphisms. *Gastroenterology* 2008; 135:91–99.

Beasley RP, Hwang LY, Stevens CE, Lin CC, Hsieh FJ, Wang KY, et al. Efficacy of hepatitis B immune globulin for prevention of perinatal transmission of the hepatitis B virus carrier state: final report of a randomized double-blind, placebo-controlled trial. *Hepatology* 1983; 3:135–141.

Beasley RP, Trepo C, Stevens CE, Szmuness W. The e antigen and vertical transmission of hepatitis B surface antigen. *Am J Epidemiol* 1977; 105:94–98.

Bukh J, Purcell RH, Miller RH. Sequence analysis of the core gene of 14 hepatitis C virus genotypes. *Proc Natl Acad Sci U S A* 1994; 91:8239–8243.

Cao GW. Clinical relevance and public health significance of hepatitis B virus genomic variations. *World J Gastroenterol* 2009; 15:5761–5769.

Chang MH, Chen CJ, Lai MS, Hsu HM, Wu TC, Kong MS, et al. Universal hepatitis B vaccination in Taiwan and the incidence of hepatocellular carcinoma in children. Taiwan Childhood Hepatoma Study Group. *N Engl J Med* 1997; 336:1855–1859.

Chang TT, Lai CL, Kew Yoon S, Lee SS, Coelho HS, Carrilho FJ, et al. Entecavir treatment for up to 5 years in patients with hepatitis B e antigen-positive chronic hepatitis B. *Hepatology* 2010; 51:422–430.

Chen HL, Chang MH, Ni YH, Hsu HY, Lee PI, Lee CY, et al. Seroepidemiology of hepatitis B virus infection in children: Ten years of mass vaccination in Taiwan. *JAMA* 1996; 276:906–908.

Chen YC, Sheen IS, Chu CM, Liaw YF. Prognosis following spontaneous HBsAg seroclearance in chronic hepatitis B patients with or without concurrent infection. *Gastroenterology* 2002; 123:1084–1089.

Cho LY, Yang JJ, Ko KP, Park B, Shin A, Lim MK, et al. Coinfection of hepatitis B and C viruses and risk of hepatocellular carcinoma: systematic review and meta-analysis. *Int J Cancer* 2011; 128:176–184.

Choi MH, Park SK, Li Z, Ji Z, Yu G, Feng Z, et al. Effect of control strategies on prevalence, incidence and re-infection of clonorchiasis in endemic areas of China. *PLoS Negl Trop Dis* 2010; 4:e601.

Choo QL, Kuo G, Weiner AJ, Overby LR, Bradley DW, Houghton M (1989) Isolation of a cDNA clone derived from a blood-borne non-A, non-B viral hepatitis genome. Science 244:359–362.

Chu CM, Yeh CT, Liaw YF. Low-level viremia and intracellular expression of hepatitis B surface antigen (HBsAg) in HBsAg carriers with concurrent hepatitis C virus infection. *J Clin Microbiol* 1998; 36:2084–2086.

Chuah SK, Tsay FW, Hsu PI, Wu DC. A new look at anti-Helicobacter pylori therapy. *World J Gastroenterol* 2011; 17:3971–3975.

Correa P. Human gastric carcinogenesis: a multistep and multifactorial process-First American Cancer Society Award Lecture on Cancer Epidemiology and Prevention. *Cancer Res* 1992; 52:6735–6740.

Correa P, Fontham ET, Bravo JC, Bravo LE, Ruiz B, Zarama G, et al. Chemoprevention of gastric dysplasia: randomized trial of antioxidant supplements and anti-helicobacter pylori therapy. *J Natl Cancer Inst* 2000; 92:1881–1888.

Dore GJ, Law M, Macdonald M, Kaldor JM. Epidemiology of hepatitis C virus infection in Australia. *J Clin Virol* 2003; 26:171–184.

Du MQ, Bacon CM, Isaacson PG. Kaposi sarcoma-associated herpesvirus/human herpesvirus 8 and lymphoproliferative disorders. *J Clin Pathol* 2007; 60:1350–1357.

Farrell GC. New hepatitis C guidelines for the Asia-Pacific region: APASL consensus statements on the diagnosis, management and treatment of hepatitis C virus infection. *J Gastroenterol Hepatol* 2007; 22:607–610.

Fattovich G, Bortolotti F, Donato F. Natural history of chronic hepatitis B: special emphasis on disease progression and prognostic factors. *J Hepatol* 2008; 48:335–352.

Fuccio L, Zagari RM, Eusebi LH, Laterza L, Cennamo V, Ceroni L, et al. Meta-analysis: can Helicobacter pylori eradication treatment reduce the risk for gastric cancer? *Ann Intern Med* 2009; 151:121–128.

Fujino Y, Mizoue T, Tokui N, Kikuchi S, Hoshiyama Y, Toyoshima H, et al. Cigarette smoking and mortality due to stomach cancer: findings from the JACC Study. *J Epidemiol* 2005; 15 Suppl 2:S113–119.

Garten RJ, Zhang J, Lai S, Liu W, Chen J, Yu XF. Coinfection with HIV and hepatitis C virus among injection drug users in southern China. *Clin Infect Dis* 2005; 41 Suppl 1:S18–24.

Gonzalez CA, Agudo A. Carcinogenesis, prevention and early detection of gastric cancer: where we are and where we should go. *Int J Cancer* 2012; 130:745–753.

Gonzalez CA, Figueiredo C, Lic CB, Ferreira RM, Pardo ML, Ruiz Liso JM, et al. Helicobacter pylori cagA and vacA genotypes as predictors of progression of gastric preneoplastic lesions: a long-term follow-up in a high-risk area in Spain. *Am J Gastroenterol* 2011; 106:867–874.

Graham CS, Baden LR, Yu E, Mrus JM, Carnie J, Heeren T, et al. Influence of human immunodeficiency virus infection on the course of hepatitis C virus infection: a meta-analysis. *Clin Infect Dis* 2001; 33:562–569.

Hamada H, Yatsuhashi H, Yano K, Daikoku M, Arisawa K, Inoue O, et al. Impact of aging on the development of hepatocellular carcinoma in patients with posttransfusion chronic hepatitis C. *Cancer* 2002; 95:331–339.

Hamajima N, Naito M, Kondo T, Goto Y. Genetic factors involved in the development of Helicobacter pylori-related gastric cancer. *Cancer Sci* 2006; 97:1129–1138.

Hara M, Mori M, Hara T, Yamamoto K, Honda M, Nishizumi M. Risk of developing hepatocellular carcinoma according to the titer of antibody to hepatitis C virus. *Hepatogastroenterology* 2001; 48:498–501.

Hayashi N, Okanoue T, Tsubouchi H, Toyota J, Chayama K, Kumada H. Efficacy and safety of telaprevir, a new protease inhibitor, for difficult-to-treat patients with genotype 1 chronic hepatitis C. *J Viral Hepat* 2012; 19:e134–142.

Hong ST, Fang Y. Clonorchis sinensis and clonorchiasis, an update. *Parasitol Int* 2012; 61:17–24.

Hsu HM, Lu CF, Lee SC, Lin SR, Chen DS. Seroepidemiologic survey for hepatitis B virus infection in Taiwan: the effect of hepatitis B mass immunization. *J Infect Dis* 1999;179:367–370.

Hsu YS, Chien RN, Yeh CT, Sheen IS, Chiou HY, Chu CM, et al. Long-term outcome after spontaneous HBeAg seroconversion in patients with chronic hepatitis B. *Hepatology* 2002; 35:1522–1527.

IARC. *Alcohol Drinking*. IARC Monographs on the Evaluation of Carcinogenic Risk to Humans Vol 44, Lyon, International Agency for Research on Cancer, 1988.

IARC. *Some Naturally Occurring Substances: Food Items and Constituents, Heterocyclic Aromatic Amines and Mycotoxins*. IARC Monographs on the Evaluation of Carcinogenic Risk to Humans Vol. 56 Lyon, International Agency for Research on Cancer, 1993.

IARC. *Schistosomes, liver flukes and Helicobacter pylori*. IARC Monographs on the Evaluation of Carcinogenic Risk to Humans Vol 61. Lyon, International Agency for Research on Cancer, 1994.

IARC. *Human Immunodeficiency Viruses and Human T-Cell Lymphotropic Viruses*. IARC Monographs on the Evaluation of Carcinogenic Risk to Humans Vol 67. Lyon, International Agency for Research on Cancer, 1996.

IARC. *Epstein-Barr Virus and Kaposi's Sarcoma Herpesvirus/Human Herpesvirus 8*. IARC Monographs on the Evaluation of Carcinogenic Risk to Humans Vol 70. Lyon, International Agency for Research on Cancer, 1997.

IARC. *Tobacco Smoke and Involuntary Smoking*. IARC Monographs on the Evaluation of Carcinogenic Risk to Humans Vol 83. Lyon, International Agency for Research on Cancer, 2004.

Ikeda K, Arase Y, Kobayashi M, Saitoh S, Someya T, Hosaka T, et al. A long-term glycyrrhizin injection therapy reduces hepatocellular carcinogenesis rate in patients with interferon-resistant active chronic hepatitis C: a cohort study of 1249 patients. *Dig Dis Sci* 2006; 51:603–609.

Inoue M, Tajima K, Kobayashi S, Suzuki T, Matsuura A, Nakamura T, et al. Protective factor against progression from atrophic gastritis to gastric cancer--data from a cohort study in Japan. *Int J Cancer* 1996; 66:309–314.

Ishiguro S, Inoue M, Tanaka Y, Mizokami M, Iwasaki M, Tsugane S. Impact of viral load of hepatitis C on the incidence of hepatocellular carcinoma: A population-based cohort study (JPHC Study). *Cancer Lett* 2011; 300:173–179.

Kamsa-Ard S, Wiangnon S, Suwanrungruang K, Promthet S, Khuntikeo N, Mahaweerawat S. Trends in Liver Cancer Incidence between 1985 and 2009, Khon Kaen, Thailand: Cholangiocarcinoma. *Asian Pac J Cancer Prev* 2011; 12:2209–2213.

Kao JH, Chen PJ, Lai MY, Chen DS. Hepatitis B virus genotypes and spontaneous hepatitis B e antigen seroconversion in Taiwanese hepatitis B carriers. *J Med Virol* 72:363–369.

Kato I, Vivas J, Plummer M, Lopez G, Peraza S, Castro D, et al. Environmental factors in Helicobacter pylori-related gastric precancerous lesions in Venezuela. *Cancer Epidemiol Biomarkers Prev* 2004; 13:468–476.

Kato S, Tsukamoto T, Mizoshita T, Tanaka H, Kumagai T, Ota H, et al. High salt diets dose-dependently promote gastric chemical carcinogenesis in Helicobacter pylori-infected Mongolian gerbils associated with a shift in mucin production from glandular to surface mucous cells. *Int J Cancer* 2006; 119:1558–1566.

Keiser J, Utzinger J. Emerging foodborne trematodiasis. *Emerg Infect Dis* 2005; 11:1507–1514.

Kneller RW, You WC, Chang YS, Liu WD, Zhang L, Zhao L, et al. Cigarette smoking and other risk factors for progression of precancerous stomach lesions. *J Natl Cancer Inst* 1992; 84:1261–1266.

Ko TM, Lin KH, Ho MM, Hwang MF, Hwang KC, Hsieh FJ, et al. Perinatal transmission of hepatitis B virus in the Taoyuan area. *Taiwan Yi Xue Hui Za Zhi* 1986; 85:341–351.

Koyama T, Matsuda I, Sato S, Yoshizawa H. Prevention of perinatal hepatitis B virus transmission by combined passive-active immunoprophylaxis in Iwate, Japan (1981-1992) and epidemiological evidence for its efficacy. *Hepatol Res* 2003; 26:287–292.

Kurbanov F, Tanaka Y, Mizokami M. Geographical and genetic diversity of the human hepatitis B virus. *Hepatol Res* 2010; 40:14–30.

Larsson SC, Wolk A. Coffee consumption and risk of liver cancer: a meta-analysis. *Gastroenterology* 2007; 132:1740–1745.

Leung WK, Lin SR, Ching JY, To KF, Ng EK, Chan FK, et al. Factors predicting progression of gastric intestinal metaplasia: results of a randomised trial on Helicobacter pylori eradication. *Gut* 2004; 53:1244–1249.

Liu J, Yang HI, Lee MH, Lu SN, Jen CL, Wang LY, et al. Incidence and determinants of spontaneous hepatitis B surface antigen seroclearance: a community-based follow-up study. *Gastroenterology* 2010; 139:474–482.

Lo KJ, Tsai YT, Lee SD, Wu TC, Wang JY, Chen GH, et al. Immunoprophylaxis of infection with hepatitis B virus in infants born to hepatitis B surface antigen-positive carrier mothers. *J Infect Dis* 1985; 152:817–822.

Lo KJ, Tsai YT, Lee SD, Yeh CL, Wang JY, Chiang BN, et al. Combined passive and active immunization for interruption of perinatal transmission of hepatitis B virus in Taiwan. *Hepatogastroenterology* 1985; 32:65–68.

Lu JJ, Cheng CC, Chou SM, Hor CB, Yang YC, Wang HL. Hepatitis B immunity in adolescents and necessity for boost vaccination: 23 years after nationwide hepatitis B virus vaccination program in Taiwan. *Vaccine* 2009; 27:6613–6618.

Madden A, Cavalieri W. Hepatitis C prevention and true harm reduction. *Int J Drug Policy* 2007; 18:335–337.

Mangia A, Ricci GL, Persico M, Minerva N, Carretta V, Bacca D, et al. A randomized controlled trial of pegylated interferon alpha-2a (40 KD) or interferon alpha-2a plus ribavirin and amantadine vs interferon alpha-2a and ribavirin in treatment-naive patients with chronic hepatitis C. *J Viral Hepat* 2005; 12:292–299.

Matsuura K, Tanaka Y, Hige S, Yamada G, Murawaki Y, Komatsu M, et al. Distribution of hepatitis B virus genotypes among patients with chronic infection in Japan shifting toward an increase of genotype A. *J Clin Microbiol* 2009; 47:1476–1483.

Mbarek H, Ochi H, Urabe Y, Kumar V, Kubo M, Hosono N, et al. A genome-wide association study of chronic hepatitis B identified novel risk locus in a Japanese population. *Hum Mol Genet* 2011; 20:3884–3892.

Mcmahon BJ. The influence of hepatitis B virus genotype and subgenotype on the natural history of chronic hepatitis B. *Hepatol Int* 2009; 3:334–342.

Moriya K, Fujie H, Shintani Y, Yotsuyanagi H, Tsutsumi T, Ishibashi K, et al. The core protein of hepatitis C virus induces hepatocellular carcinoma in transgenic mice. *Nat Med* 1998; 4:1065–1067.

Mostafa MH, Sheweita SA, O'Connor PJ. Relationship between schistosomiasis and bladder cancer. *Clin Microbiol Rev* 1999; 12:97–111.

Murphy EL, Hanchard B, Figueroa JP, Gibbs WN, Lofters WS, Campbell M, et al. Modelling the risk of adult T-cell leukemia/lymphoma in persons infected with human T-lymphotropic virus type I. *Int J Cancer* 1989; 43:250–253.

Nakamura M, Haruma K, Kamada T, Mihara M, Yoshihara M, Sumioka M, et al. Cigarette smoking promotes atrophic gastritis in Helicobacter pylori-positive subjects. *Dig Dis Sci* 2002; 47:675–681.

Nakao M, Matsuo K, Ito H, Shitara K, Hosono S, Watanabe M, et al. ABO genotype and the risk of gastric cancer, atrophic gastritis, and Helicobacter pylori infection. *Cancer Epidemiol Biomarkers Prev* 2011; 20:1665–1672.

Nelson PK, Mathers BM, Cowie B, Hagan H, Des Jarlais D, Horyniak D, et al. (2011) Global epidemiology of hepatitis B and hepatitis C in people who inject drugs: results of systematic reviews. Lancet 378:571–583.

Ng KP, Saw TL, Baki A, Rozainah K, Pang KW, Ramanathan M. Impact of the Expanded Program of Immunization against hepatitis B infection in school children in Malaysia. *Med Microbiol Immunol* 2005; 194:163–168.

Ni YH, Chang MH, Huang LM, Chen HL, Hsu HY, Chiu TY, et al. Hepatitis B virus infection in children and adolescents in a hyperendemic area: 15 years after mass hepatitis B vaccination. *Ann Intern Med* 2001; 135:796–800.

Ohki T, Tateishi R, Sato T, Masuzaki R, Imamura J, Goto T, et al. Obesity is an independent risk factor for hepatocellular carcinoma development in chronic hepatitis C patients. *Clin Gastroenterol Hepatol* 2008; 6:459–464.

Ohkusa T, Fujiki K, Takashimizu I, Kumagai J, Tanizawa T, Eishi Y, et al. Improvement in atrophic gastritis and intestinal metaplasia in patients in whom Helicobacter pylori was eradicated. *Ann Intern Med* 2001; 134:380–386.

Ohto H, Terazawa S, Sasaki N, Hino K, Ishiwata C, Kako M, et al. Transmission of hepatitis C virus from mothers to infants. The Vertical Transmission of Hepatitis C Virus Collaborative Study Group. *N Engl J Med* 1994; 330:744–750.

Orito E, Ichida T, Sakugawa H, Sata M, Horiike N, Hino K, et al. Geographic distribution of hepatitis B virus (HBV) genotype in patients with chronic HBV infection in Japan. *Hepatology* 2001; 34:590–594.

Osella AR, Misciagna G, Guerra VM, Chiloiro M, Cuppone R, Cavallini A, et al. Hepatitis C virus (HCV) infection and liver-related mortality: a population-based cohort study in southern Italy. The Association for the Study of Liver Disease in Puglia. *Int J Epidemiol* 2000; 29:922-927.

Parkin DM. The global health burden of infection-associated cancers in the year 2002. *Int J Cancer* 2006; 118:3030–3044.

Plummer M, Van Doorn LJ, Franceschi S, Kleter B, Canzian F, Vivas J, et al. Helicobacter pylori cytotoxin-associated genotype and gastric precancerous lesions. *J Natl Cancer Inst* 2007; 99:1328–1334.

Queiroz DM, Carneiro JG, Braga-Neto MB, Fialho AB, Fialho AM, Goncalves MH, et al. Natural History of Helicobacter pylori infection in childhood: eight-year follow-up cohort study in an urban community in northeast of Brazil. *Helicobacter* 2012; 17:23–29.

Robertson B, Myers G, Howard C, Brettin T, Bukh J, Gaschen B, et al. Classification, nomenclature, and database development for hepatitis C virus (HCV) and related viruses: proposals for standardization. International Committee on Virus Taxonomy. *Arch Virol* 1998; 143:2493–2503.

Sasaki F, Tanaka J, Moriya T, Katayama K, Hiraoka M, Ohishi K, et al. Very low incidence rates of community-acquired hepatitis C virus infection in company employees, long-term inpatients, and blood donors in Japan. *J Epidemiol* 1996; 6:198–203.

Sheen IS, Liaw YF, Chu CM, Pao CC. Role of hepatitis C virus infection in spontaneous hepatitis B surface antigen clearance during chronic hepatitis B virus infection. *J Infect Dis* 1992; 165:831–834.

Shiels MS, Pfeiffer RM, Gail MH, Hall HI, Li J, Chaturvedi AK, et al. Cancer burden in the HIV-infected population in the United States. *J Natl Cancer Inst* 2011; 103:753–62.

Simmonds P, Holmes EC, Cha TA, Chan SW, Mcomish F, Irvine B, et al. Classification of hepatitis C virus into six major genotypes and a series of subtypes by phylogenetic analysis of the NS-5 region. *J Gen Virol* 1993; 74 (Pt 11):2391–2399.

Songserm N, Promthet S, Sithithaworn P, Pientong C, Ekalaksananan T, Chopjitt P, et al. Risk factors for cholangiocarcinoma in high-risk area of Thailand: Role of lifestyle, diet and methylenetetrahydrofolate reductase polymorphisms. *Cancer Epidemiol* 2012; 36:e89–94.

Sumi H, Yokosuka O, Seki N, Arai M, Imazeki F, Kurihara T, et al. Influence of hepatitis B virus genotypes on the progression of chronic type B liver disease. *Hepatology* 2003; 37:19–26.

Sun CA, Wu DM, Lin CC, Lu SN, You SL, Wang LY, et al. Incidence and cofactors of hepatitis C virus-related hepatocellular carcinoma: a prospective study of 12,008 men in Taiwan. *Am J Epidemiol* 2003; 157:674–682.

Sung JJ, Lin SR, Ching JY, Zhou LY, To KF, Wang RT, et al. Atrophy and intestinal metaplasia one year after cure of H. pylori infection: a prospective, randomized study. *Gastroenterology* 2000; 119:7–14.

Suzuki Y, Kobayashi M, Ikeda K, Suzuki F, Arfase Y, Akuta N, et al. Persistence of acute infection with hepatitis B virus genotype A and treatment in Japan. *J Med Virol* 2005; 76:33–39.

Tajima K, Hinuma Y. Epidemiology of HTLV-I/ I I in Japan and the world. *Gann Monograph on Cancer Reserch* 1992; 39:129–149.

Tajima K, Kuroishi T. Estimation of rate of incidence of ATL among ATLV (HTLV-I) carriers in Kyushu, Japan. *Jpn J Clin Oncol* 1985; 15:423–430.

Tajima K, Takezaki T. Human T Cell Leukaemia Virus Type I. In: Newton R, Beral V, Weiss RA (eds) *Infections and Human Cancer*, Cancer Surveys. 1999. NewYork, 33: 191–211.

Tajiri H, Tanaka H, Brooks S, Takano T. Reduction of hepatocellular carcinoma in childhood after introduction of selective vaccination against hepatitis B virus for infants born to HBV carrier mothers. *Cancer Causes Control* 2011; 22:523–527.

Takezaki T, Tajima K, Ito M, Ito S, Kinoshita K, Tachibana K, et al. Short-term breast-feeding may reduce the risk of vertical transmission of HTLV-I. The Tsushima ATL Study Group. *Leukemia* 1997; 11 Suppl 3:60–62.

Tanaka H, Hiyama T, Tsukuma H, Okubo Y, Yamano H, Kitada A, et al. Prevalence of second generation antibody to hepatitis C virus among voluntary blood donors in Osaka, Japan. *Cancer Causes Control* 1994; 5:409–413.

Tanaka H, Tsukuma H, Hori Y, Nakade T, Yamano H, Kinoshita N, et al. The risk of hepatitis C virus infection among blood donors in Osaka, Japan. *J Epidemiol* 1998; 8:292–296.

Tanaka H, Tsukuma H, Yamano H, Oshima A, Shibata H. Prospective study on the risk of hepatocellular carcinoma among hepatitis C virus-positive blood donors focusing on demographic factors, alanine aminotransferase level at donation and interaction with hepatitis B virus. *Int J Cancer* 2004; 112:1075–1080.

Tanaka Y, Kurbanov F, Mano S, Orito E, Vargas V, Esteban JI, et al. Molecular tracing of the global hepatitis C virus epidemic predicts regional patterns of hepatocellular carcinoma mortality. *Gastroenterology* 2006a; 130:703–714.

Tanaka K, Tsuji I, Wakai K, Nagata C, Mizoue T, Inoue M, et al. Cigarette smoking and liver cancer risk: an evaluation based on a systematic review of epidemiologic evidence among Japanese. *Jpn J Clin Oncol* 2006b; 36:445–456.

Tanaka K, Tsuji I, Wakai K, Nagata C, Mizoue T, Inoue M, et al. Alcohol drinking and liver cancer risk: an evaluation based on a systematic review of epidemiologic evidence among the Japanese population. *Jpn J Clin Oncol* 2008a; 38:816–838.

Tanaka H, Imai Y, Hiramatsu N, Ito Y, Imanaka K, Oshita M, et al. Declining incidence of hepatocellular carcinoma in Osaka, Japan, from 1990 to 2003. *Ann Intern Med* 2008b; 148:820–826.

Tanaka M, Ma E, Tanaka H, Ioka A, Nakahara T, Takahashi H. Trends of stomach cancer mortality in Eastern Asia in 1950–2004: comparative study of Japan, Hong Kong and Singapore using age, period and cohort analysis. *Int J Cancer* 2012; 130:930–936.

Tanaka Y, Nishida N, Sugiyama M, Kurosaki M, Matsuura K, Sakamoto N, et al. Genome-wide association of IL28B with response to pegylated interferon-alpha and ribavirin therapy for chronic hepatitis C. *Nat Genet* 2009; 41:1105–1109.

Thomas DL. Hepatitis C and human immunodeficiency virus infection. *Hepatology* 2002; 36(Suppl 1):S201–209.

Toyoda K, Furusyo N, Ihara T, Ikezaki H, Urita Y, Hayashi J (2012). Serum pepsinogen and Helicobacter pylori infection-a Japanese population study. *Eur J Clin Microbiol Infect Dis* 2012; DOI 10.1007/s10096-011-1543-0.

Tsai YT, Lo KJ, Lee SD. Immunoprophylaxis against hepatitis B virus infection: a controlled trail in infants born to HBeAg-negative HBsAg carrier mothers in Taiwan. *Chin J Gastroenterol* 1984; 1:181–185.

Tsukuma H, Hiyama T, Tanaka S, Nakao M, Yabuuchi T, Kitamura T, et al. Risk factors for hepatocellular carcinoma among patients with chronic liver disease. *N Engl J Med* 1993; 328:1797–1801.

Ueno Y, Sollano JD, Farrell GC. Prevention of hepatocellular carcinoma complicating chronic hepatitis C. *J Gastroenterol Hepatol* 2009; 24:531–536.

Wang XQ, Terry PD, Yan H. Review of salt consumption and stomach cancer risk: epidemiological and biological evidence. *World J Gastroenterol* 2009; 15:2204–2213.

Watanabe H, Yamaguchi N, Kuwayama H, Sekine C, Uemura N, Kaise M, et al. Improvement in gastric histology following Helicobacter pylori eradication therapy in Japanese peptic ulcer patients. *J Int Med Res* 2003; 31:362–369.

West DJ, Calandra GB. Vaccine induced immunologic memory for hepatitis B surface antigen: implications for policy on booster vaccination. *Vaccine* 1996; 14:1019–1027.

Weyermann M, Rothenbacher D, Brenner H. Acquisition of Helicobacter pylori infection in early childhood: independent contributions of infected mothers, fathers, and siblings. *Am J Gastroenterol* 2009; 104:182–189.

Whittle HC, Maine N, Pilkington J, Mendy M, Fortuin M, Bunn J, et al. Long-term efficacy of continuing hepatitis B vaccination in infancy in two Gambian villages. *Lancet* 1995; 345:1089–1092.

Yang HI, Yeh SH, Chen PJ, Iloeje UH, Jen CL, Su J, et al. Associations between hepatitis B virus genotype and mutants and the risk of hepatocellular carcinoma. *J Natl Cancer Inst* 2008; 100:1134–1143.

Yang R, Gui X, Xiong Y, Gao S, Zhang Y, Deng L, et al. Risk of liver-associated morbidity and mortality in a cohort of HIV and HBV coinfected Han Chinese. *Infection* 2011; 39:427–431.

You WC, Zhang L, Gail MH, Chang YS, Liu WD, Ma JL, et al. Gastric dysplasia and gastric cancer: Helicobacter pylori, serum vitamin C, and other risk factors. *J Natl Cancer Inst* 2000; 92:1607–1612.

Young LS, Rickinson AB. Epstein-Barr virus: 40 years on. *Nat Rev Cancer* 2004; 4:757–768.

Yuen MF, Fung SK, Tanaka Y, Kato T, Mizokami M, Yuen JC, et al. Longitudinal study of hepatitis activity and viral replication before and after HBeAg seroconversion in chronic hepatitis B patients infected with genotypes B and C. *J Clin Microbiol* 2004; 42:5036–5040.

Yuen MF, Tanaka Y, Fong DY, Fung J, Wong DK, Yuen JC, et al. Independent risk factors and predictive score for the development of hepatocellular carcinoma in chronic hepatitis B. *J Hepatol* 2009; 50:80–88.

Zanetti AR, Mariano A, Romano L, D'amelio R, Chironna M, Coppola RC, et al. Long-term immunogenicity of hepatitis B vaccination and policy for booster: an Italian multicentre study. *Lancet* 2005; 366:1379–1384.

Zhang H, Zhai Y, Hu Z, Wu C, Qian J, Jia W, et al. Genome-wide association study identifies 1p36.22 as a new susceptibility locus for hepatocellular carcinoma in chronic hepatitis B virus carriers. *Nat Genet* 2010; 42:755–758.

Chapter 6
Applying Physical Activity in Cancer Prevention

Christine M. Friedenreich, Brigid M. Lynch, and Annie Langley

6.1 Introduction

Over the past two decades, epidemiological research has generated compelling data describing the benefits of physical activity in relation to cancer risk. The evidence has been systematically reviewed by national (Physical Activity Guidelines Advisory Committee 2008) and international agencies (World Cancer Research Fund and the American Institute for Cancer Research 2007), and there is broad agreement that physical activity is associated with a reduced risk of colon, breast, and endometrial and possibly other cancer sites. Despite progress in understanding the cancer-protective effects of physical activity, uncertainty still exists regarding the type, timing, and amount of physical activity required for significant benefit. In this chapter, we provide an overview of the existing epidemiological evidence relating physical activity to cancer risk.

A related area of research that has received minimal attention to date is the effect of sedentary behavior on cancer risk. Sedentary behaviors involve prolonged sitting or reclining, the absence of whole-body movement, and low (≤1.5 metabolic equivalents) energy expenditure. Emerging epidemiological evidence suggests that sedentary behavior may increase the risk of colorectal, endometrial, and ovarian cancer, although only five cancer sites have thus far been studied (results for breast and renal cell carcinoma have been null) (Lynch 2010). Here we update this review of the epidemiological literature on associations of sedentary behavior with cancer risk.

An emerging literature is now examining the biologic mechanisms whereby physical activity influences cancer risk. Observational and randomized intervention trials are examining how adiposity, endogenous sex hormones, inflammation, and

C.M. Friedenreich, PhD (✉) • B.M. Lynch, PhD • A. Langley, MSc
Department of Population Health Research, Alberta Health Services - Cancer Care, 1331 29 St NW, Calgary, AB, CANADA T2N 4 N2
e-mail: Christine.Friedenreich@albertahealthservices.ca

A.B. Miller (ed.), *Epidemiologic Studies in Cancer Prevention and Screening*, Statistics for Biology and Health 79, DOI 10.1007/978-1-4614-5586-8_6,

insulin resistance might explain the effect of physical activity and sedentary behavior on cancer risk. We provide an overview of the main findings on these mechanisms.

Finally, we highlight some of the public health implications of using physical activity as a means for cancer prevention by providing an overview of the current physical activity guidelines, the prevalence of physical inactivity, and the approaches that have been used to promote physical activity at a population level.

6.2 Epidemiological Evidence: Physical Activity and Cancer

6.2.1 Colon Cancer

The strongest evidence for an effect of physical activity on cancer prevention exists for colon cancer. To date, 85 separate studies have been published that have examined some aspect of physical activity and colon or colorectal cancer risk (Wolin and Tuchman 2011). Of these studies, 34 found a statistically significant reduced risk when comparing the most to the least active study participants, 38 studies observed a nonstatistically significant risk reduction, and 14 showed no effect of physical activity on colon cancer risk. The magnitude of the risk decrease ranges from 30% to 35%, and there is evidence of a linear dose–response with increasing physical activity and decreasing risk in 41 of 47 studies. The risk reduction is somewhat stronger in case–control studies than in cohort studies (Figs. 6.1 and 6.2). The effect of physical activity on colon cancer risk is seen equally in men and women, in different racial/ethnic groups, for all types of activity, and for activity done at different time points in life and at different intensities.

6.2.2 Breast Cancer

Nearly equally strong evidence for a role of physical activity exists for breast cancer as was found for colon cancer with 86 independent studies reported to date (Lynch et al. 2011a). A statistically significant reduced risk of breast cancer was observed in 36 studies and a nonstatistically significant reduction in 28 studies.

Only three studies found a slight, nonstatistically significant increased risk with increased physical activity levels, and 19 found no effect of activity on risk. The magnitude of the risk reduction was approximately 25% with a stronger association found in case–control than in cohort studies (Figs. 6.3 and 6.4). Breast cancer risk is decreased most with recreational and household activities and activity after the menopause. Both moderate- and vigorous-intensity activities contribute nearly equally to the risk reduction. Some effect modification by other factors has been investigated with a stronger association found in non-Caucasian populations, parous women, non-obese women, and those without a family history of breast cancer.

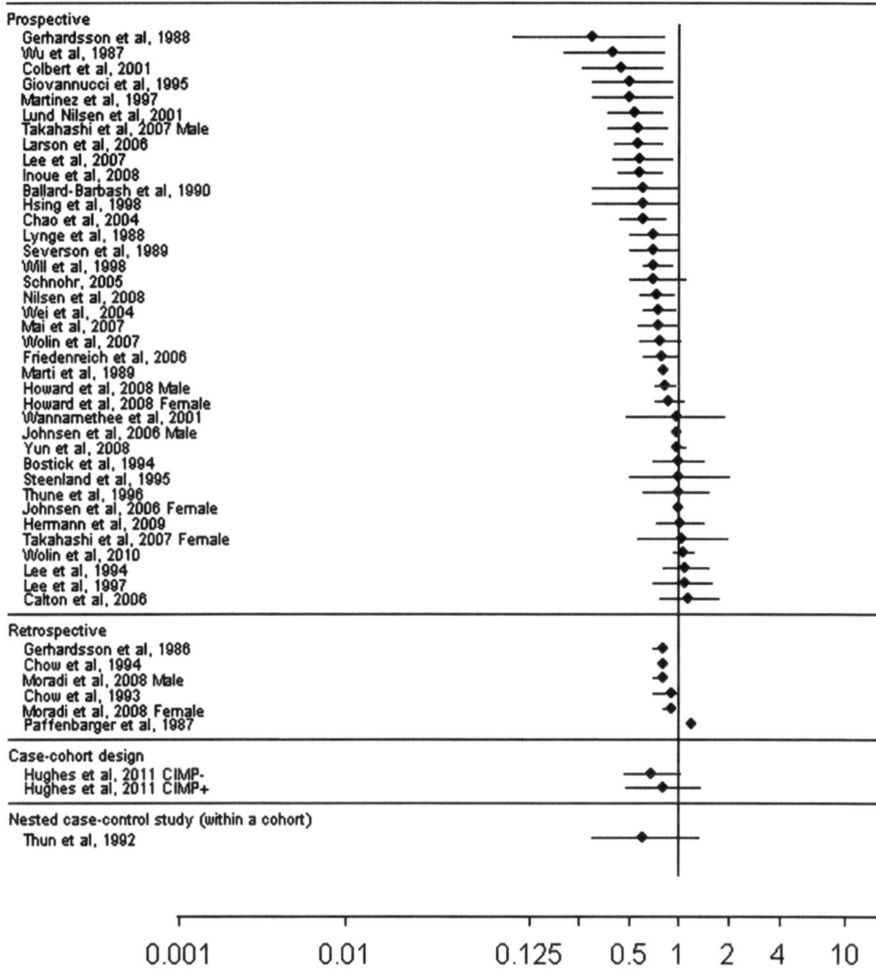

Fig. 6.1 Cohort studies of physical activity and colon cancer risk

6.2.3 Endometrial Cancer

Of the 28 studies on physical activity and endometrial cancer, half found a statistically significant risk reduction with increased activity levels and 9 of 28 a nonstatistically significant risk decrease (Cust 2011). The association is quite strong ranging from an average 38% decrease in case–control studies to a 25% decrease in cohort studies (Fig. 6.5). There is evidence for a dose–response association in 12 of 19 studies that examined this trend. There is no clear effect modification for this relationship by other factors. All types of activity, done at a moderate–vigorous intensity level, throughout lifetime, appear to be beneficial for reducing endometrial cancer risk.

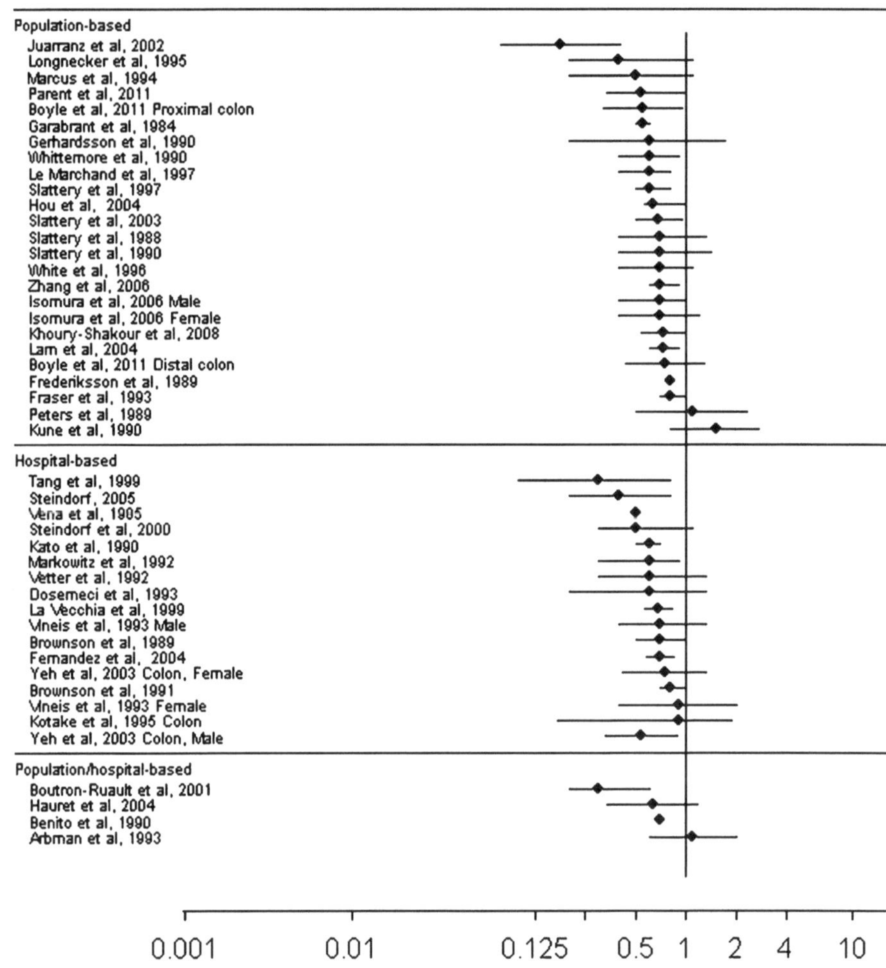

Fig. 6.2 Case–control studies of physical activity and colon cancer risk

6.2.4 Ovarian Cancer

In contrast to endometrial cancer, the epidemiological evidence for an association between physical activity and ovarian cancer is much weaker. Of the 23 studies published to date, only eight observed statistically significant risk reductions for ovarian cancer with higher levels of physical activity, four found nonstatistically significant decreases, eight showed no association, and three observed increased risks (Cust 2011). The risk reductions were, on average, less than 10%, and there was evidence for a dose–response effect in only nine of 11 studies (Fig. 6.6). There is only limited evidence thus far on any subgroup effects, and there is no clarity on whether any specific type, timing, or dose of activity is more beneficial for ovarian cancer risk reduction.

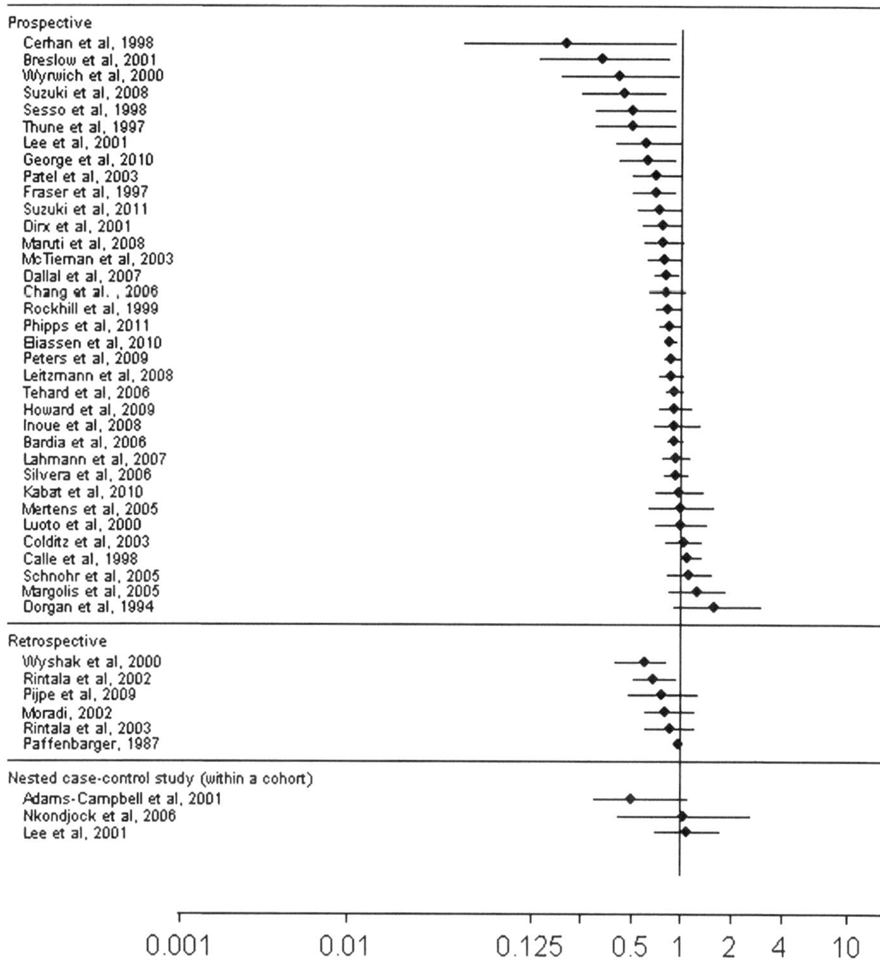

Fig. 6.3 Cohort studies of physical activity and breast cancer risk

6.2.5 *Prostate Cancer*

In total, 56 separate studies have been conducted on physical activity and prostate cancer risk (Figs. 6.7 and 6.8), of which 16 have found statistically significant risk reductions with increased activity levels, 10 nonstatistically significant decreases, 25 no effect, and five studies have detected an increased risk that was statistically significant in three studies (Leitzmann 2011). The magnitude of the risk decrease is on average about 10%. There are specific methodological challenges in studies of prostate cancer given the high prevalence of undetected prostate cancer in many men who would have served as controls in many of the case–control studies. Hence, there may have been some nondifferential misclassification bias that obstructed the ability to detect an association in these studies.

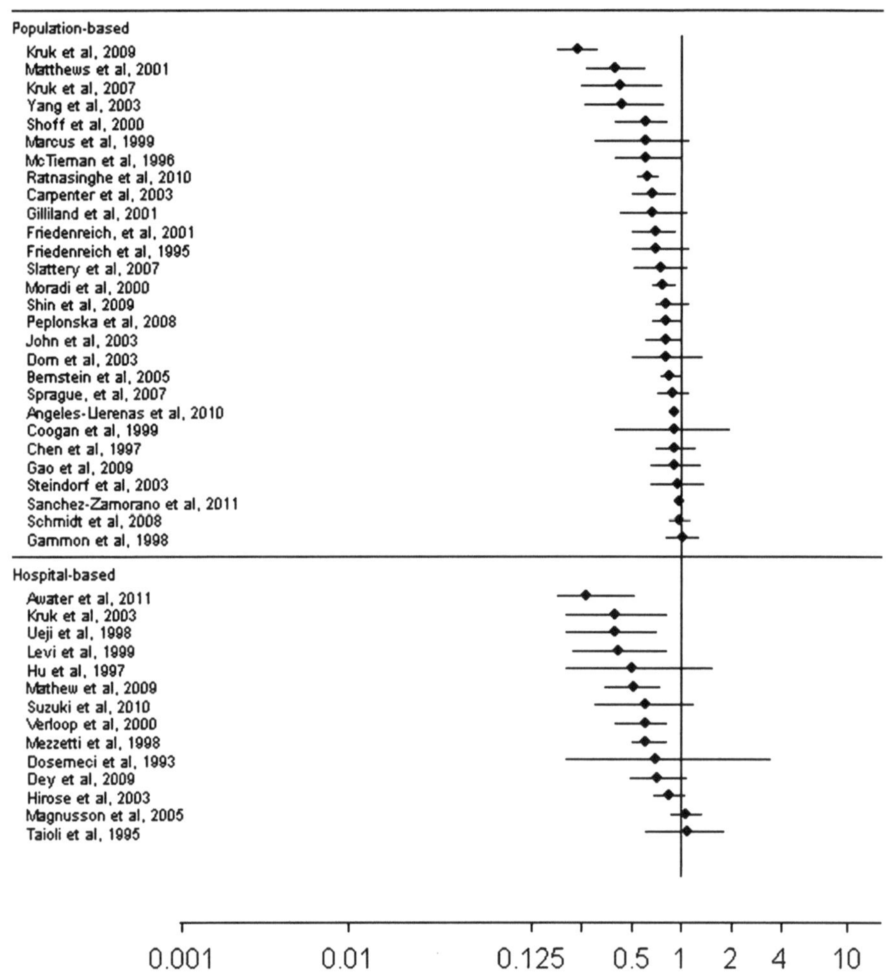

Fig. 6.4 Case–control studies of physical activity and breast cancer risk

There is not yet any clear evidence on the type, timing, and dose of activity needed to reduce prostate cancer risk nor is there any consistent evidence regarding associations specific to population subgroups.

6.2.6 Lung Cancer

Relatively few studies have been conducted on physical activity and lung cancer with 27 reported to date (Emaus and Thune 2011). Nearly half of the studies (13/27) showed a statistically significant risk reduction and six observed nonstatistically significant risk decreases among the most physically active men and women when compared to the least active. The magnitude of the risk reduction was about 25%

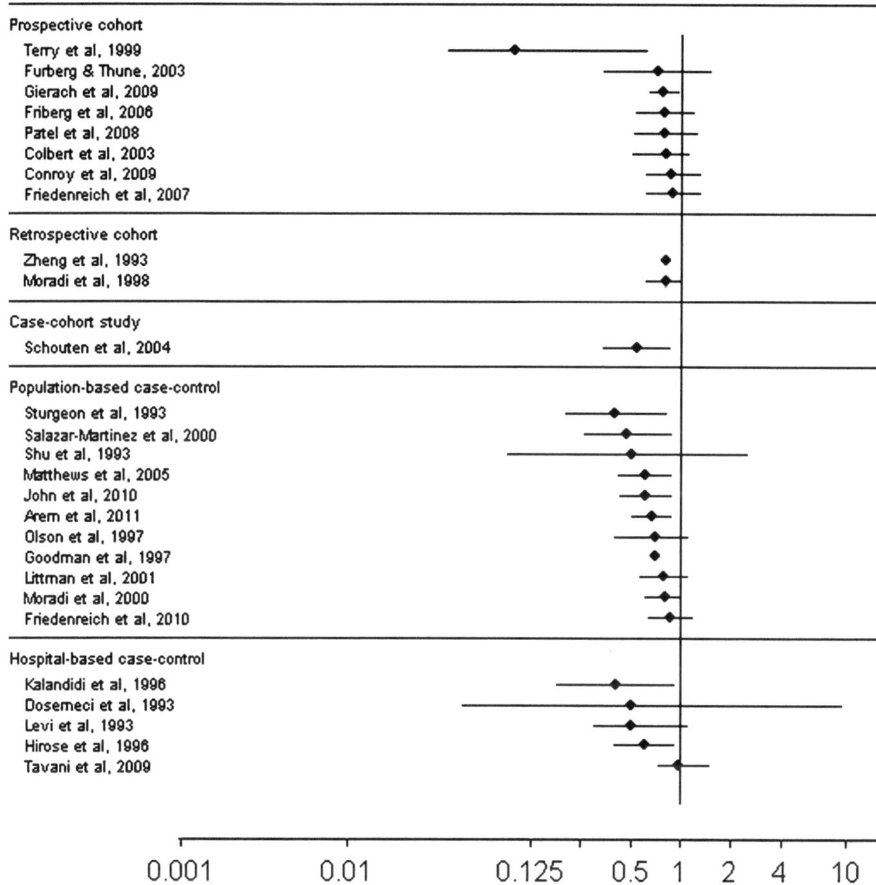

Fig. 6.5 Epidemiological studies of physical activity and endometrial cancer risk

and was observed equally in cohort and case–control studies (Figs. 6.9 and 6.10). A particular methodological issue in these studies is the ability to control for the possible confounding effect of smoking. Several of the studies examined the association separately for smokers and nonsmokers and found a stronger effect for current and former smokers compared to never smokers. Risk reductions appear to be of equal magnitude for different types of activity and for activity done at different time points in life or at different doses. There is no evidence yet of any specific effect modification within population subgroups.

6.2.7 *Other Sites*

For other cancer sites, such as the hematologic cancers (Pan and Morrison 2011), kidney, testicular, bladder cancers (Leitzmann 2011), and cervical cancers (Cust 2011),

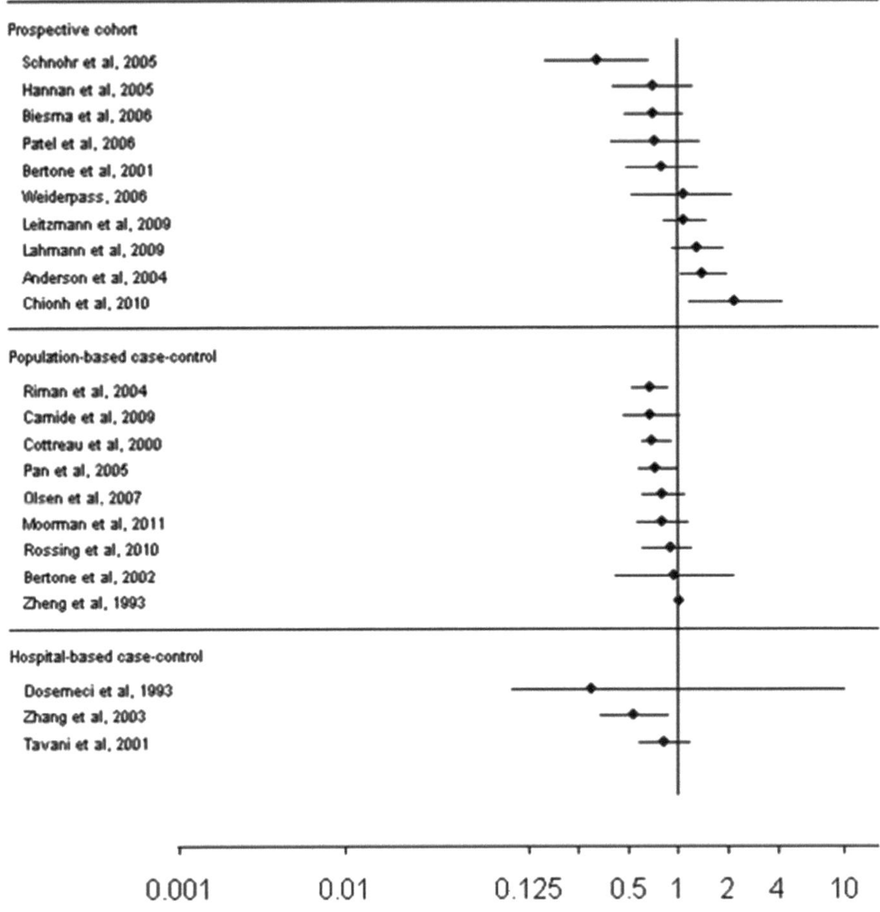

Fig. 6.6 Epidemiological studies of physical activity and ovarian cancer risk

there have been only a few studies published to date, and the data are insufficient to draw any conclusions at this time regarding the strength, dose–response, and consistency of the association between physical activity and risk of these other cancers.

6.3 Epidemiological Evidence: Sedentary Behavior and Cancer

6.3.1 Colorectal Cancer

Two studies have considered how sedentary behavior affects colorectal cancer risk (Howard et al. 2008; Steindorf et al. 2000). The National Institutes of

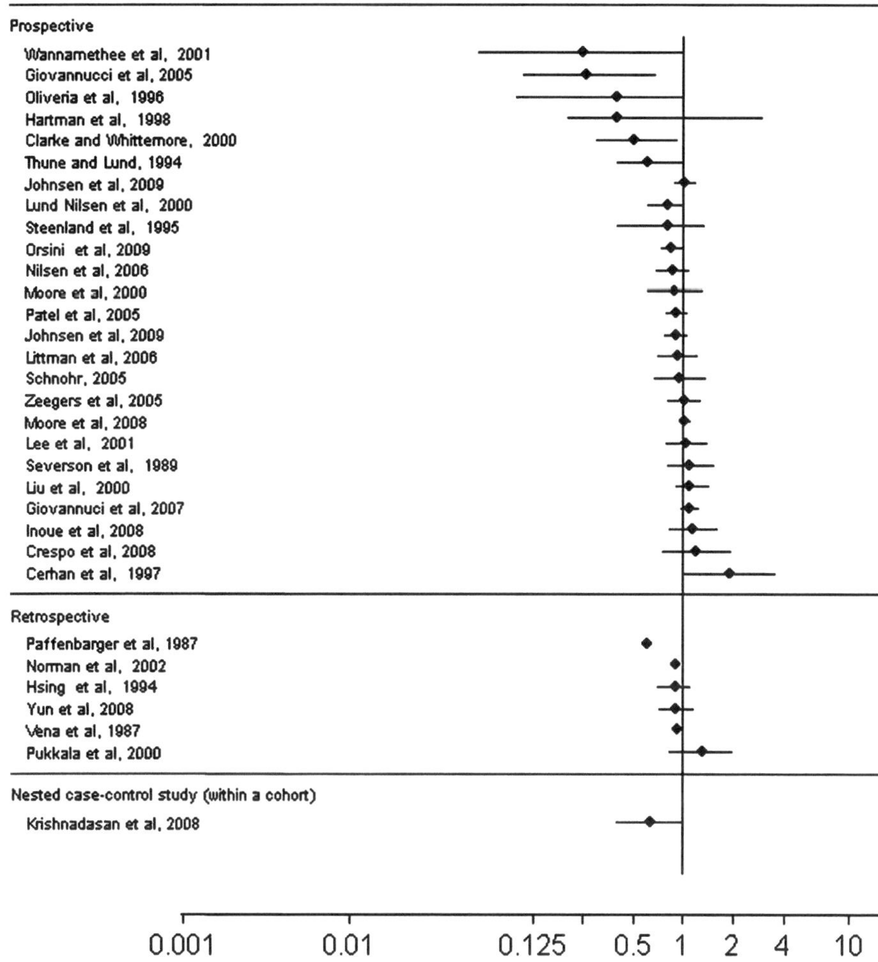

Fig. 6.7 Cohort studies of physical activity and prostate cancer risk

Health-American Association of Retired Persons (NIH-AARP) Diet and Health Study examined the associations of television viewing time and total sitting time with colorectal cancer risk in 300,673 men and women. Colorectal cancer risk increased significantly by more than 50% for men with longer television viewing times (≥9 vs. <3 h/day; RR = 1.56, 95% CI: 1.11, 2.20); for women, the risk was somewhat lower and of borderline significance (RR = 1.45, 95% CI: 0.99–2.13). About a 20% nonstatistically significant increased risk for longer total sitting time (≥9 vs. <3 h/day) was observed for both men and women (Howard et al. 2008). In a small case–control study of Polish women, Steindorf et al. (2000) found a statistically significant increased risk of colorectal cancer between the top and bottom tertiles (≥2 vs. <1.14 h/day) of television viewing (OR = 2.22, 95% CI: 1.19–4.17).

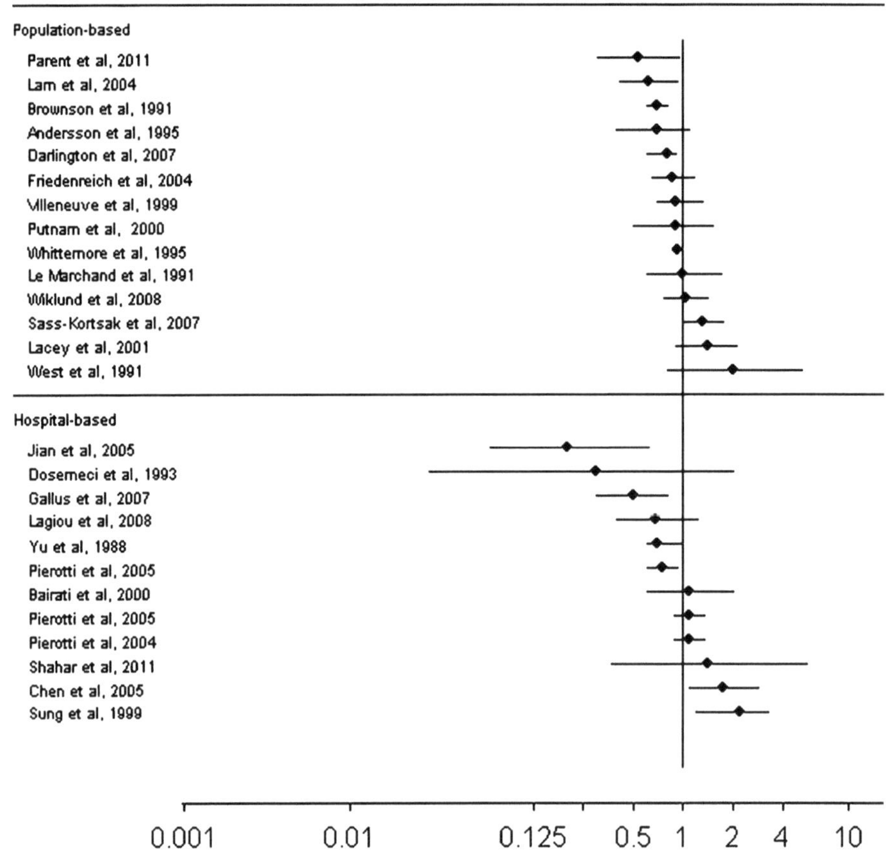

Fig. 6.8 Case–control studies of physical activity and prostate cancer risk

6.3.2 *Endometrial Cancer*

To date, three cohort studies (Friberg et al. 2006; Moore et al. 2010; Patel et al. 2008) and two case–control studies (Friedenreich et al. 2010a; Arem et al. 2011) have examined the association between sedentary behavior and endometrial cancer risk. Statistically significant increased risks were found in one cohort study (for ≥5 vs. <5 h/day television viewing RR = 1.66, 95% CI: 1.05–2.61) (Friberg et al. 2006) and in both case–control studies: OR = 1.52 (95% CI: 1.07–2.16) for ≥8 versus <4 h/day total sitting time (Arem et al. 2011) and OR = 1.11 (95% CI: 1.01–1.22) for every 5 h/week/year of lifetime occupational sitting (Friedenreich et al. 2010a). A borderline increased risk was shown in the NIH-AARP study: RR = 1.23 (95% CI: 0.96–1.57) for ≥7 versus <3 h/day total sitting time (Moore et al. 2010). A slightly increased nonsignificant risk was found in the Cancer Prevention Study II (CPS II) Nutrition Cohort for ≥6 versus <3 h/day total sitting time (Patel et al. 2008).

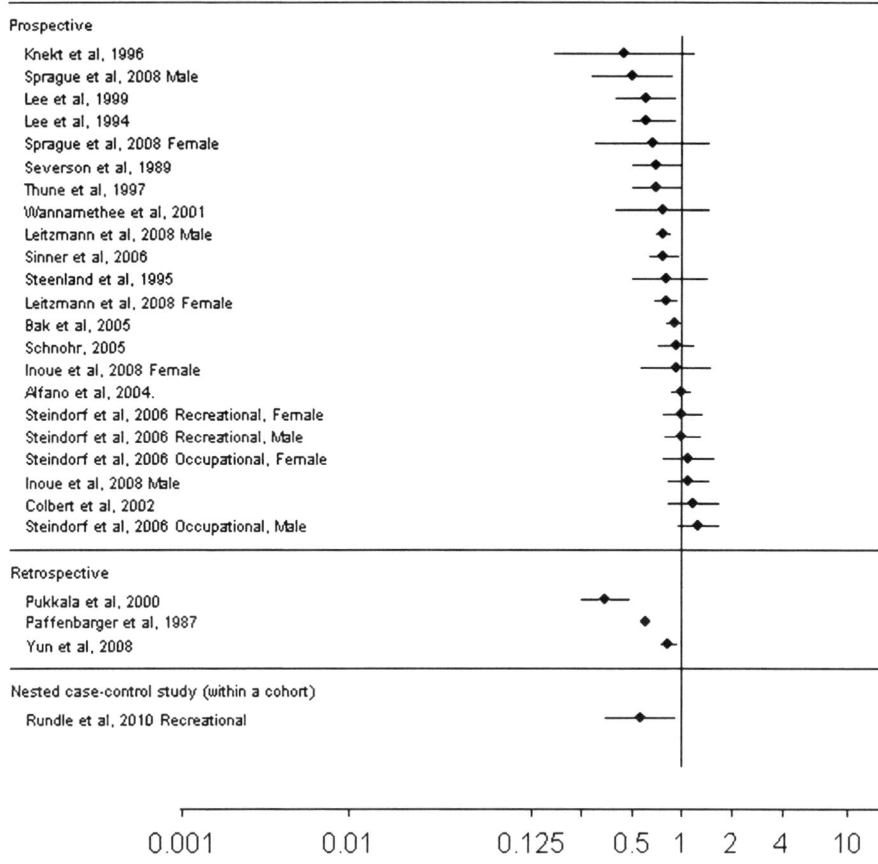

Fig. 6.9 Cohort studies of physical activity and lung cancer risk

6.3.3 *Ovarian Cancer*

Two studies have examined the role of sedentary behavior in ovarian cancer risk; both found a statistically significant association. Total sitting time (≥6 vs. <3 h/day) was associated with an RR of 1.55 (95% CI: 1.08–2.22) among women in the CPS II Nutrition Cohort (Patel et al. 2006). In a Chinese case–control study, television viewing time (>4 vs. <2 h/day) was significantly associated with ovarian cancer risk (OR = 3.39, 95% CI: 1.0–11.5), as was total sitting time (>10 vs. <4 h/day, OR = 1.77, 95% CI: 1.0–3.1) and occupational sitting time (>6 vs. <2 h/day, OR = 1.96, 95% CI: 1.2–3.2) (Zhang et al. 2003).

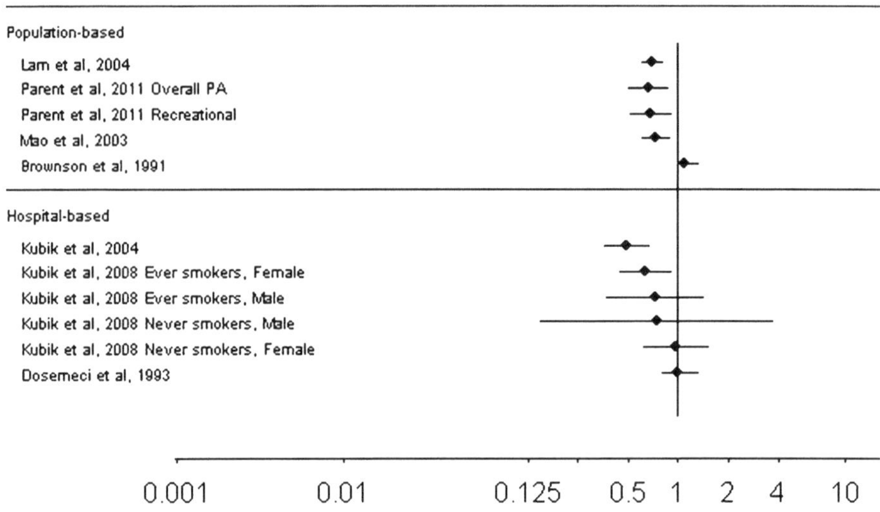

Fig. 6.10 Case–control studies of physical activity and lung cancer risk

6.3.4 Other Sites

Neither television viewing nor overall sitting time was associated with breast cancer (George et al. 2010) or with renal cell carcinoma (George et al. 2011) in the NIH-AARP Diet and Health study. Similarly, no association between television viewing and breast cancer was found in a case–control study of Indian women (Mathew et al. 2009).

6.4 Proposed Biologic Mechanisms

A number of biologic pathways relating physical activity and sedentary behavior to the development and progression of cancer have been proposed (McTiernan 2008; Friedenreich 2010; Lynch 2010) (Fig. 6.11). It is likely that these mechanisms are interrelated and that their relative contributions vary by cancer type. To become firmly established in a causal pathway, each proposed mechanism must relate significantly both to cancer risk and to physical activity/sedentary behavior.

6.4.1 Adiposity

Adiposity may facilitate carcinogenesis directly or through a number of pathways including increased levels of sex and metabolic hormones, chronic inflammation, and altered secretion of adipokines (Neilson et al. 2009; van Kruijsdijk et al. 2009).

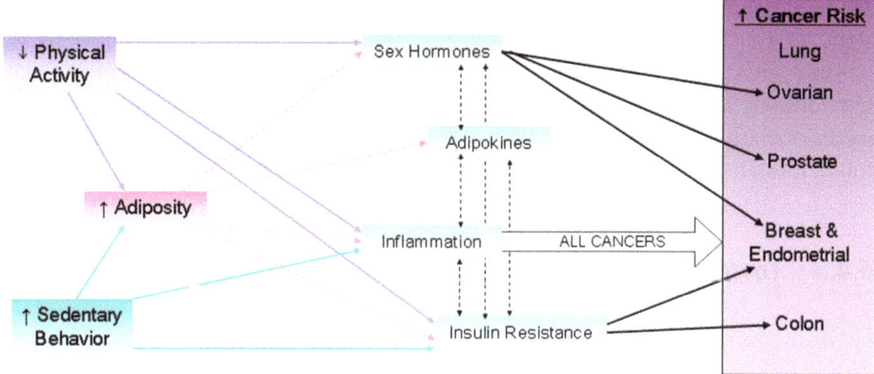

Fig. 6.11 Hypothesized biologic model relating proposed biomarkers of cancer risk to long-term physical activity and sedentary behavior

There is convincing evidence that adiposity increases colon, postmenopausal breast, endometrial, kidney, and esophageal cancer risk and cancer-related mortality (Reeves et al. 2007; Renehan et al. 2008).

There is now evidence from three randomized controlled exercise intervention trials that physical activity reduces adiposity, all of which found statistically significant reductions in adiposity levels with increased aerobic exercise as well as a dose–response effect on all body fat measures with increasing adherence to the exercise intervention (Irwin et al. 2003; Friedenreich et al. 2010c; Monninkhof et al. 2009).

Time in sedentary behavior generally displaces time spent in light-intensity physical activity (Owen et al. 2010); such a shift reduces overall cumulative daily energy expenditure. Sedentary behavior and adiposity are consistently associated in cross-sectional studies; however, results from cohort studies are mixed (Lynch 2010).

6.4.2 Sex Hormones

Exposure to biologically available sex hormones is a risk factor for hormone-related cancers, particularly breast, endometrial, and prostate cancers (McTiernan 2008; Friedenreich 2010). Sex hormone-binding globulin (SHBG) may also affect cancer risk by binding to sex hormones, rendering them biologically inactive (Neilson et al. 2009). Both physical activity and sedentary behavior may be associated with endogenous sex hormones via adiposity. In postmenopausal women, the main source of circulating estrogen is from conversion of androgens within adipose tissue (Kendall et al. 2007); hence, adiposity directly influences levels of total and bioavailable estrogen (Kaaks et al. 2002). Visceral adipose tissue is also important in the production of adipokines, which influence estrogen (Pou et al. 2007) and androgen biosynthesis (Böttner et al. 2004).

There is evidence from randomized intervention trials that exercise can reduce the level of estradiol and increase SHBG but limited evidence for an effect on estrone, testosterone, and androstenedione (McTiernan et al. 2004; McTiernan et al. 2006;

Monninkhof et al. 2009; Tworoger et al. 2007; Friedenreich et al. 2010b; Chubak et al. 2004).

Only one study has considered whether or not sedentary behavior directly affects sex hormone levels. A cross-sectional study of 565 postmenopausal women examined associations of sitting time with various estrogens, androgens, and SHBG and found no statistically significant associations (Tworoger et al. 2007).

6.4.3 Insulin Resistance

Associations between insulin levels and colorectal, postmenopausal breast, pancreatic, and endometrial cancers have been demonstrated in epidemiological studies, while fasting glucose levels have been directly associated with pancreatic, kidney, liver, endometrial, biliary, and urinary tract cancers (Becker et al. 2009). Neoplastic cells use glucose for proliferation; therefore, hyperglycemia may promote carcinogenesis by providing an amiable environment for tumor growth (Xue and Michels 2007). High insulin levels increase bioavailable insulin-like growth factor-I (IGF), which is involved in cell differentiation, proliferation, and apoptosis (Nandeesha 2009). Decreasing blood insulin levels also results in increased hepatic synthesis of SHBG; hence, insulin indirectly increases bioavailability of endogenous sex hormones (Kaaks 2001; Xue and Michels 2007).

Exercise intervention trials have found that insulin, glucose, and insulin resistance as assessed by the HOMA score are all reduced with aerobic exercise (Friedenreich et al. 2011a; Mason et al. 2011). No effect has been found for exercise on any of the IGF family of proteins (Friedenreich et al. 2011a; Irwin et al. 2005; McTiernan et al. 2005).

Sedentary behavior could plausibly affect metabolic function via increased adiposity and decreased skeletal muscle mass. The sustained periods of muscular inactivity that occur during sedentary behavior may reduce glucose uptake (Hamilton et al. 2007; Tremblay et al. 2010). Although cross-sectional studies mostly demonstrate significant associations between sedentary behavior and biomarkers of metabolic dysfunction, no clear evidence of an association has emerged from the limited prospective research to date (Thorp et al. 2011; Proper et al. 2011).

6.4.4 Adipokines and Inflammation

Chronic inflammation is acknowledged as a risk factor for most types of cancer (McTiernan 2008; Neilson et al. 2009). Inflammation may induce cell proliferation, microenvironmental changes, and oxidative stress, which in turn could deregulate normal cell growth and promote progression and malignant conversion (Coussens and Werb 2002). Obesity is considered a low-grade, systemic inflammatory state (Lee et al. 2007). Adipose tissue is a complex metabolic and endocrine organ that secretes multiple biologically active polypeptides known collectively as adipokines (Kershaw and Flier 2004; Antuna-Puente et al. 2008), including leptin, adiponectin, tumor necrosis factor-α (TNF-α), and interleukin-6 (IL-6). C-reactive protein (CRP) is an acute phase protein produced in the liver in response to TNF-α and IL-6 levels; each of these factors is a biomarker of inflammation.

The release of adipokines may play a central role in the development of insulin resistance (Antuna-Puente et al. 2008), and elevated levels of adipokines might also increase cancer risk by affecting estrogen biosynthesis and activity (Pou et al. 2007).

Exercise intervention trials have demonstrated a direct effect of exercise on CRP but no effect on TNF-α or IL-6 levels (Friedenreich et al. 2011b; Tworoger et al. 2007; Irwin et al. 2009; Campbell et al. 2009). Likewise, no direct effect on adiponectin was observed; however, the ratio of leptin/adiponectin was associated with increasing exercise levels (Friedenreich et al. 2011a).

There have been few epidemiological studies linking sedentary behavior with biomarkers of inflammation. One prospective study found a significant, positive association between average television time (four assessments over 6 years) and leptin but no association with CRP (Fung et al. 2000). In contrast, data from the National Health and Nutrition Examination Survey has demonstrated statistically significant, cross-sectional associations between accelerometer-assessed sedentary time and CRP in postmenopausal women (Lynch et al. 2011b) and in the broader adult population (Healy et al. 2011).

6.5 Public Health Implications

Despite compelling evidence for the health benefits of physical activity, including a reduced risk of several cancers, many individuals do not meet recommended activity levels. Several key areas need to be addressed to translate scientific knowledge on the health benefits of physical activity that include education of the public on these benefits through evidence-based guidelines, increased health promotion activities, coordinated efforts at different jurisdictional levels, public engagement, partnerships between governmental and nongovernmental organizations, changes in fiscal policies, and urban and rural planning (Global Advocacy for Physical Activity (GAPA) 2010).

6.5.1 Physical Activity Guidelines

Global recommendations for physical activity for health issued by the World Health Organization (WHO) currently recommend that adults 18–64 years of age engage in at least (1) 150 min of moderate intensity aerobic physical activity, or (2) 75 min of vigorous intensity aerobic physical activity, or (3) an equivalent combination of moderate and vigorous intensity activity, in intervals of 10 min or greater over the course of a week. Additional moderate–vigorous aerobic activity (of up to 300 min for moderate, 150 min for vigorous, or an equivalent combination of moderate and vigorous activities) and muscle strengthening on two or more occasions may be performed over the week for additional health benefits (World Health Organization 2010).

Through endorsements from the WHO, national physical activity guidelines have become available in many countries (World Health Organization 2008; United Nations General Assembly 2011). National guidelines in Canada (Canadian Society for Exercise Physiology 2011) and the United States (U.S. Department of Health and Human Services 2008) are similar but differ from available cancer prevention-specific guidelines from the American Cancer Society that recommends at least 30 min of moderate–vigorous activity on at least 5 days/week for adults (Kushi et al. 2006) and the World Cancer Research Fund/American Institute for Research on Cancer that recommends that adults be "physically active everyday in any way for at least 30 min" (World Cancer Research Fund and the American Institute for Cancer Research 2007).

Despite widespread and long-standing guidelines, the majority of Canadians (Bryan and Katzmarzyk 2009; Colley et al. 2011) and Americans (Troiano et al. 2008) do not meet recommended activity levels. It is estimated that if recommended all Canadians followed activity guidelines, up to 20% of colon cancer deaths and 14% of breast cancer deaths in Canada could be prevented (Warburton et al. 2007).

6.5.2 Population-Based Strategies to Increase Physical Activity Levels

Physical activity guidelines are not produced under the intention of directly eliciting behavior change, but rather offer evidence-based targets that if adhered to are associated with reduced risks of disease. To encourage uptake and adherence, physical activity guidelines must be supplemented with effective public health messaging and, where possible, population-based physical activity programs or interventions.

Effective public health messaging should address not only why physical activity is important but also how recommended levels may be achieved. Messaging should be informative and persuasive and be disseminated to the public through a multiphase social marketing campaign to target the largest possible audience (Brawley and Latimer 2007). Evaluations of messaging strategies have demonstrated only modest and short-term changes to physical activity levels with this approach alone (Kahn et al. 2002).

Publicly accessible activity programs and/or interventions may be a more direct and effective means to physical activity promotion, but available resources limit implementation. Several trials have assessed intervention-based strategies for encouraging uptake and adherence to physical activity guidelines. A critical review of this research revealed that many interventions had only modest effects on changing activity levels and that few strategies had the capacity to elicit behavioral changes that are adequate to fulfill currently recommended guidelines (Hillsdon et al. 2005).

Measurement error is one optimistic explanation for the minimal changes to physical activity levels observed with these strategies, as many studies have employed self-reported measures of activity that may not be sufficiently sensitive to detect meaningful differences between study groups. Further, it may take people time to change physical activity, and so they may occur beyond the follow-up period of a typical study. Given these limitations, comprehensive evaluation of activity promotion should also consider changes in awareness, understanding, motivation, and self-efficacy to pursue physical activity (Brawley and Latimer 2007).

An important consideration for physical activity intervention trials is the feasibility of interventions on a population level. In their review of the literature, Hillsdon et al. observed that the most effective interventions were those that included professional advice and ongoing support and which took place in a community or health-care center (Hillsdon et al. 2005). Such interventions may be too costly and complex to apply beyond the research setting. To facilitate this bridge from research to community, future trials should consider consultation with key stakeholders such as community organizations and policy makers.

The subtle changes to physical activity levels observed with public health messaging and activity interventions highlight the importance of the underlying socio-cultural, environmental, and policy influences of inactive and sedentary lifestyles, which may require transformation in order to achieve the greatest possible changes to physical activity levels. The 2010 Toronto Charter for Physical Activity and its supporting action document provide an international consensus regarding the specific steps that should be taken to promote and support physical activity on a global scale (Bull 2011). Recommendations advise that governments and organizations working to improve physical activity levels address the determinants of physical inactivity in all relevant sectors including programs targeting education, transport, sports and recreation, primary health-care systems, and urban planning.

Overall, improving physical activity participation in the future requires a concerted effort from many parties. While approaches to increasing population physical activity levels have been identified and endorsed, implementing these strategies requires serious political commitment and strong investments (Bull 2011). Continued dissemination and advocacy for the Toronto Charter and its specific recommendations and continued efforts to secure support from key governmental agencies are key priorities to increasing global physical activity levels and, ultimately, preventing cancer.

6.6 Conclusions

There is now consistent and strong evidence that physical activity reduces the risk of colon and breast cancers and fairly consistent evidence for endometrial cancer as well (Table 6.1). The evidence is somewhat weaker for lung and prostate cancers and currently insufficient for ovarian and other cancer sites.

There is also emerging evidence for an etiologic role of sedentary behavior in increasing the risk of several cancer sites. Several hypothesized biologic mechanisms have emerged for these associations of physical activity and sedentary behavior and cancer risk with the strongest evidence for a role of adiposity, insulin resistance, inflammation, and endogenous sex hormones. More research is needed,

Table 6.1 Summary of epidemiological evidence on physical activity and cancer prevention by cancer site

Cancer site	Number of studies	Number of studies with statistically significant risk reduction	Magnitude of risk reduction	Dose–response effect	Overall classification of evidence
Colon	85	72 (34)	30%	Yes	Convincing
Breast	86	64 (36)	25%	Yes	Convincing
Endometrial	28	23 (14)	30–35%	Yes	Probable
Ovarian	23	12 (4)	<10%	Limited	Weak
Prostate	56	26 (15)	10%	Limited	Weak
Lung	27	19 (7)	25%	Some	Possible

ideally from randomized controlled trials, to improve understanding of the effects of different doses and types of physical activity and sedentary behavior on the various biologic pathways. Translation of this knowledge on cancer prevention benefits to the general population has not yet occurred; concerted and coordinated efforts are needed at several jurisdictional levels to increase physical activity levels before benefit with respect to cancer risk reduction will be realized.

Acknowledgements Dr Friedenreich was supported by an Alberta Innovates-Health Solutions (AI-HS) Senior Health Scholar Award and Dr Lynch by Postdoctoral Fellowship awards from the National Health Medical Research Council and AI-HS while writing this chapter. The figures were prepared by Qinggang Wang.

References

Antuna-Puente B, Feve B, Fellahi S, Bastard JP. Adipokines: The missing link between insulin resistance and obesity. *Diabetes Metab* 2008; 34:2–11.

Arem H, Irwin M, Zhou Y, Lu L, Risch H, Yu H. Physical activity and endometrial cancer in a population-based case-control study. *Cancer Causes Control* 2011; 22:219–226.

Becker S, Dossus L, Kaaks R. Obesity related hyperinsulinaemia and hyperglycaemia and cancer development. *Arch Physiol Biochem* 2009; 115:86–96.

Böttner A, Kratzsch J, Müller G, Kapellen TM, Blüher S, Keller E et al. (2004). Gender Differences of Adiponectin Levels Develop during the Progression of Puberty and Are Related to Serum Androgen Levels. *J Clin Endocr Metab* 2004; 89: 4053–4061.

Brawley LR, Latimer AE. Physical activity guides for Canadians: messaging strategies, realistic expectations for change, and evaluation. *Appl Physiol Nutr Metab* 2007; 32:S170–S184.

Bryan SN, Katzmarzyk PT. Are Canadians meeting the guidelines for moderate and vigorous leisure-time physical activity? *Appl Physiol Nutr Metab* 2009; 34: 707–715.

Bull FC. Global Advocacy for Physical Activity - Development and Progress of the Toronto Charter for Physical Activity: A Global Call for Action. *Res Exerc Epidemiol* 2011;13:1–10.

Campbell PT, Campbell KL, Wener MH, Wood BL, Potter JD, McTiernan A et al. A yearlong exercise intervention decreases CRP among obese postmenopausal women. *Med Sci Sports Exerc* 2009; 41:1533–1539.

Canadian Society for Exercise Physiology. Canadian Physical Activity Guidelines. 2011.

Chubak J, Tworoger SS, Yasui Y, Ulrich CM, Stanczyk FZ, McTiernan A. Associations between reproductive and menstrual factors and postmenopausal sex hormone concentrations. *Cancer Epidemiol Biomarkers Prev* 2004; 13:1296–1301.

Colley RC, Garriquet D, Janssen I, Craig J, Tremblay MS. Physical activity of Canadian adults: Accelerometer results from the 2007 to 2009 Canadian Health Measures Survey. *Health Rep* 2011; 22:15–23.

Coussens LM, Werb Z. Inflammation and cancer. *Nature* 2002; 420:860–867.

Cust AE. In Courneya KS & Friedenreich CM (Eds.) *Physical activity and gynecologic cancer prevention.* Springer Berlin Heidelberg, 2011; pp. 159–185.

Emaus A, Thune I. In Courneya KS & Friedenreich CM (Eds.) *Physical activity and gynecologic cancer prevention.* Springer Berlin Heidelberg, 2011; pp. 101–133.

Friberg E, Mantzoros CS, Wolk A. Physical activity and risk of endometrial cancer: a population -based prospective cohort study. *Cancer Epidemiol Biomarkers Prev* 2006; 15:2136–2140.

Friedenreich CM. Physical activity and breast cancer risk: epidemiologic evidence and biologic mechanisms. *Eur J Cancer* 2010; Suppl 8: 5.

Friedenreich C, Norat T, Steindorf K, Boutron-Ruault MC, Pischon T, Mazuir M et al. Physical activity and risk of colon and rectal cancers: the European prospective investigation into cancer and nutrition. *Cancer Epidemiol Biomarkers Prev* 2006; 15:2398–2407.

Friedenreich CM, Cook LS, Magliocco AM, Duggan MA, Courneya KS. Case-control study of lifetime total physical activity and endometrial cancer risk. *Cancer Causes Control* 2010a; 21:1105–1116.

Friedenreich CM, Woolcott CG, McTiernan A, Ballard-Barbash R, Brant RF, Stanczyk FZ et al. Alberta physical activity and breast cancer prevention trial: sex hormone changes in a year-long exercise intervention among postmenopausal women. *J Clin Oncol* 2010b; 28:1458–1466.

Friedenreich CM, Woolcott CG, McTiernan A, Terry T, Brant R, Ballard-Barbash R et al. Adiposity changes after a 1-year aerobic exercise intervention among postmenopausal women: a randomized controlled trial. *Int J Obes* 2010c; 35:427–435.

Friedenreich CM, Neilson HK, Woolcott CG, McTiernan A, Wang Q, Ballard-Barbash R et al. Changes in insulin resistance indicators, insulin-like growth factors, and adipokines in a year-long trial of aerobic exercise in postmenopausal women. *Endocr Relat Cancer* 2011a; 18:357–369.

Friedenreich CM, Neilson HK, Woolcott CG, Wang Q, Yasui Y, Brant RF et al. Mediators and moderators of the effects of a year-long exercise intervention on endogenous sex hormones in postmenopausal women. *Cancer Causes Control* 2011b; in press.

Fung TT, Hu FB, Yu J, Chu NF, Spiegelman D, Tofler GH et al. Leisure-Time Physical Activity, Television Watching, and Plasma Biomarkers of Obesity and Cardiovascular Disease Risk. *Am J Epidemiol* 2000; 152:1171–1178.

George SM, Irwin ML, Matthews CE, Mayne ST, Gail MH, Moore SC et al. Beyond Recreational Physical Activity: Examining Occupational and Household Activity, Transportation Activity, and Sedentary Behavior in Relation to Postmenopausal Breast Cancer Risk. *Am J Public Health* 2010; 100:2288–2295.

George SM, Moore SC, Chow WH, Schatzkin A, Hollenbeck AR, Matthews CE. A Prospective Analysis of Prolonged Sitting Time and Risk of Renal Cell Carcinoma Among 300,000 Older Adults. *Ann Epidemiol* 2011; 21:787–790.

Global Advocacy for Physical Activity (GAPA). *Toronto Charter for Physical Activity: A Global Call for Action.* 2010.

Hamilton MT, Hamilton DG, Zderic TW. Role of Low Energy Expenditure and Sitting in Obesity, Metabolic Syndrome, Type 2 Diabetes, and Cardiovascular Disease. *Diabetes* 2007; 56:2655–2667.

Healy GN, Matthews CE, Dunstan DW, Winkler EAH, Owen N. Sedentary time and cardio-metabolic biomarkers in US adults: NHANES 2003–06. *Eur Heart J* 2011; 32:590–597.

Hillsdon M, Foster C, Thorogood M. Interventions for promoting physical activity. *Cochrane Database Syst Rev* 2005.

Howard RA, Freedman DM, Park Y, Hollenbeck A, Schatzkin A, Leitzmann M F. Physical activity, sedentary behavior, and the risk of colon and rectal cancer in the NIH-AARP Diet and Health Study. *Cancer Causes Control* 2008; 19:939–953.

Irwin ML, Yasui Y, Ulrich CM, Bowen D, Rudolph RE, Schwartz RS et al. Effect of exercise on total and intra-abdominal body fat in postmenopausal women: a randomized controlled trial. *JAMA* 2003; 289:323–330.

Irwin ML, McTiernan A, Bernstein L, Gilliland FD, Baumgartner R. Baumgartner K et al. Relationship of obesity and physical activity with C-peptide, leptin, and insulin-like growth factors in breast cancer survivors. *Cancer Epidemiol Biomarkers Prev* 2005; 14:2881–2888.

Irwin ML, Varma K, varez-Reeves M, Cadmus L, Wiley A, Chung GG et al. Randomized controlled trial of aerobic exercise on insulin and insulin-like growth factors in breast cancer survivors: the Yale Exercise and Survivorship study. *Cancer Epidemiol Biomarkers Prev* 2009; 18:306–313.

Kaaks R. Plasma insulin, IGF-I and breast cancer. *Gynecol Obstet Fertil* 2001; 29: 185–191.

Kaaks R, Lukanova A, Kurzer MS. Obesity, endogenous hormones, and endometrial cancer risk: a synthetic review. *Cancer Epidemiol Biomarkers Prev* 2002;11:1531–1543.

Kahn EB, Ramsey LT, Brownson RC, Heath GW, Howze EH, Powell KE et al. The effectiveness of interventions to increase physical activity - A systematic review. *Am J Prev Med* 2002: 22:73–108.

Kendall A, Folkerd EJ, Dowsett M. Influences on circulating oestrogens in postmenopausal women: relationship with breast cancer. *J Steroid Biochem Mol Biol* 2007; 103:99–109.

Kershaw EE, Flier JS. Adipose tissue as an endocrine organ. *J Clin Endocrinol Metab* 2004; 89:2548–2556.

Kushi LH, Byers T, Doyle C, Bandera EV, McCullough M, Gansler T. et al. American Cancer Society Guidelines on Nutrition and Physical Activity for Cancer Prevention: Reducing the Risk of Cancer With Healthy Food Choices and Physical Activity. *CA-Cancer J Clin* 2006; 56:254–281.

Lee TS, Kilbreath SL, Sullivan G, Refshauge KM, Beith JM. The development of an arm activity survey for breast cancer survivors using the Protection Motivation Theory. *BMC Cancer* 2007; 7:75.

Leitzmann MF. Physical activity and genitourinary cancer prevention. *Recent Res Cancer* 2011; 186:43–71.

Lynch BM. Sedentary behavior and cancer: a systematic review of the literature and proposed biological mechanisms. *Cancer Epidemiol Biomarkers Prev* 2010; 19:2691–2709.

Lynch BM, Neilson HK, Friedenreich CM. In Courneya KS & Friedenreich CM (Eds.) *Physical activity and breast cancer prevention.* Springer Berlin Heidelberg 2011a; pp. 13–42.

Lynch BM, Friedenreich CM, Winkler EAH, Healy GN, Vallance JK, Eakin EG et al. Associations of objectively assessed physical activity and sedentary time with biomarkers of breast cancer risk in postmenopausal women: findings from NHANES (2003–2006). *Breast Cancer Res Tr* 2011b; 130:183–194.

Mason C, Foster-Schubert KE, Imayama I, Kong A, Xiao L, Bain C et al. Dietary Weight Loss and Exercise Effects on Insulin Resistance in Postmenopausal Women. *Am J Prev Med* 2011; 41:366–375.

Mathew A, Gajalakshmi V, Rajan B, Kanimozhi VC, Brennan P, Binukumar, BP et al. Physical activity levels among urban and rural women in south India and the risk of breast cancer: a case-control study. *Eur J Cancer Prev* 2009; 18:368–376.

McTiernan A. Mechanisms linking physical activity with cancer. *Nat Rev Cancer* 2008; 8:205–211.

McTiernan A, Tworoger SS, Ulrich CM, Yasui,Y, Irwin ML, Rajan KB et al. Effect of exercise on serum estrogens in postmenopausal women: a 12-month randomized clinical trial. *Cancer Res* 2004; 64:2923–2928.

McTiernan A, Sorensen B, Yasui Y, Tworoger SS, Ulrich CM, Irwin ML et al. No effect of exercise on insulin-like growth factor 1 and insulin-like growth factor binding protein 3 in postmenopausal women: a 12-month randomized clinical trial. *Cancer Epidemiol Biomarkers Prev* 2005; 14:1020–1021.

McTiernan A, Wu L, Chen C, Chlebowski R, Mossavar-Rahmani Y, Modugno F et al. Relation of BMI and physical activity to sex hormones in postmenopausal women. *Obesity* 2006; 14:1662–1677.

Meijer EP, Goris AHC, van Dongen JLJ, Bast A, Westerterp KR. Exercise-induced oxidative stress in older adults as a function of habitual activity level. *J Am Geriatr Soc* 2002; 50:349–353.

Monninkhof EM, Velthuis MJ, Peeters PH, Twisk JW, Schuit AJ. Effect of Exercise on Postmenopausal Sex Hormone Levels and Role of Body Fat: A Randomized Controlled Trial. *J Clin Oncol* 2009; 27:4492–4499.

Moore SC, Gierach GL, Schatzkin A, Matthews CE. Physical activity, sedentary behaviours, and the prevention of endometrial cancer. *Br J Cancer* 2010; 103: 933–938.

Nandeesha H. Insulin: a novel agent in the pathogenesis of prostate cancer. *Int Urol Nephrol* 2009; 41:267–272.

Neilson HK, Friedenreich CM, Brockton NT, Millikan RC. Physical activity and postmenopausal breast cancer: proposed biologic mechanisms and areas for future research. *Cancer Epidemiol Biomarkers Prev* 2009; 18:11–27.

Owen N, Healy GN, Matthews CE, Dunstan DW. Too Much Sitting: The Population Health Science of Sedentary Behavior. *Exerc Sport Sci Rev* 2010; 38:105–113.

Pan SY, Morrison H. Physical Activity and Hematologic Cancer Prevention. In K.S.Courneya & C. M. Friedenreich (Eds.) *Physical Activity and Cancer.* Springer Berlin Heidelberg. 2011; pp. 135–158.

Patel AV, Rodriguez C, Pavluck AL, Thun MJ, Calle EE. Recreational physical activity and sedentary behavior in relation to ovarian cancer risk in a large cohort of US women. *Am J Epidemiol* 2006; 163:709–716.

Patel AV, Feigelson HS, Talbot JT, McCullough ML, Rodriguez C, Patel RC et al. The role of body weight in the relationship between physical activity and endometrial cancer: results from a large cohort of US women. *Int J Cancer* 2008; 123: 1877–1882.

Physical Activity Guidelines Advisory Committee. *Physical Activity Guidelines Advisory Committee Report,* 2008. Washington, DC: U.S. Department of Health and Human Services.

Pou KM, Massaro JM, Hoffmann U, Vasan RS, Maurovich-Horvat P, Larson MG et al. Visceral and Subcutaneous Adipose Tissue Volumes Are Cross-Sectionally Related to Markers of Inflammation and Oxidative Stress. *Circulation* 2007: 116: 1234–1241.

Proper KI, Singh AS, van Mechelen W, Chinapaw MJM. Sedentary Behaviors and Health Outcomes Among Adults: A Systematic Review of Prospective Studies. *Am J Prev Med* 2011; 40:174–182.

Reeves GK, Pirie K, Beral V, Green J, Spencer E, Bull D. Cancer incidence and mortality in relation to body mass index in the Million Women Study: cohort study. *BMJ* 2007; 335:1134.

Renehan AG, Tyson M, Egger M, Heller RF, Zwahlen M. Body-mass index and incidence of cancer: a systematic review and meta-analysis of prospective observational studies. *Lancet* 2008; 371:569–578.

Steindorf K, Tobiasz-Adamczyk B, Popiela T, Jedrychowski W, Penar A, Matyja A et al. Combined risk assessment of physical activity and dietary habits on the development of colorectal cancer. A hospital-based case-control study in Poland. *Eur J Cancer Prev* 2000; 9:309–316.

Thorp AA, Owen N, Neuhaus M, Dunstan DW. Sedentary Behaviors and Subsequent Health Outcomes in Adults: A Systematic Review of Longitudinal Studies, 1996–2011. *Am J Prev Med* 2011 41:207–215.

Tremblay MS, Colley RC, Saunders TJ, Healy GN, Owen N. Physiological and health implications of a sedentary lifestyle. *Appl Physiol Nutr Metab* 2010; 35: 725–740.

Troiano RP, Berrigan D, Dodd KW, Masse LC, Tilert T, Mcdowell M. Physical activity in the United States measured by accelerometer. *Med Sci Sport Exerc* 2008; 40:181–188.

Tworoger SS, Missmer SA, Eliassen AH, Barbieri RL, Dowsett M, Hankinson SE. Physical activity and inactivity in relation to sex hormone, prolactin, and insulin-like growth factor concentrations in premenopausal women - exercise and premenopausal hormones. *Cancer Causes Control* 2007; 18:743–752.

U.S.Department of Health and Human Services. *Physical Activity Guidelines.* Advisory Committee Report, 2008.

United Nations General Assembly. *Political declaration of the High-level Meeting of the General Assembly on the Prevention and Control of Non-communicable Diseases*, 2011.

van Kruijsdijk RCM, van der Wall E, Visseren FLJ. Obesity and Cancer: The Role of Dysfunctional Adipose Tissue. *Cancer Epidemiol Biomarkers Prev* 2009; 18: 2569–2578.

Warburton DE, Katzmarzyk PT, Rhodes RE, Shephard R J. Evidence-informed physical activity guidelines for Canadian adults. *Can J Public Health* 2007; 98: Suppl 2, S16–S68.

Wolin KY, Tuchman H. Physical activity and gastrointestinal cancer prevention. *Rec Res Cancer* 2011; 186:73–100.

World Cancer Research Fund and the American Institute for Cancer Research. *Food, Nutrition, Physical Activity, and the Prevention of Cancer: a Global Perspective*. Washington, DC: American Institute for Cancer Research, 2007.

World Health Organization. *2008–2013 Action Plan for the Global Strategy for the Prevention and Control of Non-communicable Diseases.* World Health Organization, Geneva, 2008.

World Health Organization. Recommended Population Levels of Physical activity for Health. In *Global Recommendations on Physical activity for Health* World Health Organization, Geneva, 2010; pp. 15–34.

Xue F, Michels KB. Diabetes, metabolic syndrome, and breast cancer: a review of the current evidence. *Am J Clin Nutr* 2007; 86:s823–s835.

Zhang M, Lee AH, Binns CW. Physical activity and epithelial ovarian cancer risk: a case-control study in China. *Int J Cancer* 2003; 105:838–843.

Chapter 7
Cancer Prevention in the United States

Otis W. Brawley and Barnett S. Kramer

7.1 Introduction

Surveys show that the American public is very interested in cancer prevention. Unfortunately, cancer prevention is not consistently practiced. It is estimated that 50–60 % of the cancers occurring today could have been prevented if currently known prevention interventions had been applied years ago (Table 7.1). Many mitigating interventions are not widely employed today and represent important areas for future implementation or dissemination research.

In the United States, tobacco use, the condition of being overweight or obese, poor nutrition and overnutrition, and physical inactivity are highly prevalent modifiable risk factors for cancer. Evidence-based programs and policies championing interventions designed to modify these risk factors have the potential of preventing more than 350,000 deaths per year (American Cancer Society 2011). Ironically, a number of interventions that are widely used by the American public under the *assumption* that they prevent cancer, such as multivitamin and dietary supplement use, have not been proven to be effective.

O.W. Brawley, MD (✉)
American Cancer Society, Emory University, 250 Williams Street,
Suite 600, Atlanta, GA 30303, USA
e-mail: otis.brawley@cancer.org

B.S. Kramer, MD, MPH
Division of Cancer Prevention, National Cancer Institute,
Bethesda, MD, USA

A.B. Miller (ed.), *Epidemiologic Studies in Cancer Prevention and Screening*,
Statistics for Biology and Health 79, DOI 10.1007/978-1-4614-5586-8_7,

Table 7.1 Causes of Cancer and potential reduction in the cancer burden in the U.S. through preventive measures

Cause	Percentage of cancer causes	Number of deaths in the USA	Magnitude of possible reduction	Time to effect (in years)	Evidence and example of interventions
Smoking	33	188,700	75	10–20	Comparisons of populations' smoking habits and lung cancer mortality by state (Kenfield et al. 2008)
Overweight and obesity	20	114,400	50	2–20	Bariatric surgery and observations in markers after weight change (Chang et al. 2011)
Diet	5	28,600	50	5–20	Folate and colorectal cancer (Lee et al. 2011)
Lack of exercise	5	28,600	85	5–20	Adolescent physical activity (Maruti et al. 2008)
Occupation	5	28,600	50	20–40	Asbestos workplace regulation (Peto et al. 1995)
Viruses	5	28,600	100	20–40	Hepatitis B vaccine (Chang, 2009); HPV vaccine (Bogaards et al. 2011)
Family history	5	28,600	50	2–10	Bilateral oophorectomy for BRCA 1/2 (Rebbeck et al. 2009); aspirin for Lynch syndrome (Burn et al. 2011)
Alcohol	3	17,200	50	5–20	Regulation (Room et al. 2005)
UV and ionizing radiation	2	11,400	50	5–40	Reduced medical exposures (Brenner and Hricak 2010); reduced sun exposure (Saraiya et al. 2004)

Total potential reduction = 54.5 %*

7.2 Tobacco Use

The American Cancer Society estimates that 189,700 Americans died of cancer due to tobacco use in 2011. Tobacco use causes a third of all cancer deaths in the USA (American Cancer Society 2011), representing by far the number one cause of preventable cancer deaths. It causes even more deaths from lung and cardiovascular disease.

7.2.1 Cigarette Smoking

Most smokers take on the habit between the ages of 14 and 16 years despite laws barring sale of tobacco products to children. Given that it is unlikely for someone who has not started smoking by the age of 18 to ever become a regular smoker, educational and policy strategies aimed at the vulnerable teen years could have an enormous impact on cancer mortality. To counter childhood smoking, the US Surgeon General recommends that school-based tobacco prevention programs begin by sixth grade (U.S. DHHS 2000).

The National Youth Tobacco Survey (NYTS) found that 5.2 % of middle school students (age 12–14 years) were current smokers in 2009; susceptibility to start cigarette smoking (never-smokers who reported an openness to trying cigarettes) was 21.2 % in middle school students and 24 % in high school students. Between 2000 and 2009, there was no overall change (Jordan and Delnevo 2010). Even subtle exposures during the vulnerable ages of 10–14 years, such as images of smoking in movies, may be associated with subsequent uptake and persistence of cigarette smoking (Primack et al. 2012).

The 2009 Youth Risk Behavior Survey (YRBS) showed that 19.5 % of high school students (age 14–18 years) reported current cigarette smoking (smoking on at least one day in the past 30 days) and 7.3 % reported frequent smoking (smoking on 20 or more of the past 30 days) (U.S. DHHS 2010). According to the National Youth Tobacco Survey (NYTS), about 23.9 % of high school students reported current use of some tobacco products (cigarettes, cigars, pipes, kreteks, bidis, and smokeless tobacco) (CDC 2010). The percentage of high school students who reported current cigarette smoking decreased from 1997 to 2003, but the prevalence did not change substantially between 2003 and 2009 (Johnston et al. 2009). The stall in the decline in youth smoking since 2000 may be related to increased marketing by the tobacco industry and declines in state and federal governmental funding for comprehensive tobacco control programs.

According to the National Health Interview Survey (NHIS), an estimated 20.6 % of adults (men: 23.5 %, women: 17.9 %) smoked cigarettes in 2009. About 78 % of smokers (36.4 million) used cigarettes daily (US FDA 2009). Between 1997 and 2004, the percentage of adults who smoked decreased from 27.6 % to 23.4 % in men and from 22.1 % to 18.5 % in women. Adult smoking rates were steady between 2004 and 2006, declined in 2007, and remained unchanged between 2007 and 2009 (US FDA 2009).

7.2.2 Other Tobacco Products

The tobacco industry markets smokeless tobacco products, a source of nicotine, in smoke-free settings. The public may mistakenly view smokeless tobacco products as a low-risk option for smokers who are unable to quit. However, smokeless tobacco products may turn out to be a bridge to cigarettes for many people (Gray and Henningfield 2006; Morrison et al. 2008).

While cigarettes remain the primary tobacco product used by youth, other forms of tobacco use, including cigars, smokeless tobacco products, and hookahs (tobacco water pipes), have grown in popularity. Current use estimates for these cigarette alternatives range from 10 % to 17 % among adolescents (Connolly and Alpert 2008; American Legacy Foundation 2009; Campaign for Tobacco-Free Kids 2007; Primack et al. 2008).

Small cigars are similar in shape and size to cigarettes, but they are not regulated like cigarettes. Between 1997 and 2007, overall sales of small cigars and cigarillos rose at a much faster rate than sales of large cigars (240 %, 45 %, and 6 %, respectively) (American Legacy Foundation 2009).

The US Department of Health and Human Services has been in the forefront in emphasizing that the use of tobacco in any form can induce nicotine dependence and harm health. They stress that prevention and cessation programs should address all tobacco products, not just cigarettes (US DHHS 2000).

7.2.3 Comprehensive Tobacco Control Programs

Comprehensive tobacco control programs aim to reduce tobacco use by applying evidence-based economic, policy, regulatory, educational, social, and clinical strategies (CDC 2007). Tobacco dependence is a chronic addictive disease, hence the focus on preventing the addiction. Interventions that effectively prevent initiation of tobacco use include increases in tobacco taxes, restrictions on smoking in public places, prevention and cessation programs, and antitobacco media campaigns (US DHHS 2000).

According to the US Centers for Disease Control and Prevention's (CDC's) *Best Practices for Comprehensive Tobacco Control Programs*, a complete program has:

- State and community interventions (e.g., support of tobacco prevention and control coalitions, implementation of evidence-based policy interventions to reduce overall tobacco use, funding of community-based organizations, and development of community coalitions to strengthen partnerships between local agencies, grassroots, and voluntary and civic organizations)
- Health communication interventions (e.g., audience research to develop high-impact campaigns, market research to motivate behavior change, and marketing surveillance to counter tobacco messaging)
- Cessation interventions (e.g., increase of services available through population-based cessation programs, public and private insurance coverage of evidence-based

tobacco treatments, and elimination of cost barriers for underserved populations, including the uninsured)

- Surveillance and evaluation (e.g., regular monitoring of tobacco-related attitudes, behaviors, and health outcomes; measurement of short-term and intermediate indicators of program effectiveness, including policy changes and changes in social norms; and counter-marketing surveillance) (CDC 2007)

Several states have documented the benefits of such programs. For example, the state of California comprehensive tobacco control program is associated with a marked drop in adolescent smoking initiation as well as reduced adult consumption and increased adult cessation rates when compared to those states without a comprehensive program (Messer and Pierce 2010). This program included hard-hitting antitobacco advertising, cigarette tax increases, and smoking cessation counseling. California has experienced substantial reductions in tobacco usage and reductions in tobacco-related cancers since the implementation of the program (Barnoya and Glantz 2004).

The price of cigarettes is inversely and predictably related to consumption: A 10 % increase in price reduces overall cigarette consumption by 3–5 % (US DHHS 2000). This approach is especially effective in young people who smoke. They are up to three times more responsive to price increases than are adults (Pacula and Chaloupka 2001). State cigarette taxes vary widely, ranging from 17 cents per pack in Missouri to $4.35 per pack in New York. The wide differences in taxes have had an apparent impact on cigarette use. Missouri has a high smoking prevalence, whereas New York's prevalence is among the lowest.

A number of comprehensive smoking bans (also referred to as clean indoor air laws) have been implemented at state and local levels. Today, 79.4 % of the US population is covered by a 100 % smoke-free provision in workplaces, restaurants, and bars versus 46.1 % in 1992 (American Nonsmokers' Rights Foundation 2011; Giovino et al. 2009).

As the options for traditional advertising venues have narrowed, the tobacco industry has turned to Internet and point-of-sale advertising. However, there is also increasing use of sustained mass media campaigns that highlight the negative consequences of tobacco use, to some effect (NCI 2008). States that have combined mass media campaigns with other antitobacco activities have seen declines in youth and adult smoking prevalence (NCI 2008; CDC 2007). For example, a Florida "truth" antismoking campaign developed messages that countered the perception of smoking as cool and rebellious by highlighting the tobacco industry's advertising practices (NCI 2008). It has been widely replicated.

Effective tobacco control can be envisioned as a series of obstacles: make it hard for the nonsmoker to start smoking and then make it hard for the smoker to smoke and easier for the smoker to quit. Increasing the price of cigarettes makes them less affordable. Smoke-free laws make smoking less convenient. If the smoker finds a place to smoke, advertising on the tobacco pack, on billboards, from electronic media, and even messages from friends can encourage the smoker to quit. Tobacco quit lines and a wealth of on-line tobacco cessation information are readily available to the large number of smokers who are trying to break their addiction (1-877-44U-QUIT; see http://www.cancer.gov/cancertopics/tobacco/smoking).

While states have traditionally been at the forefront of tobacco control efforts, the US federal government has recently enacted some tobacco control legislation. In 2009, federal tobacco taxes were increased on cigarettes (from $0.39 to $1.01 per pack). In concert with this increase, per-capita cigarette consumption fell to 969 cigarettes per person in 2011—the lowest figure since the 1920s—and a 17 % decline since 2008 (the last full year before the tax increase). The tax also serves as a revenue source for federally funded cessation and tobacco control programs.

The Family Smoking Prevention and Tobacco Control Act of 2009 for the first time granted the US Food and Drug Administration (FDA) the authority to regulate the manufacturing, marketing, and sale of tobacco products (US FDA 2009). To date, the following are banned:

- Fruit or candy flavorings in cigarettes
- Use of potentially misleading or misunderstood advertising descriptors such as "light," "low," and "mild"
- Tobacco brand name sponsorship of sports and entertainment events
- Free tobacco and nontobacco item giveaways
- Sale of cigarettes in packs of less than 20 (Connolly and Alpert 2008)

The law requires the tobacco industry to disclose the ingredients of their products to the FDA, and stores are required to make tobacco products less accessible to children by placing them behind counters. The law also mandates new, larger, warning labels on both cigarettes and on smokeless tobacco products. As this chapter is being written, the tobacco industry is contesting the legality of this part of the legislation in the US courts.

While other flavorings have been banned from cigarettes, menthol was specifically not banned. However, in March 2011, the FDA's Tobacco Products Scientific Advisory Committee found that menthol cigarettes increase youth experimentation and initiation (Benowitz and Samet 2011). The committee concluded that removing menthol cigarettes from the marketplace would benefit public health. This conclusion could provide a legal basis for the FDA to try to limit, phase out, or even ban menthol in cigarettes.

7.2.4 Tobacco Cessation

While it is easier and more effective to prevent smoking, we must help those who are addicted to tobacco. The US Public Health Service has published guidelines for smoking cessation treatment. These include use of over-the-counter nicotine replacement treatment (NRT), prescription medications, or combinations of these medications and counseling (individual, group, or by telephone) (Clinical Practice Guideline 2008). The combined use of counseling and medication appears to be more effective than the use of any individual treatment. Nationally, the receipt and use of recommended cessation services remains low. In 2005, about 35 % of then-current smokers tried to quit (Cokkinides et al. 2008).

However, there have been successes: The State of Massachusetts is providing its Medicaid beneficiaries access to two 90-day courses of pharmacotherapy and up to 16 individual or group counseling sessions, with minimum cost barriers; co-payments are as low as $1 to $3. This benefit has been associated with a decline in smoking prevalence by 10 percentage points between the pre- and post-benefit time period (38.3–28.3 %), with an estimated annual decline of 15 % (Land et al. 2010).

At the federal level, provisions in the Affordable Care Act, signed into law on March 23, 2010, assure insurance coverage for evidence-based cessation treatments for almost all Americans by 2014. These treatments include pharmacotherapy and cessation counseling.

Tobacco control is the most obvious focus area for cancer prevention and overall health promotion. Tobacco in any form is an addictive and harmful drug. When used as intended, tobacco causes the premature death of at least half its users. While it is the cause of at least 30 % of all cancer deaths, it also causes lung and cardiovascular disease and is the cause of one in every five American deaths (ACS 2011).

7.3 Obesity, Physical Inactivity, and Poor Nutrition

The triad of obesity, physical inactivity, and poor nutrition are estimated to cause 172,000 cancer deaths in the USA per year, though these estimates are very imprecise and require a number of assumptions (ACS 2011). Together they are associated with increased risk for developing cancer of the breast (postmenopausal), colon, endometrium, esophagus, and kidney. In addition, observational studies suggest that they are correlated with increases in the risk for cancers of the pancreas, gallbladder, thyroid, ovary, cervix, multiple myeloma, Hodgkin lymphoma, and aggressive prostate cancer (ACS 2011; Doll and Peto 1981; McGinnis and Foege 1993; IARC 2002; Brawer et al. 2009).

The proportion of obese adults aged 20–74 was small and varied little from 1960 to 1980; in contrast, obesity rates more than doubled between 1980 and 2000 from 15.1 % to 31 %. Today, 35 % of Americans are obese, as defined by a body mass index (BMI) of ≥ 30 kg/m^2 and more than two-thirds are overweight (BMI = 25–29.9) or obese (Ogden et al. 2007).

Between 1980 and 2000, the prevalence of obesity among adolescents aged 12–19 tripled from 5 % to 15.5 %. More than half of all children who are overweight will remain overweight in adulthood (US DHHS 2011), hence the importance of a focus on obesity prevention for children and adolescents (White House Taskforce on Childhood Obesity 2010; Kumanyika et al. 2008). Historical changes that likely contributed to this obesity epidemic include reduced leisure time for physical activity, shifts from using walking as a mode of transportation to increased reliance on automobiles, shifts to more sedentary work, more meals eaten away from home, increased marketing and availability of cheap, energy-dense processed foods, and increased consumption of larger portion sizes (Darmon and Drewnowski 2008; Koplan et al. 2005; Krebs-Smith et al. 2010; Kushi et al. 2012). Socio-environmental factors include the lack of access to full-service grocery stores, relatively high costs of healthy foods compared to processed foods, and lack of access to safe places to play and exercise.

In a 2009 survey, only 24 % of American adults consumed five or more servings of fruits or vegetables per day, and 25 % reported no leisure-time physical activity at all (ACS 2011).

As with tobacco control, emphasis is placed on preventing children from becoming overweight or obese. However, few studies to date have sufficient evidence suggesting that weight loss reduces the risk of cancer. There are some data showing that surgery to treat extreme obesity improves insulin sensitivity and hormone metabolism and reduces risk of some cancers (Adams et al. 2007; Sjöström et al. 2009, and see James, this volume).

Obesity is a complex problem that requires a broad range of effective approaches (Koplan et al. 2005; Kushi et al. 2012), underscoring the need for addressing healthy lifestyles not only at the individual but also at the community level. The CDC, the Institute of Medicine, and others have outlined a variety of approaches in schools, worksites, and communities to mitigate or reverse obesity trends (Institute of Medicine 2009; Koplan et al. 2005; Task Force on Community Preventive Services 2001; Waxman 2004; World Cancer Research Fund 2007).

Much as with tobacco control, the approach to weight control efforts is rooted in providing information on the harms of poor nutrition and lack of exercise and the need to maintain an ideal body weight. The aim is also to be positive and encourage healthy eating and healthy activity. Although the effectiveness of specific recommendations is not known with precision, public education campaigns usually advise people to:

Balance caloric intake with physical activity.

- The goal should be to maintain a healthy weight throughout life.
- Try to lose weight if currently overweight or obese.

Consume a healthy diet, with an emphasis on plant sources.

- Eat a variety of fruits and vegetables each day.
- Choose whole grains in preference to processed (refined) grains.

Limit consumption of processed and red meats.

- Select lean cuts of meat and eat smaller portions.
- Prepare meat by baking, broiling, or poaching rather than by frying or charbroiling.
- Choose fish, poultry, or beans as an alternative to beef, pork, and lamb.

Limit consumption of alcoholic beverages.

- No more than 1 drink per day for women.
- No more than 2 per day for men.

Adopt a physically active lifestyle.

- Adults should engage in at least 30 min of moderate to vigorous physical activity, above usual activities, on 5 or more days of the week; 45–60 min of intentional physical activity is preferable.
- Children and adolescents should engage in at least 60 min per day of moderate to vigorous physical activity at least 5 days per week.

In 2010, the President of the United States issued an executive order creating the White House Task Force on Childhood Obesity. This task force of experts has published some strategies to control childhood obesity:

Strategies to promote the availability of affordable healthy food and beverages

- Limit availability, advertising, and marketing of foods and beverages of low nutritional value, particularly in schools.
- Strengthen nutritional standards in schools for foods and beverages served as part of the school meal program and for foods and beverages served outside of the program.
- Encourage restaurants to provide nutrition information on menus, especially calories.

Strategies to encourage physical activity or limit sedentary activity among children and youth

- Invest in community design that supports the development of sidewalks, bike lanes, and access to parks and green space.
- Increase and enforce physical education requirements in all grades of schools.

Soon after this announcement, First Lady Michelle Obama launched the Let's Move initiative, an awareness campaign focused on engaging parents, caregivers, youth, educators, industry, and policy makers at all levels of government.

7.4 Conclusion

The knowledge and tools to prevent many cancers and cancer deaths now exist, as a result of research efforts. It has been estimated that cancer prevention interventions, if fully implemented, could potentially prevent several hundred thousand cancer deaths per year (McCullough et al. 2011; Colditz et al. 2012). If we are to achieve this, much of the emphasis should be on children as most prevention interventions are most useful when deployed early in life.

Numerous obstacles stand in the way of fully applying cancer preventive interventions. Consistent application of cancer prevention may not occur without effective interventions at the individual, clinical, community, and policy levels. This is a public health challenge at national and local levels.

Disclaimer The opinions expressed in this chapter do not represent official positions of the US Federal Government or the Department of Health and Human Services.

References

Adams TD, Gress RE, Smith SC, Halverson RC, Simper SC, Rosamond WD et al. Long terms mortality after gastric bypass surgery. *N Engl J Med.* 2007; 357:753–761.

American Cancer Society. *Cancer Facts & Figures 2011*. Atlanta, GA: American Cancer Society; 2011.

American Legacy Foundation. *Cigars, Cigarillos & Little Cigars Fact Sheet. 2009*. Available at: legacyforhealth.org/PDF/Cigars-Cigarillos-and-Little-Cigars_FactSheet.pdf. Accessed December 21, 2010.

American Nonsmokers' Rights Foundation. *Overview List – How Many Smokefree Laws? 2010*; Available at: no-smoke.org/pdf/mediaordlist.pdf. Accessed April 6, 2011.

Barnoya J, Glantz S. Association of the California tobacco control program with declines in lung cancer incidence. *Cancer Causes Control.* 2004; 15:689–695.

Benowitz NL, Samet JM. The Threat of Menthol Cigarettes to U.S. Public Health. *N Engl J Med* 2011; 364:2179–2181.

Bogaards JA, Coupe VM, Xiridou M, Meijer CJ, Wallinga J, Berkhof J. Long-term impact of human papillomavirus vaccination on infection rates, cervical abnormalities, and cancer incidence. *Epidemiology.* 2011; 22:505–515.

Brawer R, Brisbon N, Plumb J. Obesity and cancer. *Prim Care.* 2009; 36:509–531.

Brenner DJ, Hricak H. Radiation exposure from medical imaging: time to regulate? *JAMA*. 2010; 304:208–209.

Burn J, Gerdes AM, Macrae F, Mecklin JP, Moeslein G, Olschwang S et al. Long-term effect of aspirin on cancer risk in carriers of hereditary colorectal cancer: an analysis from the CAPP2 randomised controlled trial. *Lancet.* 2011; 378:2081–2087.

Campaign for Tobacco-Free Kids. Smokeless Tobacco in the United States: *An Overview of the Health Risks and Industry Marketing Aimed at Children and the Compelling Need for Effective Regulation of All Tobacco Products by the FDA*. 2007; Available at: tobaccofreekids.org/research/factsheets/pdf/0231.pdf. Accessed October 9, 2007.

Centers for Disease Control and Prevention. *Best Practices for Comprehensive Tobacco Control Programs – 2007*. Atlanta, GA: US Department of Health and Human Services, Centers for Disease Control and Prevention, National Center for Chronic Disease Prevention and Health Promotion, Office of Smoking and Health; 2007.

Centers for Disease Control and Prevention. Tobacco Use Among Middle and High School Students - United States, 2000–2009. *MMWR Morb Mortal Wkly Rep*. 2010; 59:1063–1068.

Chang MH, You SL, Chen CJ, Liu CJ, Lee CM, Lin SM et al. Taiwan Hepatoma Study Group. Decreased incidence of hepatocellular carcinoma in hepatitis B vaccinees: a 20-year follow-up study. *J Natl Cancer Inst*. 2009; 101:1348–55.

Chang SH, Stoll CR, Colditz GA. Cost-effectiveness of bariatric surgery: should it be universally available? *Maturitas*. 2011; 69:230–238.

Clinical Practice Guideline Treating Tobacco Use and Dependence 2008 Update Panel, Liaisons, and Staff. A clinical practice guideline for treating tobacco use and dependence: 2008 update. A U.S. Public Health Service report. *Am J Prev Med*. 2008; 35:158–176.

Cokkinides VE, Halpern MT, Barbeau EM, Ward E, Thun MJ. Racial and ethnic disparities in smoking-cessation interventions: analysis of the 2005 National Health Interview Survey. *Am J Prev Med*. 2008; 34:404–412.

Colditz GA, Wolin KY, Gehlert S. Applying what we know to accelerate cancer prevention. *Sci. Transl.Med.* 2012; 4:127rv4.

Connolly GN, Alpert HR. Trends in the use of cigarettes and other tobacco products, 2000–2007. *JAMA*. 2008; 299:2629–2630.
Darmon N, Drewnowski A. Does social class predict diet quality? *Am J Clin Nutr*. 2008; 87:1107–1117.
Doll R, Peto R. *The Causes of Cancer*. New York, NY: Oxford Press; 1981.
Giovino GA, Chaloupka FJ, Hartman AM, Joyce KG, Chriqui J, Orleans CT et al. Cigarette Smoking Prevalence and Policies in the 50 States: An Era of Change-The Robert Wood Johnson Foundation ImpacTeen Tobacco Chart Book. Buffalo, NY: University of Buffalo, State University of New York; 2009.
Gray N, Henningfield J. Dissent over harm reduction for tobacco. *Lancet*. 2006; 368:899–901.
Institute of Medicine and National Research Council of the National Academies. *Local Government Actions to Prevent Childhood Obesity*. Available at: iom.edu/Reports/2009/ChildhoodObesityPreven-tionLocalGovernments.aspx2009.
International Agency for Research on Cancer. IARC Handbooks of Cancer Prevention. Volume 6: Weight Control and Physical Activity. Lyon, France: IARC Press; 2002.
Johnston L, O'Malley P, Bachman J, Schulenberg J. *Smoking continues gradual decline among U.S. teens, smokeless tobacco threatens a come-back. 2009*. Available at: monitoringthefuture.org Accessed December 14, 2009
Jordan HM, Delnevo CD. Emerging tobacco products: Hookah use among New Jersey youth. *Prev Med*. 2010; 51:394–396.
Kenfield SA, Stampfer MJ, Rosner BA, Colditz GA. Smoking and smoking cessation in relation to mortality in women. *JAMA*. 2008; 299:2037–2047.
Koplan JP, Liverman CT, Kraak VI. Preventing childhood obesity: health in the balance: executive summary. *J.Am.Diet.Assoc*. 2005; 105:131–138.
Krebs-Smith SM, Guenther PM, Subar AF, Kirkpatrick SI, Dodd KW. Americans do not meet federal dietary recommendations. *J Nutr*. 2010; 140:1832–1838.
Kumanyika SK, Obarzanek E, Stettler N, Bell R, Field AE, Fortmann SP et al. Population-based prevention of obesity: the need for comprehensive promotion of healthful eating, physical activity, and energy balance: a scientific statement from American Heart Association Council on Epidemiology and Prevention, Interdisciplinary Committee for Prevention (formerly the expert panel on population and prevention science). *Circulation*. 2008; 118:428–464.
Kushi LH, Doyle C, McCullough M, Rock CL, Demark-Wahnefried W, Bandera EV, Gapstur S et al. American Cancer Society Guide-lines on Nutrition and Physical Activity for cancer prevention: reducing the risk of cancer with healthy food choices and physical activity. *CA Cancer J Clin*. 2012; 62:30–67.
Land T, Warner D, Paskowsky M, Cammaerts A, Wetherell L, Kaufmann R et al. Medicaid coverage for tobacco dependence treatments in Massachusetts and associated decreases in smoking prevalence. PLoS One. 2010; 5(3):e9770.
Lee JE, Willett WC, Fuchs CS, Smith-Warner SA, Wu K, Ma J et al. Folate intake and risk of colorectal cancer and adenoma: modification by time. *Am.J.Clin.Nutr*. 2011; 93:817–825.
Maruti SS, Willett WC, Feskanich D, Rosner B, Colditz GA. A prospective study of age-specific physical activity and premenopausal breast cancer. *J.Natl.Cancer Inst*. 2008; 100:728–737.
McCullough ML, Patel AV, Kushi LH, Patel R, Willett WC, Doyle C et al. Following cancer prevention guidelines reduces risk of cancer, cardiovascular disease, and all-cause mortality. *Cancer Epidemiol. Biomarkers Prev*. 2011; 20:1089–1097.
McGinnis JM, Foege WH. Actual causes of death in the United States. *JAMA*. 1993; 270:2207–2212.
Messer K, Pierce JP. Changes in age trajectories of smoking experimentation during the California Tobacco Control Program. *Am J Public Health*. 2010; 100:1298–1306.
Morrison MA, Krugman DM, Park P. Under the Radar: Smokeless Tobacco Advertising in Magazines With Substantial Youth Readership. *Am J Public Health*. 2008; 98: 543–548.
National Cancer Institute. *The Role of the Media in Promoting and Reducing Tobacco Use. Tobacco Control Monograph No. 19*. Bethesda, MD: U.S. Department of Health and Human Services, National Institutes of Health, National Cancer Institute; June 2008.

Ogden CL, Carroll MD, McDowell MA, Flegal KM. *Obesity among Adults in the United States – no statistically significant change since 2003–2004: NCHS data brief no 1*. National Center for Health Statistics, Hyattsville, MD; 2007.

Pacula RL, Chaloupka FJ. The effects of macro-level interventions on addictive behavior. *Subst. Use.Misuse*. 2001; 36:1901–1922.

Peto J, Hodgson JT, Matthews FE, Jones JR. Continuing increase in mesothelioma mortality in Britain. *Lancet*. 1995; 345:535–539.

Primack BA, Longacre MR, Beach ML, Adachi-Mejia AM, Titus LJ, Dalton MA. Association of Established Smoking Among Adolescents With Timing of Exposure to Smoking Depicted in Movies. *J Natl Cancer Inst* 2012; 104:549–555.

Primack BA, Sidani J, Agarwal AA, Shadel WG, Donny EC, Eissenberg TE. Prevalence of and Associations with Waterpipe Tobacco Smoking among U.S. University Students. *Ann Behav Med*. 2008: 36:81–86.

Rebbeck TR, Kauff ND, Domchek SM. Meta-analysis of risk reduction estimates associated with risk-reducing salpingo-oophorectomy in BRCA1 or BRCA2 mutation carriers. *J.Natl.Cancer Inst*. 2009; 101:80–87.

Room R, Babor T, Rehm J. Alcohol and public health. *Lancet*. 2005; 365:519–530.

Saraiya M, Glanz K, Briss PA, Nichols P, White C, Das D et al. Interventions to prevent skin cancer by reducing exposure to ultraviolet radiation: a systematic review. *Am J Prev Med*. 2004; 27:422–466.

Sjöström L, Gummesson A, Sjöström CD, Narbro K, Peltonen M, Wedel H et al. Effects of bariatric surgery on cancer incidence in obese patients in Sweden (Swedish Obese Subjects Study): a prospective, controlled intervention trial. *Lancet Oncol*. 2009; 10:653–662.

Task Force on Community Preventive Services. Increasing physical activity – a report on recommendations of the Task Force on Community Preventive Services. *MMWR Morb Mortal Wkly Rep*. 2001; 50 (RR-18):1–1.

US Department of Health and Human Services. *Reducing Tobacco Use: A Report of the Surgeon General*. Atlanta, GA: US Department of Health and Human Services, Centers for Disease Control and Prevention, National Center for Chronic Disease Prevention and Health Promotion, Office on Smoking and Health; 2000.

USDHHS. Dietary guidelines for Americans, 2010. 2005 (revised 2010 Dec). NGC:008657 Department of Agriculture (U.S.) - Federal Government Agency [U.S.]; Department of Health and Human Services (U.S.) - Federal Government Agency [U.S.].

US Food and Drug Administration. *FDA & Tobacco Regulation. 2009*; Available at: fda.gov/NewsEvents/PublicHealthFocus/ucm168412.htm. Accessed July 30, 2009.

Waxman A, World Health Assembly. WHO global strategy on diet, physical activity and health. *Food Nutr Bull*. 2004; 25:292–302.

White House Task Force on Childhood Obesity Report to the President. *Solving the problem of childhood obesity within a generation*. Available at: letsmove.gov/pdf/TaskForce_on_Childhood_Obesity_May2010_FullReport.pdf2010.

World Cancer Research Fund/American Institute for Cancer Research. *Food, Nutrition, Physical Activity, and the Prevention of Cancer: A Global Perspective*. Washington, DC. AICR 2007.

Chapter 8
The Role of Nutrition in Cancer Prevention

W. Philip T. James

8.1 Introduction

Diet has been cited as making a contribution to the development of cancer ever since Doll and Peto (1981) scanned the global prevalence of cancer and estimated that diet could contribute anything from 25% to 75% to the global incidence of cancer based on what they recognized were crude ecological analyses combined with what was already known from more detailed epidemiological studies of the carcinogenicity of smoking and other environmental contaminants. They then summarized their findings by assuming for the time being that about a third of all cancers were of dietary origin. By the late 1970s far more analyses were underway by epidemiologists, based mostly in Europe and North America and relying on case–control studies to assess the likelihood of diet being involved (Miller 1977; Morgan et al. 1978; Howe 1981). However, more general claims started to be made, for example, by Burkitt, the missionary surgeon whose relatively simple analyses had already highlighted the infective nature of Burkitt's lymphoma (Burkitt 1962) based on his observations of cases coming to hospitals in East Africa. Given this success he was emboldened to suggest that the startlingly different rates of cancers in Europeans and Africans were probably due to their very different diets, and in characteristic style he chose dietary fiber as the most likely food ingredient as of major interest because of the completely different nature of the abdominal organs when he operated on Europeans and Africans (Burkitt 1988). He already recognized the far greater daily fecal output in Africans and then linked this to a variety of differences in intestinal pathologies including the rarity of appendicitis, Crohn's disease, and ulcerative colitis as well as colorectal cancer in Africans.

W.P. T. James (✉)
London School of Hygiene and Tropical Medicine, International Association for the Study of Obesity, Charles Darwin House, 12 Roger Street, WC1N 2JU London, UK
e-mail: Jeanhjames@aol.com

A.B. Miller (ed.), *Epidemiologic Studies in Cancer Prevention and Screening*, Statistics for Biology and Health 79, DOI 10.1007/978-1-4614-5586-8_8,

This set in train far more detailed cross-sectional analyses of dietary patterns in communities with different cancer rates (Bingham 1985; Chen et al. 1991) together with metabolic studies attempting to discern which dietary factors might produce or induce dietary-derived or endogenously induced carcinogens. Soon, the explosion of interest in the molecular basis of disease took over major funding with the carcinogenic process being considered in ever greater detail and with a focus on DNA repair as it became clearer that cancer was a multistaged process which might be affected by dietary factors at any stage in the sequence of molecular changes. Then epidemiologists, having recognized early on that case-control studies had their severe limitations in attempting to evaluate dietary practices years or even decades before, began to undertake prospective studies with a very big increase in the numbers involved and with varying emphases on the need to improve the accuracy and detail of the dietary studies (Lipnick et al. 1986; Monroe et al. 2003). Given the problems of first assessing the dietary intake of ingredients accurately and then also taking account of the unknown intraindividual and probably genetic-based differences in the metabolic responses along the dietary-cancer inducing pathways (see later), a greater emphasis is now being given to detailed metabolic epidemiological studies in different environments with far more marked differences in dietary habits than can be expected within any one country as in the wide-ranging European EPIC studies (Riboli 2001). Migration studies have also helped to emphasize the dynamic nature of the processes (Haenszel and Kurihara 1968). Now, however, the worlds of toxicology and nutrition are interacting with new analyses showing, for example, that polycyclic hydrocarbons come not only from smoking and other environmental factors but can contaminate as well as be derived from food which provides an important source for their intake, and these polycyclic hydrocarbons can then be metabolically amplified in their effects by specific factors in foods, for example, fatty acids (Diggs et al. 2011).

8.2 The Magnitude of Potential Dietary Factors: Perspectives from Global and Migrant Studies

Table 8.1 shows the difference between breast, colon/rectum, and prostate cancer incidence rates in different parts of the world. This shows that for each cancer it is possible to find rates which vary 6–30-fold between centers but with more affluent countries such as those in North America or Western Europe having much higher rates. These differences, of course, could be related to genetic differences between the ethnic groups or major differences in a variety of environmental exposures. Nevertheless, these remarkable differences, if not related to genetic factors, suggest that Doll and Peto's (1981) range of estimates for cancers of 10–70% attributed to dietary factors may indeed be closer to their upper limit of 70% for the proportion of cancers caused by diet than their crude preliminary average figure of 35%.

There is increasing interest in the genetic differences between different ethnic groups with substantial evidence emerging of the progressive changes in the

Table 8.1 Breast cancer in women, prostate cancer, and colorectal cancer (all rates age standardized yearly incidence per 100,000 for the years 1983–1987)

Place	Breast (total)	Prostate	Colon/rectum men	Colon/rectum women
China (Shanghai)	21.2	1.7	17.8	15.6
Thailand (Chang Mai)	13.7	4.0	9.9	7.7
India (Madras)	19.9	2.1	3.9	3.4
Belarus	24.7	9.0	17.9	13.3
Poland (Warsaw)	18.7	11.9	21.2	18.1
Hungary (Szabolcs)	29.6	14.3	20.8	16.6
Italy (Florence)	65.4	22.0	38.7	27.8
Germany (Saarland)	56.3	28.9	40.5	29.4
UK(B'ham)	63.4	25.0	38.0	25.4
Cuba	35.0	27.3	13.7	14.6
Brazil (Golania)	40.5	29.0	13.4	12.7
Peru (Trujillo)	28.3	19.9	6.0	9.0
USA Whites (10 regions);	89.2	61.8	46.5	33.2

Data derived from WCRF/AICR (1977) but based on data from specific cancer registries presented by the World Health Organization's International Agency for Research on Cancer

Table 8.2 Examples of the magnitude of change in cancer incidence or mortality in response to migration

Cancer	Population	Male	Female
Colon	Japanese to USA	Incidence/10^5	
	In USA	142.5	90.1
	In Japan	69.3	63.5
Colon	Greeks to Australia	Relative risk death versus native Australians	
	<16 years residence	0.36	
	>16 years residence	0.69	
Colon	Iran to British Columbia (BC) Canada	Incidence/10^5	
	Iran (Kerman Province)	5.9	
	Iranians in BC	11.6	
	Residents in BC	26.6	
Breast	Iranian Women to BC	Incidence/10^5	
	Kerman Province	16.9	
	Iranians in BC	68.5	
	BC Residents	81.4	

Data extracted from WCRF/AICR (2007)

retention of "primate" genes derived from nonhuman primate analyses as one tracks our current understanding of the migration of homo sapiens from Africa to the Middle East and Europe, then on to India, China, and Japan, then to the aborigines in Australia, through to the North American Indians, and finally to the Mayans and Incas of Latin America (Li et al. 2008). Table 8.2 gives examples of some analyses of cancer incidence relating to immigrants in North America and Australia where it is difficult to suppose that there are substantial differences in the genetics of those groups who for one reason or another choose to migrate. The data are selected from those collated for the World Cancer Research Fund (WCRF) second report WCRF/AICR (2007) and are used to highlight the way in which cancer rates can change, often quite dramatically. Furthermore, the incidence of cancer in immigrants comes much closer to those of the host population the longer they have lived in the country. This emphasizes the dominance of environmental factors with twin studies also showing that, although there may be some susceptibility to cancers related to genes, the effect is not usually very impressive (Risch 2001). Changing cancer trends within a country also emphasize the flexibility in the carcinogenic process.

8.3 Establishing the Validity of a Causal Link Between Diet and Cancer

Given this complexity, how can one begin to establish a robust understanding of dietary factors in the carcinogenic process? One approach, much favored by those in public health, is to rely on epidemiological studies because these studies are far more likely to provide an indication of the quantitative importance and relevance of any relationship in public health terms. Thus, those fascinated with molecular mechanisms or cellular studies of factors which promote DNA changes still have to establish how much this is relevant either in vivo or in overall metabolic terms on a long-term basis. There was therefore often a disjunction between cell biologists and epidemiologists with the former group confident in the precision and comparative speed of their methods at the molecular or cellular level and dismayed by the error-ridden vague approach to dietary surveys and the complexity of seemingly endless statistical adjustments for confounding factors such as age, smoking habits, and the assumptions made about delay times in the carcinogenic process. The epidemiologists, however, comforted themselves by recognizing that the molecular understanding of the process of DNA change was highlighting the multistaged nature of the process but providing only a limited perspective of what the overall significance is of any one dietary factor in the chain of events, leading to the actual induction of cancer.

Any coherent overview of the relationship between diet and cancer has been driven by the challenge of how to assess the validity of different avenues of research in developing suitable evidence of sufficient reliability to justify changes in policy whether in medical practice or government policies. By the late 1980s the US National Academy of Sciences was already attempting to synthesize different approaches to the diet-cancer link so that by the time the WCRF established its first analysis in 1994 it was accepted that a variety of approaches were needed. But now greater emphasis was being given to cohort studies and to meta-analyses and pooled studies with intervention trials being seen as the ultimate desirable basis for reaching firm conclusions. Then the WCRF brought together cancer and nutritional experts in the 1990s and set out an overall analysis of the relationship between food and the principal cancers found worldwide and began to try to assess the relationships between diet and cancer on a global basis and with a systematic approach. It was accepted that Bradford Hill's criteria of consistency, unbiased, strong, graded, coherent, repeatable, and plausible relationships were necessary before one could reasonably assume a substantial causal link between an exposure such as diet and cancer.

The basis for inferring causation in the relationship of diet and cancer was now proposed by the WCRF panel as being "confidently inferred when epidemiological evidence, and experimental and other biological findings, is consistent, unbiased, strong, graded, coherent, repeated, and plausible." More detailed requirements were then given with the convincing category now needing at least two independent cohort studies. Furthermore, there was a very clear requirement for a plausible biological dose–response gradient with strong and plausible experimental evidence either from human studies or suitable animal models showing that typical human exposures can lead to relevant outcomes

With this array of evidence, the WCRF/AICR (1997) first report on diet and cancer developed a scheme whereby they described their criteria for specifying whether a relationship was convincing, probable, possible, or insufficient and displayed the data as shown in Table 8.1 which includes their conclusions on the risks for postmenopausal breast cancer. It was concluded that only the convincing and probable relationships should be considered sufficiently powerful to justify policy making. To take the criteria for convincing evidence as an example, they specified that the "epidemiological studies show consistent associations, with little or no evidence to the contrary. There should be a substantial number of acceptable studies (that is, for dietary variables more than 20 studies) preferably to include prospective designs, conducted in different populations, controlled for confounding factors. Dietary intake data should refer to the time preceding occurrence of cancer. Any dose–response relationship should be supportive of a causal relationship. Associations should be biologically plausible. Laboratory evidence is usually supportive or strongly supportive." Thus, it is already evident that the epidemiological evidence was dominating the decision making, and a series of studies in different countries with a preference for prospective studies were the cornerstone of decision making with laboratory evidence being relegated to a supporting role. This approach led to a very big surge in new studies on diet and cancer but with a far greater emphasis on prospective studies. The WCRF approach to assessing the dietary basis of cancer was in effect endorsed by WHO in its technical report in 2003 (WHO 2003) which formed the basis of the current WHO action plan on diet and physical activity for the prevention of the non-communicable diseases (NCDs) (WHO 2008). However, this WHO technical report in 2003, on the basis of the earlier WCRF report and analyses by the WHO's International Agency for Research in Cancer (IARC), highlighted that there were "few definite relationships between diet and cancer."

A decade after its original 1997 report, the WCRF again reviewed the evidence but now, after often fraught debates, the same categories were used but with different criteria and all the epidemiological analyses were based on a novel and very time-consuming process (WCRF/AICR 2007). A statistical design for all the epidemiological analyses was first developed by an independent group of epidemiologists and statisticians, and then the specified categories of diet were assessed for each cancer according to this protocol by a group of specialists (nine successful groups in all) who had bid successfully for each contract on the basis of having a full complement of expertise. Externally appointed monitors of the whole process as well as independent evaluators from the main WCRF panel were also involved in ensuring that the process was followed properly. Then their conclusions had to pass further scrutiny by the whole WCRF panel of global experts. This is undoubtedly the most exhaustive review of the evidence to date, and the WCRF has continued to progressively update and present online the latest analysis of individual diet-cancer relationships since their major analyses were completed in December 2005. The choice of dietary factors, ingredients, and nutrients for analysis was not easy, and in all 60 foods, drinks or nutrients were considered with being breastfed considered separately. Even this is very crude when in molecular terms we know that specific minor changes to the molecular structure of compounds alter markedly their biological properties, but until we have fool-proof biological tools to asses each component of the carcinogenic process and specifically of factors modifying their activity, we will have to move incrementally forward in our understanding.

Table 8.3 gives an example of the assessment of the convincing and probable factors inducing or protecting against premenopausal and postmenopausal breast cancer as determined by the WCRF process, which considered a wide range of foods and nutrients in relation to the development of the breast cancer. Early life events seem to have an impact because breast cancers are more likely in taller women, and this is not only genetically determined but has a very important environmental component with the WCRF analyses also showing that rapid growth in childhood seems to promote the process. Furthermore, greater birth weights seem to promote premenopausal breast cancer with overweight and obesity having opposite effects depending on whether the cancer develops before or after the menopause.

The overall analysis of diet related to 20 different cancers (pre- and postmenopausal breast cancer being considered separately) and this range included some cancers, for example, lung, where there seemed to be overwhelming evidence of the far greater importance of other factors such as smoking. What came through most powerfully compared with the first WCRF report was that now obesity was seen to be a particular risk and the evidence for the protective role of vegetables and fruit was less robust. In terms of specific cancers, red meat was seen to be linked more powerfully with colon/rectal cancer with processed meats having an even greater risk.

Figure 8.1 reproduces the abbreviated summary of the links between diet and cancer as set out in the subsequent policy report of the WCRF/AICR (2009). Since then, there has been a WCRF update which shows a more powerful effect of meat and processed meat on colon cancer induction, so this is now a convincing relationship. It is clear that some factors are promoting cancers and others are protective. In the 2009 policy report, WCRF/AICR estimated the potential preventability of cancers from changes in nutrition, physical activity, and reduction in body weight, that is, in body fatness.

Table 8.4 reproduces a table from the WCRF/AICR (2007) report based on the prevalence of different cancers in four countries for which there were comparatively clear nationally representative data about the incidence of cancers, dietary patterns, physical activity levels, and body fatness, that is, USA, UK, Brazil, and China. Clearly where there are powerful agents involved, for example, alcohol, in inducing cancers of the mouth, pharynx, larynx, and esophagus, then clearly the majority of these cancers are preventable by not drinking alcohol. Similarly, endometrial cancer is highly preventable if one does not increase one's body fat mass.

Table 8.3 Causal factors in the development of pre-menopausal and postmenopausal breast cancer

	Premenopausal		Postmenopausal	
Level of evidence	Decreases risk	Increases risk	Decreases risk	Increases risk
Convincing	Lactation	Alcoholic drinks	Lactation	Alcoholic drinks, body fatness, adult-attained height
Probable	Body fatness	Adult-attained height, greater birth weight	Physical activity	Abdominal fatness Adult weight gain
Limited suggestive	Physical activity			Total fat

From WCRF/AICR (2007)

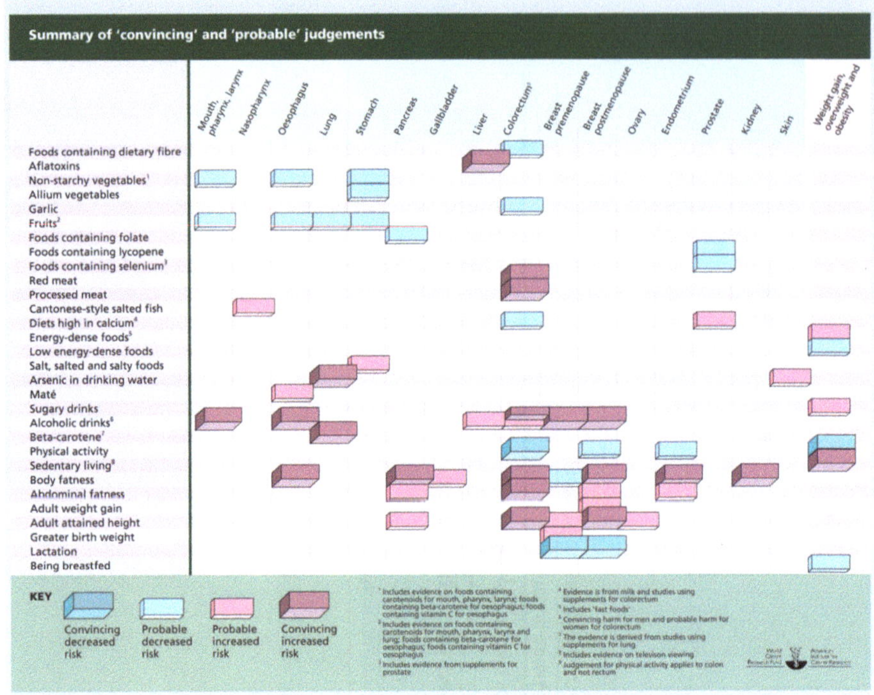

Fig. 8.1 Food, nutrition, physical activity, and the prevention of cancer: overview of the Panel's key judgements

Nevertheless, the analyses suggested that even for lung cancer about a third is preventable by dietary means. Indeed their overall estimates came surprisingly close to the original ones of Doll and Peto (1981). When body fatness was assessed in terms of its contribution to this preventable figure, then the report took the cancers previously identified as being promoted by being overweight/obese, that is, esophagus pancreas, gallbladder, colon/rectum, breast, endometrium, and kidney, and assessed the role of body fatness in preventing these cancers in men and women separately. Because the level of obesity is far higher in the USA and UK, this component proved more important than in Brazil and China.

8.4 Intervention Studies to Demonstrate the Impact of Reducing Obesity on Cancer Induction

Traditionally, this has rarely been considered because it is so difficult to imagine major trials which induce marked changes in diet, physical activity, or body fatness, but recently, some evidence in this regard has been collated. The first relates to the impact

Table 8.4 The WCRF/AICR estimates of preventability of different cancers in the USA, UK, Brazil, and China by an appropriate diet, level of physical activity, and appropriate level of body fatness (from WCRF/AICR (2009))

Estimates[1] of cancer preventability by appropriate food, nutrition, physical activity, and body fatness in four countries[2]

	USA	UK	BRAZIL	CHINA
Mouth, pharynx, larynx	63	67	63	44
Oesophagus	69	75	60	44
Lung	36	33	36	38
Stomach	47	45	41	33
Pancreas	39	41	34	14
Gallbladder	21	16	10	6
Liver	15	17	6	6
Colorectum	45	43	37	17
Breast	38	42	28	20
Endometrium	70	56	52	34
Prostate	11	20	N/A[3]	N/A[3]
Kidney	24	19	13	8
Total for these cancers combined	34	39	30	27
Total for all cancers	24	26	19	20

1. These values are percentages rounded to the nearest whole number and are based on several assumptions. There is a range of likely plausible figures around these point estimates, but they represent the most likely estimates.
2. Based on the conclusions of the 2007 WCRF/AICR Diet and Cancer Report.
3. Exposure data not available

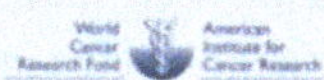

of marked reductions in obesity by the use of bariatric surgery. A preliminary study was reported by Christou et al. (2004) who used predominantly by-pass surgery and found a 76% reduction in new cancer cases with even greater falls in total mortality in a Quebec sample of over 1,000 patients undergoing bariatric surgery where health care use was meticulously monitored for a defined 5-year period in comparison with a sixfold greater number of age-, sex-, and BMI-matched Quebec residents. They later reported that breast cancer was significantly reduced with a trend to lower cancer rates

Table 8.5 The impact of intentional weight changes on cancer incidence or mortality

Type of study/ Author	Cancer site	Population studied	Body weight loss	Cancer risk reduction (%)
Cohort studies				
Parker	All sites	Postmenopausal Iowa women	≥16.4%	11
Eliassen	Breast	US nurses	≥14.5%	57
Harvie	Breast	Postmenopausal Iowa women	≥5%	64
Bariatric surgery studies				
Sjöström	All sites	Women	31.9%	42
		Men	19.3	3
Adams	All sites	Women	31.1%	24
		Men		2
Christou	All sites	Men and women	31.9%	78
Dietary RCTs				
Pierce	Breast	Women	0.5% group difference	4
Prentice	Breast	Women	1.0% group difference	9
Chlebowski	Breast	Women	3.7% group difference	24

See Byers and Sedjo (2011) for more details

in all other cancers, but the surgical group was too small for detailed analyses of individual cancer sites (Christou et al. 2008). Adams et al. (2007) also set out their comparison of the impact of marked weight loss after gastric by-pass surgery by comparing their data from a state cancer registry of the causes of death in their surgical patients with sex-, age-, and weight-matched data from very obese adults in Utah who had to specify their weights and heights (from which BMIs corrected for the self-report values were calculated) when they took out their driving licenses. Comparing the two groups over an 18-year period showed that the surgical group had within only 7 years a 46% reduction in total death rates with 58.6% lower rates of death from cancer, type and sex relationships unspecified. Later Adams and Hunt (2009) set out cancer incidence to weight loss in more detail with six times the number of cases assessed in Quebec. They found a 24% reduction in cancer incidence with a 46% lower cancer death rate and with the apparent reduction affecting all cancers, not just those considered normally related to obesity. The Swedish Obese Subjects Study (Sjostrom et al. 2009) with more modest weight losses from lap banding observed a surprising female only reduction in the incidence of cancer (HR 0.58 95% CI 0.44–0.77 p=0.0001) with detailed follow-up of both their surgical and control groups. Again, a broad range of cancers seemed to be affected and the results seemed unrelated to that expected from the usual obesity-cancer relationships. They also could not relate the reduction in cancer incidence to the degree of weight loss nor to a crude assessment of the fall in long-term energy intake after the surgical procedures.

From this we might conclude that surgically induced weight loss has a profound effect on cancer incidence with perhaps an even greater fall in cancer mortality. These data also suggests that the reduction affects a whole range of cancers and not just those which the WCRF analyses of prospective studies suggest as related to obesity. This finding may relate to the traditional findings in so many animal models that semi-starvation reduces the incidence of a wide range of both spontaneous and carcinogen-induced cancers (Hursting et al. 2010). Recently Byers and Sedjo (2011) reviewed this field of body weight and added the data relating to nonsurgical weight loss. Their analyses are included in Table 8.5, and on this basis Byers suggested that the degree of intentional weight loss seems to relate to a proportionate reduction in cancer incidence and that the effect does occur surprisingly quickly.

8.5 Body Weight, Diet, and Physical Activity in Relation to Cancer Progression

The distinction between factors which influence the incidence of cancers and those which promote or inhibit the proliferation of cancers is now being explored. The 2007 WCRF analyses recognized that thinner people may be more readily diagnosed with preexisting cancer, and this difference in ready diagnosis may therefore reduce the apparent relationship between obesity and the incidence of cancer, but once diagnosed the question then is whether changes in body weight, physical activity, or diet as such affect the recurrence or progression of the disease. On the basis of their systematic analyses, the WCRF concluded that higher body fatness *before* diagnosis resulted in a worse outcome, but they noted only one intervention where weight was deliberately lost in patients with early breast cancer placed on a low-fat diet, namely, the WINS trial where there was a 24% reduction in breast cancer recurrence (Blackburn and Wang 2007). Additionally, when subgroups were analyzed, it appeared that the dietary intervention had a greater effect on relapse-free survival in women with hormone-receptor-negative (estrogen, progesterone, or both) disease than in women with receptor-positive disease; the relapse-free survival rate was 42% greater than in the control group, corresponding to a relapse-free survival rate of 9.5% after 8 years. However, the groups were not strictly comparable in that the intervention group had had more radical surgery. A similar study on dietary change without weight loss, the WHEL study (Thiébaut et al. 2007), showed no effect of a more prudent diet without weight loss. More recent analyses of weight gain after diagnosis of breast cancer (Hauner et al. 2011) found that 5 of 6 studies showed not only a clear association with total mortality but also breast cancer-specific mortality; recurrence rates as such were clearly related to weight increases. These studies strongly suggest that weight status is important in determining the outcome of breast cancer with the latest analyses contradicting the earlier WCRF conclusions that obesity was protective of premenopausal breast cancer. Eighteen of the 20 studies on physical activity showed an improvement in the quality of life, but only a third of all studies reported mortality rates, and these were not significantly affected.

Perhaps what is surprising about these studies is the relatively small number of studies relating to survival after diagnosis when, as a recent US Institute of Medicine workshop highlighted (IOM 2012), patients once diagnosed are extremely anxious and willing to alter their diet and physical activity if that would help their prognosis, and there is now reasonable evidence that changes can be achieved in both dietary patterns and weight loss in these patients (Befort et al. 2012).

8.6 Distinguishing Intake Effects from Body Weight Differences or Changes

The problem with studies of differences in body weight or weight change is that there is an automatic association between total energy intake and the size of the individual. So, increases in body weight mean an increase in basal energy needs and the cost of physical activity. In practice the basal metabolic rate (BMR), that is, basal energy requirements, is predominantly related to total body weight with height adding very little to the predicted relationship and the physical activity level (PAL). This is usually about 1.6–1.8 times the BMR value for the individual, range 1.4–2.1 depending on the amount and intensity of physical activity. The BMR multiplied by the PAL gives a value which is a far more reliable prediction of what subjects in practice eat on average than food frequency questionnaires. So we know that when subjects lose weight after surgery or after dieting, then their food requirements fall by about 30–40 kcals/kg body weight loss, greater than the normal relationship predicted from body composition (Rosenbaum et al. 2010). So distinguishing between the effects of body weight or BMI per se and total energy intake or total fat, carbohydrate, or other intake is not easy unless there are drastic changes in the composition of the food eaten as part of the slimming program.

8.7 Emerging Specific Dietary Relationships

Apart from those dietary relationships highlighted in Fig. 8.1 and relating to data collected up to 2006 by WCRF, some additional analyses have been made and emphasize the likely impact of specific macronutrients or dietary components on the development of cancers.

8.7.1 Fat Intake Relating to Breast Cancer Obscured by Imprecise Dietary Methods

This has been a much disputed subject for some time with animal studies, cross-country comparisons, and case–control studies all showing a relationship between fat intake and the incidence of breast cancer. This led the first WCRF group's analyses to conclude (with one dissenting eminent epidemiologist) that fat intake did probably relate to breast cancer. However, prospective studies with their routine reliance on food frequency have led to a great debate as to the validity of the food frequency questionnaire (FFQ), particularly when adjusted for estimated energy intake. This author discovered major discrepancies when first applying the now universally accepted method of calculating basal metabolic rates for the individual women with a range of possible physical activity levels to estimate their probable energy intake (assuming reasonably that this will be within <10% of their expenditure). These analyses showed that an embarrassingly large number of subjects must be underestimating their food intakes because they could not survive long on their purported food frequency intakes without a profound and rapid loss of weight. These analyses led several epidemiologists to express all their intakes per 1,000 kcals. Bingham et al. (2003) then showed that if she used her carefully biomarker validated recorded 7-day dietary records as well as a FFQ similar to that developed for the nurses and physicians study that there was a very clear statistical relationship between total fat and saturated fat intakes and the development of breast cancer, whereas this was not seen when using the FFQ. This led to a much bigger study with dietary records in the USA which came to a similar conclusion (Freedman et al. 2006), and a second US study which tried to correct for methodological problems with the dietary methodology also found a significant relationship of invasive postmenopausal breast cancer with both total and subtypes of fatty acid intake (Thiebaut et al. 2007). One feature of large multinational studies with a far larger range of fat intakes than those seen within a national cohort has also allowed the European EPIC studies to see a statistically significant relationship between saturated fat intake and the incidence of invasive breast cancer with a nonsignificant trend observed with total fat intake (Sieri et al. 2008), while another analysis looking at dietary patterns associated with high fat intakes showed a doubling of risk of breast cancer irrespective of BMI status in the EPIC studies (Shulz et al. 2008). There have been several other powerful statistical analyses highlighting the spurious positive as well as negative results which may be obtained with FFQs (Day et al. 2004; Thiébaut et al. 2008). A US intervention trial (Prentice et al. 2006) has also been conducted and is interesting because the investigators were trying to assess the impact of only an 8% reduction in fat intake expressed as a proportion of presumed energy intake, whereas globally we have to remember that the Northern Europe and American fat intakes have traditionally been well over 40% compared with intakes of less than 10% in many Asian and African countries before the 1980s and with Japanese and Chinese studies by the 1980s still showing fat intakes of about 15%. So international comparisons and migration studies are dealing with far greater ranges of intakes than we see in most national epidemiological studies and particularly in intervention trials where the validity of the dietary change is even more questionable. Finally, a careful statistical review of all the different types of studies, that is, animal studies, international comparisons, case-control, prospective, and an intervention trial, has led to the conclusion that dietary measurement errors are of great importance and there is a modest but real association between fat intake and breast cancer (Freedman et al. 2008). This then is a different conclusion from the latest WCRF update to May 2008 relating to cancer of the breast (Norat et al. 2008) which in effect continued to consider the evidence as only suggestive. This analysis is dominated by systematic analyses of all prospective studies without assessing in detail the errors involved in the dietary questionnaire methods. So if we take the more rigorous analyses of diet, they fit the other forms of evidence, suggesting that fat intake is probably related to the development of breast cancer and specific measures need to be taken to limit the fat intake in the diet.

8.7.2 Red Meat, Processed Meat, and Fiber Intakes in Relation to Colon Cancer

This has been well documented in the second WCRF report, but more recently the WCRF update (Norat et al. 2010) has not only confirmed the relationship but shown that not only red meat but also processed meat is even more strongly related with the panel, concluding that the relationships are convincing. The panel also noted that the evidence for fiber intakes was more protective than hitherto noted. When a prospective nested case-control study with a reasonable number of cases, namely, 579, was undertaken in seven major cohort studies in the UK with both food frequency methods and dietary records, then again a very significant protective relationship with non-starch polysaccharide intake measured by the Englyst method was observed with the recorded measures of intake but not with the food frequency questionnaire (Dahm et al. 2010). Other major studies, albeit sometimes focusing on the less appropriate AOAC method for assessing dietary fiber as typically used in the US, did not look so robust, but extensive meta-analyses of all the cohort data showed a statistically significant 10% decreased risk in colorectal cancer per 10 g/day of dietary fiber intake, and this was even clearer if the potential preventive effects of folate intake were taken into account. The potential overall effect may be inferred from the UK study where the benefit of the highest fiber quintile intake compared to the lowest quintile amounted to a 39% (95% CI 10–58%) reduction in risk. The evidence for colon cancer looked more impressive than for rectal cancer.

8.8 Challenges in Determining the Dietary Impact on Carcinogenesis

Two features of these latest analyses are significant. First that the more robust the methods for measuring dietary intake, the more apparent the diet-cancer relationship. Thus, the validity of the frequently used food frequency questionnaire seems increasingly in doubt. This is not what epidemiologists want to hear because with the need to monitor intakes of preferably hundreds of thousands of subjects over a long period of time, it has always been accepted that the weighed intake method would be impossible. However, one might reasonably conclude that methods involving dietary records or direct careful history taking by a nutritionist with dietary modules for assessing portions sizes as introduced by Jean Hankin (Kolonel et al.

1981) have been shown to be more valid in relation to biomarkers of food intake than food frequency questionnaires and should be preferred, with the need to obtain biomarkers whenever possible as is now emphasized in the EPIC studies.

The second feature of current conclusions is the emphasis given to ever more complex meta-analyses of cohort studies with seemingly little notice being taken of biological mechanistic views. This is perhaps almost inevitable given the need to ensure that population data are robust if one is contemplating policies which involve advocating changes in societal food intake. However, as many expert groups are dominated by epidemiologists involved in cohort studies, it seems reasonable to highlight the value of including if possible human metabolic studies where changes in diet are tested for their effects on markers relating to the carcinogenic processes themselves.

8.9 The Value of Physiological and Metabolic Studies of Potential Carcinogenesis

A good example of this is the question of the impact of diets on free estrogen concentrations, bearing in mind the striking and largely ignored circadian cycle of free estrogens which also depend on the stage of the menstrual cycle (Bao et al. 2004). This would seem worthwhile in studies on diet and breast cancer given the clear association between the unbound levels of sex hormones and the likelihood of postmenopausal breast cancer. A clear association with BMI and with alcohol intake is already evident for these two known strong risk factors for this cancer (Endogenous Hormones and Breast Cancer Collaborative Group 2011), but it would be valuable to document carefully whether fat intakes per se have an independent effect on free sex hormone levels. Japanese studies show a clear relationship to saturated fat intakes (Tsuji et al. 2012), but these associations do not seem to have been backed up by controlled metabolic feeding studies in energy balance (Crighton et al. 1992) which may need to evaluate the effects of fat/fiber ratios (Aubertin-Leheudre et al. 2011) since fiber intakes are known to affect the endogenous recycling of steroids. It is important to distinguish between the effects of low-fat/high-fiber diets and changes in energy balance in carefully controlled feeding studies since without care subjects being monitored tend to reduce their energy intake, and then negative balance inducing a reduction in free estrogen levels is difficult to distinguish from fat intakes per se (Heber et al. 1991).

Another example is the elegant series of metabolic feeding experiments undertaken by the late Sheila Bingham (Bingham et al. 1996) where in a metabolic ward she studied the effects of meat intake on fecal nitroso compound excretion. These compounds increased with meat intake, and the concentration was diluted by the additional feeding of non-starch polysaccharide-rich wheat bran. Fecal nitrite levels also increased when changing white meat to red meat, so these metabolic results are entirely in keeping with the epidemiological studies. Later, she showed that vegetables through their effects on transit and fecal weight would also reduce the colonic mucosal contact with nitroso compounds (Hughes et al. 2002).

More recently, there has been a tendency to search, for example, for biomarkers of inflammation or antioxidant status, but what is really required are more sophisticated studies of the carcinogenesis process itself and the specific tissue DNA repair mechanisms. More direct studies are easier to do if direct access to the cells involved can be achieved, for example, with colonic, prostatic, or breast cells. So far, few studies have been undertaken because they involve a range of sophisticated skills as well as volunteers willing to undergo potentially unpleasant procedures which then have to be conducted under meticulously controlled conditions such as those established by Bingham and colleagues.

8.10 Background Metabolic and Genetic Research

WCRF/AICR (1997, 2007) summarized a whole range of processes that are involved in carcinogenesis, and it is not appropriate to highlight these here but a careful study of the multiple steps involved and how, for example, obesity can play a part at different stages in the process helps us to understand that the new findings of surprisingly rapid reductions in risk and indeed in the progression of cancer can reasonably be ascribed to effects during the later stages of carcinogenesis. So the process of developing cancers may take many years, but this finding is still compatible with a fairly rapid fall in the actual incidence and progression of established cancer by dietary measures and particularly by reductions in overall energy intake and a fall in body weight.

8.11 Conclusions

Although Doll and Peto's (1981) original seemingly crude but in practice erudite analyses based on ecological studies suggested perhaps a value of 35% for the dietary contributions to carcinogenesis, this value was greater than their 30% value for the impact of smoking which was their normal focus. Yet they also indicated that this dietary figure might be as great as 70%. After 30 years of endeavor, we can now be far more confident that the average value of 35% is a conservative figure as Doll and Peto (1981) considered likely, but we are still bedeviled by the fact that assessing diet accurately and being able to do this repeatedly over a number of years in prospective cohort studies are exceptionally difficult. The more accurate the methods and the greater the use of biomarkers of dietary intake, the more likely it seems that consistent significant dietary relationships are found.

Exhaustive Cochrane searches with independently specified statistical analytical protocols have come up with a host of dietary factors as in Fig. 8.1. Probable or convincing relationships are apparent for specific tissue cancers in relation to the intake of individual dietary groups of foods, for example, vegetables and fruit, fiber-rich foods, smoked and salted fish, red meats and processed meats, and alcohol. However, body weight and obesity are becoming ever more clearly a risk factor, in part, because it so easily measured with accuracy and consistency. A reduced state of energy balance with weight reduction by dietary means and/or physical activity also seems independently related to cancer prevention. However, there is a need to have more effective methods of combining metabolic studies with more refined indices of carcinogenesis, and then we may well find that dietary factors explain closer to the 70% of cancers as specified by Doll and Peto (1981) from ecological studies.

Already trial data are suggesting that interventions in cancer survivors may be beneficial, particularly when this involves weight loss in overweight/obese subjects. The range of cancers gaining benefit from this seems to be more wide ranging than that predicted from our current prospective studies relating to obesity, and there is now clearly an advantage of conducting more refined studies across a range of cultures so that the full range of potential intakes can be properly studies in a robust way.

References

Adams T D, Gress R E, Smith S C, Halverson R C, Simper S C, Rosamond W D et al. Long-Term Mortality after Gastric Bypass Surgery. *N Engl J Med* 2007; 357:753–761.

Adams TD, Hunt SC. Cancer and obesity: effect of bariatric surgery. *World J Surg* 2009; 33:2028–2033.

Aubertin-Leheudre M, Hämäläinen E, Adlercreutz H. Diets and hormonal levels in postmenopausal women with or without breast cancer. *Nutr Cancer* 2011; 63:514–524.

Bao AM, Ji YF, Van Someren EJ, Hofman MA, Liu RY, Zhou JN. Diurnal rhythms of free estradiol and cortisol during the normal menstrual cycle in women with major depression. *Horm Behav* 2004; 45:93–102.

Befort CA, Klemp JR, Austin HL, Perri MG, Schmitz KH, Sullivan DK et al. Outcomes of a weight loss intervention among rural breast cancer survivors. *Breast Cancer Res Treat* 2012; 132:631–639.

Bingham SA. Epidemiology of dietary fibre and colorectal cancer: current status of the hypothesis. *Nutr Health* 1985; 4:17–23.

Bingham SA, Pignatelli B, Pollock JR, Ellul A, Malaveille C, Gross G et al, Does increased endogenous formation of N-nitroso compounds in the human colon explain the association between red meat and colon cancer? *Carcinogenesis* 1996 17:515–523.

Bingham SA, Luben R, Welch A, Wareham N, Khaw KT, Day N. Are imprecise methods obscuring a relation between fat and breast cancer? *Lancet* 2003; 362:212–214.

Blackburn GL, Wang KA. Dietary fat reduction and breast cancer outcome: results from the Women's Intervention Nutrition Study (WINS) *Am J Clin Nutr* 2007; 86:878S–881S.

Burkitt D. A lymphoma syndrome in African children. *Ann R Coll Surg Engl* 1962; 30:211–219.

Burkitt DP. Dietary fiber and cancer. *J Nutr* 1988; 118:531–533.

Byers T, Sedjo RL. Does intentional weight loss reduce cancer risk? *Diabetes Obes Metab* 2011; 13:1063–1072.

Chen J., Campbell T.C., Li J., Peto R. *Diet, Life-style and Mortality in China. A Study of the Characteristics of 65 Chinese Counties*. Oxford University Press, (Oxford, U.K.), Cornell University Press, (Ithaca, NY), People's Medical Publishing House (Beijing PRC), 894 pp. 1991.

Christou NV, Sampalis JS, Liberman M, Look D, Auger S, McLean AP et al. Surgery decreases long-term mortality, morbidity, and health care use in morbidly obese patients. *Ann Surg* 2004; 240:416–423; discussion 423–424.

Christou NV, Lieberman M, Sampalis F, Sampalis JS. Bariatric surgery reduces cancer risk in morbidly obese patients. *Surg Obes Relat Dis* 2008; 4:691–695. Comment in: *Surg Obes Relat Dis* 2008; 4:696–697.

Crighton IL, Dowsett M, Hunter M, Shaw C, Smith IE. The effect of a low-fat diet on hormone levels in healthy pre- and postmenopausal women: relevance for breast cancer. *Eur J Cancer* 1992; 28A:2024–2027.

Dahm CC, Keogh RH, Spencer EA, Greenwood DC, Key TJ, Fentiman IS et al. Dietary fiber and colorectal cancer risk: a nested case-control study using food diaries. *J Natl Cancer Inst* 2010; 102:614–626. Erratum in: *J Natl Cancer Inst* 2010; 103:1484.

Day NE, Wong MY, Bingham S, Khaw KT, Luben R, Michels KB et al. Correlated measurement error--implications for nutritional epidemiology. *Int J Epidemiol* 2004; 33:1373–1381.

Diggs DL, Huderson AC, Harris KL, Myers JN, Banks LD, Rekhadevi PV et al. Polycyclic aromatic hydrocarbons and digestive tract cancers: a perspective. *J Environ Sci Health C Environ Carcinog Ecotoxicol Rev* 2011; 29:324–357.

Doll R, Peto R. The causes of Cancer *J Natl Cancer Inst* 1981; 66: 1191–1308.

Endogenous Hormones and Breast Cancer Collaborative Group, Key TJ, Appleby PN, Reeves GK, Roddam AW, Helzlsouer KJ, Alberg AJ et al. Circulating sex hormones and breast cancer risk factors in postmenopausal women: reanalysis of 13 studies. *Br J Cancer* 2011; 105:709–722.

Freedman LS, Potischman N, Kipnis V, Midthune D, Schatzkin A, Thompson FE et al. A comparison of two dietary instruments for evaluating the fat-breast cancer relationship. *Int J Epidemiol* 2006; 35:1011–1121.

Freedman LS, Kipnis V, Schatzkin A, Potischman N. Methods of epidemiology: evaluating the fat-breast cancer hypothesis--comparing dietary instruments and other developments. *Cancer J* 2008; 14:69–74.

Haenszel W, Kurihara M. Studies of Japanese migrants. I. Mortality from cancer and other diseases among Japanese in the United States. *J Natl Cancer Inst* 1968; 40:43–68.

Hauner D, Janni W, Rack B, Hauner H. The effect of overweight and nutrition on prognosis in breast cancer. *Dtsch Arztebl Int* 2011; 108:795–801.

Heber D, Ashley JM, Leaf DA, Barnard RJ. Reduction of serum estradiol in postmenopausal women given free access to low-fat high-carbohydrate diet. *Nutrition* 1991; 7:137–139.

Howe GR. Some methodological issues in epidemiological studies of fat and cancer. *Cancer Res* 1981; 41(Pt 2):3731–3732.

Hughes R, Pollock JR, Bingham S. Effect of vegetables, tea, and soy on endogenous N-nitrosation, fecal ammonia, and fecal water genotoxicity during a high red meat diet in humans. *Nutr Cancer* 2002; 42:70–77.

Hursting SD, Smith SM, Lashinger LM, Harvey AE, Perkins SN. Calories and carcinogenesis: lessons learned from 30 years of calorie restriction research. *Carcinogenesis* 2010; 31:83–89.

IOM (Institute of Medicine). *The role of obesity in cancer survival and recurrence*. Workshop summary. 2012. Washington, DC: The National Academies Press.

Kolonel LN, Hankin JH, Nomura AM, Chu SY. Dietary fat intake and cancer incidence among five ethnic groups in Hawaii. *Cancer Res* 1981; 41:3727–3728.

Li JZ, Absher DM, Tang H, Southwick AM, Casto AM, Ramachandran S et al. Worldwide human relationships inferred from genome-wide patterns of variation. *Science* 2008; 319:1100–1104.

Lipnick RJ, Buring JE, Hennekens CH, Rosner B, Willett W, Bain C et al. Oral contraceptives and breast cancer. A prospective cohort study. *JAMA* 1986; 255:58–61.

Miller AB. Role of nutrition in the etiology of breast cancer. *Cancer* 1977; 39(Suppl): 2704–2708.

Monroe KR, Hankin JH, Pike MC, Henderson BE, Stram DO, Park S et al. Correlation of dietary intake and colorectal cancer incidence among Mexican-American migrants: the multiethnic cohort study. *Nutr Cancer* 2003; 45:133–147.

Morgan RW, Jain M, Miller AB, Choi NW, Matthews V, Munan L et al. A comparison of dietary methods in epidemiologic studies. *Am J Epidemiol* 1978; 107:488–498.

Norat T, Chan D, Lau R, Vieira R The Associations between Food, Nutrition and Physical Activity and the Risk of Breast Cancer. WCRF Update. http://www.dietandcancerreport.org/cancer_resource_center/downloads/cu/cu_breast_cancer_report_2008.pdf

Norat T, Chan D, Lau R, Vieira R. WCRF/AICR Systematic Literature Review. Continuous Update Project Report. The Associations between Food, Nutrition and Physical Activity and the Risk of Colorectal Cancer. October 2010 WCRF/ AICR cancer update http://www.wcrf.org/cancer_research/cup/index.php

Prentice RL, Caan B, Chlebowski RT, Patterson R, Kuller LH, Ockene JK et al. Low-fat dietary pattern and risk of invasive breast cancer: the Women's Health Initiative Randomized Controlled Dietary Modification Trial. *JAMA* 2006; 295:629–642.

Riboli E. The European Prospective Investigation into Cancer and Nutrition (EPIC): plans and progress. *J Nutr* 2001; 131:170S–175S.

Risch N. The genetic epidemiology of cancer: interpreting family and twin studies and their implications for molecular genetic approaches. *Cancer Epidemiol Biomarkers Prev* 2001; 10:733–741.

Rosenbaum M, Kissileff HR, Mayer LE, Hirsch J, Leibel RL. Energy intake in weight-reduced humans. *Brain Res* 2010; 1350:95–102.

Schulz M, Hoffmann K, Weikert C, Nöthlings U, Schulze MB, Boeing H. Identification of a dietary pattern characterized by high-fat food choices associated with increased risk of breast cancer: the European Prospective Investigation into Cancer and Nutrition (EPIC)-Potsdam Study. *Br J Nutr* 2008; 100:942–946.

Sieri S, Krogh V, Ferrari P, Berrino F, Pala V, Thiébaut AC et al. Dietary fat and breast cancer risk in the European Prospective Investigation into Cancer and Nutrition. *Am J Clin Nutr* 2008; 88:1304–1312.

Sjöström L, Gummesson A, Sjöström CD, Narbro K, Peltonen M, Wedel H et al. Swedish Obese Subjects Study. Effects of bariatric surgery on cancer incidence in obese patients in Sweden (Swedish Obese Subjects Study): a prospective, controlled intervention trial. *Lancet Oncol* 2009; 10:653–662.

Thiébaut AC, Kipnis V, Chang SC, Subar AF, Thompson FE, Rosenberg PS et al . A. Dietary fat and postmenopausal invasive breast cancer in the National Institutes of Health-AARP Diet and Health Study cohort. *J Natl Cancer Inst* 2007; 99:451–462.

Thiébaut AC, Kipnis V, Schatzkin A, Freedman LS. The role of dietary measurement error in investigating the hypothesized link between dietary fat intake and breast cancer--a story with twists and turns. *Cancer Invest* 2008; 26:68–73.

Tsuji M, Tamai Y, Wada K, Nakamura K, Hayashi M, Takeda N, Yasuda K, Nagata C. Associations of intakes of fat, dietary fiber, soy isoflavones, and alcohol with levels of sex hormones and prolactin in premenopausal Japanese women. *Cancer Causes Control.* 2012 Mar 8. [Epub ahead of print]

World Cancer Research Fund/American Institute for Cancer Research. *Food, Nutrition and the Prevention of Cancer: a Global Perspective.* Washington, DC: AICR, 1997.

World Cancer Research Fund/American Institute for Cancer Research. *Food, Nutrition, Physical Activity, and the Prevention of Cancer: a Global Perspective.* Washington DC: AICR, 2007.

World Cancer Research Fund/American Institute for Cancer Research. *Policy and Action for Cancer Prevention. Food, Nutrition and Physical Activity: a Global Perspective.* Washington AICR, 2009.

World Health Organization. *Diet, nutrition and the prevention of chronic diseases.* Report of a Joint WHO/FAO Expert Consultation. WHO Technical Report Series No. 916, 2003. WHO, Geneva

WHO 2008-2013 action plan for the global strategy for the prevention and control of noncommunicable diseases: prevent and control cardiovascular diseases, cancers, chronic respiratory diseases and diabetes. WHO, 2008.Geneva

Chapter 9
Chemoprevention of Cancer: From Nutritional Epidemiology to Clinical Trials

Mary Reid and James Marshall

9.1 Introduction

The impressive successes of chemotherapy have led to the hope that cancer might be prevented by use of drugs: chemoprevention. Sporn (1980) was an early advocate and continued to support chemoprevention. (Sporn and Hong 2008) Chemoprevention may be defined as the use of a drug, nutrient, or other bioactive compound or, more broadly, as the emphasis of certain dietary components over others, as a means of preventing cancer's initial occurrence. A related approach has been to use dietary manipulation as a form of chemoprevention. The feasibility of chemoprevention has been supported by the intriguing findings of nutritional epidemiology; a plethora of studies have suggested that various dietary practices are associated with diminished risk of various cancers (World Cancer Research Fund/American Institute for Cancer Research 2007). It is tempting to suspect that, if the active substances within the diets associated with decreased risk could be identified, these substances might be administered to healthy people to decrease their vulnerability to cancer.

Few active chemical agents, however, have only one effect or act only on a single metabolic pathway. Thus, a drug that blocks a given pathway in the colon may have any number of cardiovascular or renal effects. Since chemoprevention would be administered to healthy people, the safety standard must be quite high for chemoprevention. Cancer patients may face an imminent threat to their continued survival; a cancer drug or treatment can be highly toxic, but, if its overall effect is to decrease

M. Reid
Department of Medicine, Roswell Park Cancer Institute,
Buffalo, NY 14263, USA

J. Marshall (✉)
Department of Cancer Prevention and Population Sciences,
Roswell Park Cancer Institute, Elm and Carlton Streets,
Buffalo, NY 14263, USA
e-mail: james.marshall@roswellpark.org

A.B. Miller (ed.), *Epidemiologic Studies in Cancer Prevention and Screening*,
Statistics for Biology and Health 79, DOI 10.1007/978-1-4614-5586-8_9,

mortality by even a modest degree, it may be considered useful. However, a chemopreventive agent, to be administered to people for whom the risk of any one life-threatening cancer is relatively low, must be extremely safe. It must impart essentially no toxicity. An agent that decreases the risk of certain cancers but increases those of other cancers or of other serious illnesses is not likely to be adopted for chemoprevention. Dietary substances, such as vitamins and minerals, already in the food supply and common, widely used medications may be attractive for chemoprevention, as there is reason to expect that the probability of noteworthy toxicity is low.

The pathway to drug testing and adoption is not as well defined for chemoprevention as for chemotherapy. The latter begins with in vitro, then in vivo preclinical models, followed by phase I, II, and III clinical trials. A particularly vexing question for potential chemoprevention agents is assessing the importance of observational epidemiology data—in deciding how the evidence from epidemiologic studies fits with evidence from in vitro and in vivo studies, as well as from phase I and II clinical trials.

The definitive evaluation of a chemoprevention agent is the controlled clinical trial in which a given cancer is focal and named as the object to be prevented. A critical element of this evaluation is toxicity; toxicity must be extremely low and extremely uncommon. The number of chemoprevention trials to date is relatively small, in part, because interest in chemoprevention is relatively new. In addition, chemoprevention trials in which a single set of cancers is focal have to be extremely large to be adequately powered. Often, such trials have to include several thousand subjects. This chapter will focus on chemoprevention trials targeted toward the four major cancers: breast, colon, lung, and prostate.

9.2 Breast Cancer

9.2.1 Dietary Change

The geographic distribution of breast cancer, with greater risk in the western industrialized countries, has given rise to the suspicion that the western diet, possibly dietary fat, is responsible for this excess of risk. Ecologic data suggest that countries in which a high-fat, western diet is prevalent experience increased breast cancer risk (World Cancer Research Fund/American Institute for Cancer Research 2007). However, the findings of individual-based dietary epidemiologic studies of breast cancer, whether focused on dietary fat or on other components of the diet, have been disturbingly inconsistent. Some epidemiologic studies show diet, especially dietary fat, to be associated with breast cancer risk, but other studies show no such association (World Cancer Research Fund/American Institute for Cancer Research 2007). Because of suspicion that limitations of the epidemiologic study design and method might be obscuring associations, several large experimental interventions have been launched. In these, subjects in one group have been assigned to a diet change program, while those in another group have been assigned to receive advice, but no assistance in diet change.

In the Women's Health Initiative, experimental women whose diet was assessed to be relatively high in fat were randomized to a diet modification program designed to decrease their fat intake and increase their fruit and vegetable intake, or to a comparison group. After an average follow-up of over 8 years, the breast cancer incidence of subjects in this group was essentially equal to that of the control subjects (Prentice et al. 2006). A smaller study, the Women's Intervention Nutrition Study (WINS), focused on dietary fat reduction, was carried out among 2,437 women who had undergone treatment for early stage breast cancer. The participants were randomly assigned to a diet intervention or to a comparison group. An interim report indicated that intervention subjects reported greater decreases in fat intake and weight loss, and decreased breast cancer recurrence or new primary tumor risk, compared to subjects assigned to the control condition (Chlebowski et al. 2006). The final report has yet to be released. The Women's Healthy Eating and Living Study (WHEL) followed a similar, randomized design, with experimental subjects encouraged by an intensive intervention program to substantially increase their intake of fruits and vegetables. As in the WINS, the participants were breast cancer patients, enrolled after the completion of definitive therapy, and the outcome was a recurrent or new primary breast cancer; unlike the WINS, WHEL did not focus on fat intake. WHEL experimental subjects significantly increased their intake of vegetables, fruits, and fiber, and they decreased their fat intake, while comparison subjects did not change their dietary practices. The experimental subject changes in fruit and vegetable intake were confirmed by changes in blood carotenoids. Nonetheless, after a follow-up period of over 7 years, the risks of recurrent or second primary breast cancers among intervention and comparison subjects were virtually the same (Pierce et al. 2007).

9.2.2 Calcium Plus Vitamin D

One component of the Women's Health Initiative was a test of calcium 1,000 mg per day plus vitamin D 400 IU per day (Chlebowski et al. 2008). Over 36,000 women were enrolled in this trial, and they were followed for some 7 years. Breast cancer was a secondary endpoint of this component of the trial. Invasive breast cancer was approximately equal in the experimental and the control arms of the trial.

9.2.3 Selective Estrogen Response Modifiers

Tamoxifen and raloxifene are selective estrogen response modifiers with an impressive safety profile that makes them likely candidates for the chemoprevention of breast cancer (Fisher et al. 2005). Although the trial of tamoxifen for prevention of breast cancer showed a substantial decrease in the rate of breast cancer—approximately 3.6 cases per thousand among women assigned to tamoxifen against 6.3 per thousand among women assigned to placebo—the trial illustrates the complexity of evaluating the impact of a chemoprevention drug. Tamoxifen substantially decreased the risk of estrogen receptor-positive breast cancers, but it increased the rate of estrogen receptor-negative breast cancers (Fisher et al. 2005). Although tamoxifen decreased the risk of hip fracture, it more than tripled the risk of endometrial cancer. It also increased the risk of several forms of cardiac and vascular disease mortality: heart disease other than of the arteries and ischemic heart disease, lung disease other than lung cancer, and a large number of deaths assigned to unknown causes. Thus, the overall mortality rate for participants assigned to tamoxifen was essentially the same as that of participants assigned to placebo (Fisher et al. 2005). A second trial comparing raloxifene to tamoxifen showed that raloxifene was about 50 % less effective in decreasing the risk of breast cancer, but it also induced less risk of endometrial cancer. The numbers of hip fractures in the two groups were similar. The subjects assigned to raloxifene experienced approximately the same overall mortality rate as those assigned to tamoxifen (Vogel et al. 2006).

9.3 Colon Cancer

The ecologic data suggesting that the diet prevailing in much of the western industrial world might encourage colon carcinogenesis has given rise to a number of hypotheses: that the consumption of fat or of animal products might increase risk, or that dietary fiber or consumption of fruits, vegetables, or grain products could decrease risk. Nonetheless, the epidemiologic evidence has proven disappointingly inconsistent. Thus, trials may show the best means of testing the most likely hypotheses.

The identification of a sequence in which the adenomatous polyp is transformed over time to become increasingly dysplastic and eventually develop into colon cancer (Lev 1990) has led to a plethora of interventions focused on individuals with adenomatous polyps. The outcome of these studies in general is polyp recurrence or new polyp development. As adenomatous polyps are much more common than colon cancers, and as they take much less time than colon cancer to develop, studies designed to prevent polyp recurrence or occurrence can be more efficiently executed than studies targeted to colon cancer (Schatzkin et al. 1990). Thus, the number of chemoprevention trials directed at colon cancer, but with the adenomatous polyp as the biomarker of colon cancer risk, is larger than that directed at any other cancer.

9.3.1 Diet Change

One of the earlier experimental efforts involving diet change was carried out among some 2,000 adenoma patients (Schatzkin et al. 2000). The patients were randomized to an intensive, in-person dietary intervention, directed by a trained nutritionist, or to a comparison nonintervention group. The goal of the intervention was for experimental subjects to increase their fruit and vegetable intake to 5 servings per day, decrease their dietary fat intake to 20 % of calories, and increase their fiber intake to 30 g per day. Although subjects did not in general succeed in achieving those goals, they did make substantial, statistically significant changes in their dietary practice. Comparison subject diets changed, but by miniscule amounts; the changes in experimental subject diets were far greater, by a statistically significant degree, than those of the comparison subjects. Nonetheless, these changes had no bearing on the probability of polyp recurrence: polyp recurrence was essentially the same among experimental and comparison subjects (Schatzkin et al. 2000).

9.3.2 Antioxidants

The evidence that oxidative stress is critical to the genesis of cancer led to one of the earliest dietary interventions focused on adenomatous polyps: a trial of vitamin C, beta-carotene, and vitamin E (Greenberg et al. 1994). It was hypothesized that these agents were at least partly responsible for any protection against colon cancer afforded by fruit and vegetable intake. Subjects were confirmed by pathology to have had colonoscopically ablated adenomatous polyps. Agent compliance among the 864 subjects, confirmed by plasma biomarkers, was high. Nonetheless, none of these agents had any impact in decreasing the risk of adenomatous polyp recurrence. In a much larger study of the effects of a regimen involving two antioxidants—beta-carotene and alpha-tocopherol were studied among 29,000 male cigarette smokers and colorectal cancer was a secondary endpoint. Beta-carotene was associated with no alteration of risk, but alpha-tocopherol was associated with a slight, statistically nonsignificant decrease in colorectal cancer (Albanes et al. 2000). The evidence to date, then, suggests that antioxidants do not impart appreciable chemopreventive effects on adenomatous polyps.

9.3.3 Aspirin

Epidemiologic evidence indicating that long-term use of aspirin is associated with decreased risk of colon cancer mortality (Thun et al. 1992) led to two important trials of aspirin use. The trials of Baron et al. (2003) and Sandler et al. (2003) were focused on adenoma occurrence. Baron et al. (2003) followed 1,121 adenoma patients randomized to placebo, 81 mg or 325 mg of aspirin daily. Patients, scheduled to be followed for 3 years, were examined colonoscopically at least 1 year after randomization. The surprising result of this trial is that 81 mg/day decreased adenoma incidence by 20 %, but that 325 mg/day had no effect. Sandler et al. (2003) conducted a trial among colorectal cancer patients after curative surgical treatment. Patients were randomized to receive either 325 mg of aspirin or placebo daily. Aspirin decreased the incidence of new adenomas by approximately 35 %. Thus, although Sandler et al. (2003) found that 325 mg aspirin decreased risk by over a third, Baron et al. (2003) found that aspirin at that dose does not alter the risk of adenoma but found that aspirin at 81 mg/day is protective. Nonetheless, a meta-analysis of randomized, double-blind, placebo-controlled trials indicates that aspirin decreases the risk of adenoma in general by approximately 17 % and advanced adenoma by almost 30 % among people who have already been shown to have at least one adenomatous polyp (Cole et al. 2009).

9.3.4 Cyclooxygenase II Inhibitors

Concern over gastric erosion and bleeding disorders induced by aspirin led to the search for other nonsteroidal anti-inflammatory drugs that might have anticarcinogenic effects similar to those of aspirin (Bertagnolli et al. 2006). A class of agents, cyclooxygenase II inhibitors that act to reduce inflammation, were also suspected to have anticarcinogenic effects. In one of the largest of these trials, patients previously treated for adenomatous polyps were randomized to placebo, celecoxib 200 mg or celecoxib 400 mg, both of these doses twice per day. Celecoxib 200 mg decreased total and advanced adenoma incidence by 33 % and 57 %, respectively, while 400 mg decreased total and advanced adenoma incidence by 45 % and 66 %, respectively. Unfortunately, the incidence of adjudicated, prespecified serious cardiovascular events was increased 2.6 and 3.4 times among those assigned to 200 and 400 mg celecoxib, respectively. In addition, the incidence of nonadjudicated, investigator-reported cardiovascular disorders was increased 1.5 and 1.8 times among those assigned to 200 and 400 mg celecoxib, respectively. Bertagnolli et al. (2006) concluded that, although celecoxib is clearly effective for prevention of colorectal adenomas, it increases the risk of cardiovascular disease enough to render it unsuitable for general use.

9.3.5 Folate

Folate intake is associated with decreased colon cancer risk and decreased risk of colorectal cancer (Giovannucci et al. 1998). Alcohol consumption, which lowers plasma folate, is associated with increased colorectal cancer risk (Baron et al. 1998). This evidence led Cole et al. (2007) to test whether adenoma patients randomized to folic acid 1 mg/day or placebo experienced decreased adenoma risk. The trial protocol called for patients to be followed for 3 years; a second follow-up, 3–5 years after the protocol period, was added to the protocol. The trial provided no evidence that folic acid supplementation decreased the risk of adenoma formation. Indeed, the relative risks of adenoma during the first and second follow-up periods, respectively, were 1.04 and 1.13; neither of these is statistically significant. The relative risks of advanced lesions during the first and second follow-up periods, respectively, were 1.32 and 1.67; the latter relative risk is statistically significant. The relative risk of multiple adenomas during the second follow-up period was a statistically significant 2.32. Cole et al. (2007) pointed out that the subjects of this study were folate replete at the beginning of the study. Thus, folic acid supplementation of folate-replete subjects is not likely to protect against colorectal adenoma (Cole et al. 2007). It has been generally assumed that folic acid in supplements has the same effects as folate from foods. Whether folate supplementation other than by folic acid might be possible and impart protective effects is not entirely clear.

9.3.6 Calcium

In light of epidemiologic evidence that diet may affect bile acids, which may be carcinogenic to the large bowel, and basic scientific evidence that calcium may bind bile acids and thus reduce their carcinogenic effects, Alberts et al. (1997) conducted a randomized, placebo-controlled phase II trial among 93 adenomatous polyp patients. This study also evaluated the importance of dietary fiber and calcium supplementation 1,500 mg/day on rectal mucosal proliferation; the study revealed no change in rectal mucosal cellular proliferation. In a phase III trial, Baron et al. (1999) randomized 930 adenoma patients to placebo or to 3 g/day of calcium carbonate. Adenoma risk was reduced approximately 15 % by calcium supplementation. In addition, the number of adenomas among those assigned to calcium supplementation was reduced by approximately 24 %. It is not yet clear how calcium might actually work in humans to decrease colon cancer risk. Although calcium supplementation in this randomized trial significantly reduced the risk of adenoma formation, the effect of such supplementation is only modest. The best use of calcium may be in conjunction with other protective agents.

9.3.7 Dietary Fiber

There is indirect epidemiologic evidence that dietary fiber is protective against colorectal cancer. International ecological studies have played a prominent role, showing that populations with substantial dietary fiber intake have much lower colorectal cancer incidence and mortality than populations with less intake (Burkitt 1971; Wynder et al. 1967; Wynder and Reddy 1973). It is difficult, however, to distinguish the importance of fiber from that of protein, fat, or any of myriad other compounds found in the diet. Experimentalists have attempted to identify the specific importance of dietary fiber (McKeown-Eyssen et al. 1988). Evaluating the possibility that dietary fiber might lessen cellular proliferation and thus decrease the likelihood of genetic mutations that might contribute to carcinogenesis, Alberts et al. (1997) randomized 93 adenoma patients, in the already-mentioned factorial phase II trial of calcium supplementation, to either 2 or 13.5 g per day of wheat bran fiber. The disappointing result of this trial was that the fiber supplement had no impact on what was at the time regarded as the signal indicator of carcinogenesis: cellular proliferation within the rectal crypts. In a larger, phase III trial, Alberts et al. (2000) randomized 1,429 adenoma patients to 3 years of supplementation by either 2 or 13.5 g per day of wheat bran fiber. Study assignment was double blinded. The study was plagued by a high dropout rate among patients assigned to the high-fiber supplement. A number of participants found a supplement of even 13.5 g of fiber to be quite unpleasant so that the randomization scheme had to be changed to increase the number of patients completing the study on the high-fiber supplement. Assignment to the wheat bran fiber supplement made no difference to the incidence of new polyps; the probabilities of new polyp formation were essentially equal in the high- and low-fiber supplement groups. The probabilities of multiple polyps and of polyps in more than one region of the colorectum were greater in the group assigned to the high-fiber supplement. Noteworthy gastrointestinal effects, including nausea, abdominal pain, diarrhea, intestinal gas, and bloating, were also more frequent among those assigned to the high-fiber supplement. Thus, it has proven difficult to confirm by epidemiology or by clinical trials the intriguing data emerging from international ecologic studies.

9.3.8 Ursodeoxycholic Acid

A common bile acid found in the large bowel, deoxycholic acid, is highly carcinogenic, but one of the less common bile acids, ursodeoxycholic acid (UDCA), may counter the impact of deoxycholic acid (Alberts et al. 2005). There is ample preclinical evidence, including in vitro and in vivo studies, that UDCA suppresses signaling pathways associated with deoxycholic acid. UDCA is attractive as a chemopreventive agent, as it is already in wide use as a safe treatment for gall stones (Alberts et al. 2005). Alberts et al. (2005) randomized 1,285 adenomatous polyp patients to 3 years of treatment with UDCA or placebo. The impact of UDCA on overall polyp incidence was not statistically significant. Although UDCA induced a 39 % decrease in polyps with high-grade dysplasia, it had no effect on a broader category of advanced or aggressive adenomas; this category included adenomas with diameter 10 mm or more, those with high-grade dysplasia and with villous or tubulovillous histology or carcinoma.

9.3.9 Vitamin D

Although there is strong evidence that vitamin D protects against carcinogenesis (Trump et al. 2010) and although a great deal of epidemiologic research has considered vitamin D, that research has provided only limited evidence that dietary vitamin D protects against cancer (Giovannucci 2005). However, vitamin D in people comes not just from diet but also from supplements and from sunlight exposure. The effects of sunlight can be affected by regional ultraviolet B radiation and by skin tone, and the effects of both sunlight and intake from food and supplements can be conditioned by body mass index. A study of vitamin D status focused only on diet could well fail to account for major sources of vitamin D exposure variance. The strongest attempt to account for all these sources, reported by Giovannucci et al. (2006), was based on the experience of a cohort of 47,800 health professionals. Giovannucci et al. (2006) estimated, using sunlight exposure, regional ultraviolet B radiation, skin tone, body mass index, and vitamin D from foods and supplements, the blood level of each subject. He found that those with elevated levels of estimated vitamin D, compared to those with the lowest levels, had substantially decreased colorectal cancer incidence and mortality. Giovannucci et al. (2006) estimated that supplementation with at least 1,500 IU per day would be necessary to achieve the levels of vitamin D associated with substantially decreased cancer risk.

One of the components of the Women's Health Initiative was a placebo-controlled trial of calcium 1,000 mg per day and vitamin D 400 IU per day among 36,000 postmenopausal women (Wactawski-Wende et al. 2006). The study provided no evidence that vitamin D at a dose of 400 IU per day decreases colorectal cancer incidence. Nor did the grade of the diagnosed cancers differ among the subjects receiving placebo and those receiving vitamin D. A possible reason for this null result is that the dose of vitamin D might have been too low or that a 7-year follow-up period might not have been long enough to reveal true effects (Wactawski-Wende et al. 2006). The analysis by Giovannucci et al. (2006) suggests that a supplement of 400 IU per day would not be nearly enough to induce decreased cancer risk.

9.3.10 DFMO/Sulindac

A major disappointment of research into nonsteroidal anti-inflammatory drugs has been that, although celecoxib is associated with a substantial decrease in the risk of colorectal adenoma recurrence, it also induced unacceptable coronary toxicity. Meyskens et al. (2008) used a combination of difluoromethylornithine (DFMO) 500 mg per day and a commonly used nonsteroidal anti-inflammatory drug—sulindac—150 mg per day, as these two agents interact in vivo to lessen the growth and viability of colon cancer cells. In this relatively small clinical trial, the combination of DFMO and sulindac decreased adenoma formation by

70 %; the combination also decreased the formation of advanced adenomas by over 90 %. Although some excess of serious adverse events, including cardiovascular toxicity, was observed in the group assigned to DFMO and sulindac, this excess was not statistically significant. In a follow-up analysis, Zell et al. (2009) showed that the excess cardiovascular toxicity was confined to individuals with elevated baseline cardiac risk.

9.3.11 Statins

The data suggesting that colorectal cancer is more common in the affluent, industrialized western countries has led to the search for agents that might counter some of the effects of over nutrition in these countries: drugs, for example, that are targeted at hypercholesterolemia or insulinemia. One class of drug frequently used to address hypercholesterolemia is the statins. An observational study which considered the association of statin use with colorectal cancer risk, however, found little evidence that statins are associated with decreased risk (Lee et al. 2011).

9.4 Lung Cancer

9.4.1 Beta-carotene

One of the earliest chemoprevention leads to come from epidemiology involved vitamin A and its precursor, beta-carotene. Mettlin et al. (1979), analyzing data from a case–control study carried out at Roswell Park Cancer Institute, showed that, even with statistical adjustment for the effects of smoking, those with greater vitamin A intake were at decreased lung cancer risk. Subsequent analysis of these data showed that the most important component of vitamin A intake was probably that which originated in plant products: beta-carotene. A spate of additional epidemiologic inquiries, largely confirming these observations followed; the negative association of beta-carotene intake with cancer risk appeared particularly strong for lung cancer. These studies led to a number of large chemoprevention trials. In a trial conducted among 22,071 physicians in the USA, randomized to beta-carotene or to placebo, no effect of beta-carotene was observed (Hennekens et al. 1996). In a trial conducted in Finland among 29,000 smokers randomized to beta-carotene or to placebo, those randomized to beta-carotene experienced an 18 % increase in lung cancer incidence (Albanes et al. 1995). Closely following these results, a trial of beta-carotene and retinol (CARET) showed that high-risk lung cancer subjects randomized to beta-carotene and retinol experienced a 36 % increase in lung cancer incidence (Omenn et al. 1996). This study was conducted among 18,000 individuals with a history of either smoking or of exposure to asbestos; subjects were randomized to both beta-carotene 30 mg per day and 25,000 IU per day or retinyl palmitate or to placebo. The intent of the addition of retinol to beta-carotene was that, as beta-carotene is metabolized to retinol, the presence of retinol might slow this metabolism and cause a beta-carotene effect to persist longer.

9.4.2 Retinoic Acid

In an Intergroup trial, 1,166 patients treated for stage 1 non-small cell lung cancer were randomized to the retinoid isotretinoin at 30 mg per day or to placebo for 3 years. Overall, no benefit was observable for the treatment with regard to second primary tumors (SPT), or recurrence of lung cancer or mortality. Subgroup analysis showed that isotretinoin increased the risk of recurrence in current smokers but was protective in never smokers.(Lippman et al. 2001).

9.4.3 Selenium

A trial of selenium supplementation, conducted among 1,200 men and women with nonmelanoma skin cancer (NMSC), was originally designed to evaluate the prevention of NMSC recurrence by a 200 mcg per day dose of selenium supplementation as selenized yeast. Several secondary cancer endpoints including lung cancer were added during the course of the trial. The original results showed a 40 % decrease in lung cancer risk (Clark et al. 1996), based on a 10-year follow-up period. Subsequent results based on the entire period of supplementation (1983–1996) showed an attenuation of this association (Reid et al. 2002). Responding to the original results from the trial, Karp et al. (2010) led a cooperative group trial of early stage lung cancer patients randomized to placebo or to 200 mcg per day of selenium. The trial was terminated early after an interim analysis indicated that benefit from supplementation was extremely unlikely.

9.4.4 Other Agents

Several phase II trials of lung cancer chemopreventive agents have been completed. In a randomized trial of the synthetic retinoid etretinate in moderate risk smokers, sputum atypia was the primary endpoint (Arnold et al. 1992). There was no significant impact on sputum atypia from the intervention. In a study of N-(4-hydroxyphenyl) retinamide (4 HPR) among high-risk individuals, with reversal of squamous metaplasia as the endpoint, 4-HPR produced no histologic, genetic, or phenotypic changes in bronchial tissue (Kurie et al. 2000). In a study of cis retinoic acid vs. 13 cis retinoic acid plus vitamin E, the endpoint was changed in the expression of retinoic acid receptor beta (RAR beta). Upregulation of RAR beta with 9 cis retinoic acid was shown (Kurie et al. 2003). An evolution of retinyl palmitate, with lung cancer recurrence as the endpoint, showed that the treatment group had a longer disease-free interval than the placebo group (Pastorino et al. 1993). Lam et al. (2002) evaluated anethole dithiolethione among patients with dysplasia; the treatment decreased the formation of new lesions in smokers. Former smokers treated with Iloprost experienced positive results (Keith et al. 2011). In a phase IIb trial lasting 6 months, 112 smokers with bronchial dysplasia were randomized to a placebo or budesonide as an inhaler (800 mcg twice a day). Budesonide had no effect on dysplastic lesions, but a higher rate of resolution of CT-detected lung nodules was found (Lam et al. 2004). In phase I trials presently under way at Roswell Park Cancer Institute, lung cancer patients after definitive treatment are being evaluated by bronchoscopy, then reevaluated by bronchoscopy after 3–6 months. Biopsies are taken during each bronchoscopy. In one study, calcitriol (1,25 dihydroxy vitamin D3) at an oral dose of 45 mcg, once every other week, is being tested. The outcome of the study includes toxicity, change in the expression of vitamin D receptor in the bronchial tissue, cellular proliferation, and the expression of several genes linked to the vitamin D receptor. In another similarly designed study, erlotinib, an epidermal growth factor receptor (EGFR) antagonist, is being evaluated at doses of 25, 50, 75, and 100 mg per day. Subjects are placed on the dose for 3 months, with pharmacokinetics and pharmacodynamics evaluated at baseline. The primary endpoint is change in the ratio of activated EGFR to total EGFR expression in the bronchial tissue. Other endpoints include toxicity from the treatment and changes in markers of proliferation and apoptosis.

As the search for agents that might prevent lung cancer continues, it is important to remember that antismoking medications are potential chemopreventive agents. As there is excellent evidence that continued smoking continues to increase lung cancer risk, and that cessation decreases it, an agent that helps people to discontinue smoking is likely to prove beneficial.

9.5 Prostate Cancer

9.5.1 Leads from Epidemiology

Although prostate cancer mortality is higher in the industrialized western world than in the emerging nations, it has been difficult to identify the source of this disparity. It is clear that the residents of the more affluent industrialized countries—especially North America and Western Europe—are more affluent and abundantly nourished than are those in the rest of the world; energy intake appears to be greater and obesity much greater. Prostate cancer incidence and mortality are identified much more frequently in these countries than in the rest of the world. However, the extent to which the excesses are functions of actual incidence and mortality—as opposed to screening and diagnostic practices— is not entirely known. It has been known for some time that the prevalence of a probably indolent form of prostate cancer uncovered only in postmortem examinations is appreciable even in the developing world (Breslow et al. 1977). Variance in the prevalence of prostate cancer identified only as incidental at postmortem examination is much less than variance in the prevalence of the aggressive disease that comes to clinical attention. Evidence emerging from a large clinical trial in which the protocol called for subjects to be biopsied indicated that the prevalence of undiagnosed, asymptomatic, and apparently largely indolent prostate cancer among men who were understood to be at relatively low risk at study initiation was approximately 24 % (Thompson et al. 2003). Even among those at lowest risk—those whose prostate-specific antigen never exceeded 4 ng/ml and who had neither a suspicious digital rectal examination nor symptoms during the 7-year duration of the trial—the prevalence of undiagnosed prostate cancer was 15 % (Thompson et al. 2004).

It has been hypothesized that a major biomarker of excess food intake, elevated body mass index (BMI), or obesity is related to the excess cancer risk observed in high-risk countries. However, careful studies have led to doubts about this hypothesis. It is possible that obesity is linked to only the more aggressive forms of prostate cancer; it may be negatively related to the risk of more indolent forms. As noted, a large observational study of a major anticholesterol agent showed that statin has no noteworthy association with diminished colon cancer risk (Lee et al. 2011). Nonetheless, early phase prostate cancer investigations are underway, as statins and drugs used to treat insulinemia are considered.

9.5.2 *Vitamin E*

Investigators have long suspected that vitamin E as an antioxidant could have a number of health benefits. However, an unexpected outcome of a 2×2 factorial Finnish trial in which vitamin E 50 mg per day was tested as preventive against coronary heart disease and beta-carotene 20 mg per day was tested as preventive against lung cancer was that the diagnosis of prostate cancer was decreased by 40 % in the group assigned to vitamin E (The Alpha-Tocopherol, Beta Carotene Cancer Prevention Study Group 1994). This decrease in risk was statistically significant, and it helped lead to a massive 2×2 factorial trial: the Selenium and E Chemoprevention Trial (SELECT), in which over 35,000 North American men were randomized to vitamin E 400 mg per day and selenium 200 mcg per day (Lippman et al. 2009). One fourth of the subjects received vitamin E and a selenium placebo, one fourth received selenium and a vitamin E placebo, one fourth received both vitamin E and selenium, and one fourth received a double placebo. The disappointing result of this trial was that vitamin E resulted in no decrease in prostate cancer. Extended analysis of the group assigned to vitamin E showed that the slight, statistically nonsignificant excess of prostate cancer observed at the end of the prespecified study period became, after all data had been collected, statistically significant (Klein et al. 2011).

9.5.3 Lycopene

As one of the most powerful antioxidants among the carotenoids, lycopene has received a good deal of attention within epidemiologic research circles. Giovannucci and Clinton (1998) observed in a cohort of health professionals that the intake of tomato products was associated with decreased risk of prostate cancer and especially of aggressive prostate cancer. Both of these associations were statistically significant. The associations were in general stronger for cooked than for raw tomato products. A lycopene index, comprised of foods with lycopene content, was also associated with decreased prostate cancer risk. Gann et al. (1999) also observed in a cohort of physicians that blood lycopene levels were associated with decreased risk of prostate cancer; the association was statistically significant. Again, the associations were stronger for aggressive than for more indolent, screening-derived prostate cancer. Earlier-phase trials in which lycopene is administered have also suggested that it may hinder the development of prostate cancer (Bowen et al. 1993; Küçük et al. 1994). To date, phase III trials of lycopene to block the development or progress of prostate cancer have yet to be started.

9.5.4 Selenium

As a key to human antioxidant defenses, selenium has received a good deal of attention as protective against cancer and a number of other chronic diseases (Combs 2001). In a 1,200-man trial of selenium supplementation to prevent recurrence of nonmelanoma skin cancer in which prostate cancer was a secondary endpoint, selenium supplementation was associated with a 50 % decrease in the diagnosis of prostate cancer (Clark et al. 1996). This trial was largely responsible for a number of follow-up clinical trials. The largest of these, SELECT, considered the impact of 200 mcg per day selenium supplementation. The disappointing result of this trial, which enrolled over 35,000 average-risk men, was that selenium had absolutely no effect on the risk of prostate cancer diagnosis (Lippman et al. 2009). In a much smaller study, selenium was administered to 460 men understood to be at elevated risk of prostate cancer; all had been diagnosed with high-grade prostatic intraepithelial neoplasia (HGPIN) (Marshall et al. 2011). The results of this trial paralleled those of SELECT; selenium had no effect on the progression of HGPIN to prostate cancer. In a similar study, selenium was one of three agents in a prevention "cocktail" administered to men with HGPIN; those assigned to this cocktail had essentially the same risk of prostate cancer diagnosis as those assigned to the placebo (Fleshner et al. 2011).

9.5.5 5-Alpha-Reductase Inhibitors

Interest in androgen signaling led to the development of testosterone blockade for the treatment of prostate cancer (Huggins and Hodges 1941). A linked approach involved drugs that block the enzyme, 5-alpha-reductase, that catalyzes the conversion of the major male hormone, testosterone, to its more active form of dihydrotestosterone. The first of these agents, finasteride, blocks the most common form of 5-alpha-reductase. A large trial, conducted among 18,882 men understood to be at low risk of prostate cancer, with all participants expected to undergo biopsy at the end of the trial, showed that finasteride decreased the period prevalence of prostate cancer by 25 % (Thompson et al. 2003). Finasteride also decreased the risk of what is believed to be the most significant premalignant lesion leading to prostate cancer: high-grade prostatic intraepithelial neoplasia (Thompson et al. 2007). A major drawback was that the identification of high-grade, more aggressive disease was increased among the subjects assigned to finasteride (Thompson et al. 2003). In total, 800 cancers were detected among finasteride patients, while over 1,150 were detected among placebo patients. The concern is that 280 of the cancers detected among the finasteride group and 240 of those detected among the placebo group were high grade: Gleason sum 7, 8, 9, or 10. Thompson and others have argued that this increased risk of high-grade disease is an artifact, caused by finasteride increasing the sensitivity of the prostate-specific antigen and the digital rectal examination in the presence of prostate cancer screening and diagnosis among men receiving finasteride (Cohen et al. 2007). A chemoprevention trial of dutasteride, which results in more complete 5-alpha-reductase inhibition and thus may be more effective in blocking the conversion of testosterone to dihydrotestosterone, showed similar results Andriole et al. (2010). The protocol called for all 6,729 participants to be biopsied prior to randomization, at 2 years and 4 years on trial. Relative risk was reduced by approximately 23 %. Whereas the finasteride trial revealed the excess of high-grade cancer to have appeared early in the trial and then to have decreased slightly, the dutasteride trial showed an excess of high-grade disease that increased over time (Andriole et al. 2010). Thus, although there is still active debate about the interpretation of these results, the apparent excess of high-grade disease has led prominent clinical groups to voice serious reservations about chemoprevention based on the use of finasteride and dutasteride (Kramer et al. 2009).

9.5.6 Folate

Although the role in supporting DNA repair makes folate seem a likely candidate to protect against most cancers, including prostate cancer, the human-based evidence is limited. Epidemiology has not shown folate to be protective, and a systematic review and meta-analysis indicates that it is probably associated with increased prostate cancer risk (Collin et al. 2010). In the only folate experiment conducted among average-risk, folate-replete subjects (Baron et al. 1998), folate supplementation by 1 mg per day was associated with a 2.7-fold increase in prostate cancer diagnoses (Figueiredo et al. 2009). Whether this resulted from increased detection of prostate cancer, from an increase in the formation of cancers from premalignant lesions, or from accelerated progression of early cancers is not yet known.

9.5.7 Dietary Change

As interest in diet as a risk factor for prostate cancer persists, so has interest in a means of firmly identifying diet's importance. Whether epidemiology is likely to provide definitive evidence is not entirely clear so that it may be necessary to confirm the role of diet experimentally. Limitations of experimentation with diet include first the difficulty of inducing people to change their diets. In addition, it is not readily possible to blind people to their treatment group, and being part of a treatment group—or a comparison group—could have other effects on behavior. Being part of an experimental as opposed to a control or comparison group could affect taking vitamins or other supplements, physical activity, or screening. These changes would not be addressed by randomization.

The follow-up of the Polyp Prevention Trial (Schatzkin et al. 2000; Shike et al. 2002) focused on prostate cancers identified among participants after 4 years of follow-up. As already noted, this trial effected substantial change in dietary behavior of intervention subjects, including their fat, fiber, and fruit and vegetable intake. It resulted, however, in no change in the course of the mean prostate-specific antigen or in the likelihood of prostate cancer identification.

In a more recent, presently ongoing investigation (Newman et al. 2006; Parsons et al. 2008a, b), a randomized trial of intensive dietary intervention among men with very early and probably indolent prostate cancer has been undertaken. As the prevalence of what appears to be an indolent form of prostate cancer is high relative to that of more aggressive or lethal forms, it has been hypothesized that interventions to retard the progress of this form would be likely to block its initial formation as well. The strategy of Parsons et al. (2008a, b) is to recruit prostate cancer patients who have chosen to manage their early stage, probably indolent cancer by monitoring it carefully and by reserving radical medical intervention until the cancer shows evidence of progression to a more invasive and metastatic phenotype. The study seeks to induce experimental subjects to adopt a diet in which they consume nine or more servings of vegetables and fruits per day. Vegetables that are emphasized include tomatoes and such cruciferous vegetables as broccoli, cabbage, and cauliflower. The diet also encourages reliance upon whole grains. To date, some 100 patients have been recruited, toward an accrual goal of 460: 230 randomized to the dietary intervention, 230 randomized to receive a copy of the US Department of Agriculture dietary guidelines. The study should be completed around 2016.

9.6 Conclusion

Sporn's (1980) vision of chemoprevention as a widely adopted strategy for cancer control continues to hold the attention of many cancer researchers. The attractiveness of chemoprevention is that it might forestall the unpleasantness of becoming a cancer patient and of dealing with the consequences of therapy. However, the identification of a single agent that could be administered to entire populations to decrease their vulnerability to all cancer remains little more than a dream. Epidemiology, and the search for dietary constituents that decrease risk, has been less effective than was hoped 3 decades ago.

What appears more likely to prove fruitful is the discovery of agents that halt or delay the progress of premalignant lesions or other high-risk conditions to frank cancer. There is clearly a premalignant lesion, the adenomatous polyp, that leads to colon cancer; there is believed to be a premalignant lesion that leads to prostate cancer. The evidence is less strong for premalignant lesions of the lung and breast. In any case, we have yet to identify agents that consistently block the progress of any premalignant lesions or states to cancer. Another possibility is that we will be able to extract chemoprevention leads from chemotherapeutic trials. The allure of chemoprevention remains; the findings to date remain modest. We have a good deal of work to do.

References

Albanes D, Heinonen OP, Huttunen JK, Taylor PR, Virtamo J, Edwards BK et al. Effect of alpha-tocopherol and beta-carotene supplements on cancer incidence in the alpha-tocopherol beta-carotene cancer prevention study. *Am J Clin Nutr* 1995; 62:1427S–1430S.

Albanes D, Malila N, Taylor PR, Huttunen JK, Virtamo J, Edwards BK et al. Effects of supplemental a-tocopherol and B-carotene on colorectal cancer: Results from a controlled trial (Finland). *Cancer Causes Control* 2000; 11:197–205.

Alberts DS, Martinez ME, Hess LM, Einspahr JG, Green SB, Bhattacharyya AK et al. Phase III trial of ursodeoxycholic acid to prevent colorectal adenoma recurrence. *J Natl Cancer Inst* 2005; 97:846–853.

Alberts DS, Einspahr J, Ritenbaugh C, Aickin M, Rees-McGee S, Atwood J et al. The effect of wheat bran fiber and calcium supplementation on rectal mucosal proliferation rates in patients with resected adenomatous colorectal polyps. *Cancer Epidemiology Biomarkers & Prevention* 1997; 6:161–169.

Alberts DS, Martinez ME, Roe DJ, Guillén-Rodríguez JM, Marshall JR, van Leeuwen B et al. Lack of effect of a high-fiber cereal supplement on the recurrence of colorectal adenomas. *N Engl J Med* 2000; 342:1156–1162.

Andriole GL, Bostwick DG, Brawley OW, Gomella LG, Marberger M, Montorsi F et al. Effect of dutasteride on the risk of prostate cancer. *New Eng J Med* 2010; 362:1192–1202.

Arnold AM, Browman GP, Levine MN, D'Souza T, Johnstone B, Skingley P et al. The effect of the synthetic retinoid etretinate on sputum cytology: Results from a randomised trial. *Br J Cancer* 1992; 65:737–743.

Baron JA, Sandler RS, Haile RW, Mandel JS, Mott LA, Greenberg ER. Folate intake, alcohol consumption, cigarette smoking, and risk of colorectal adenomas 371. *J Natl Cancer Inst* 1998; 90:57–62.

Baron JA, Beach M, Mandel JS, van Stolk RU, Haile RW, Sandler RS et al. Calcium supplements for the prevention of colorectal adenomas. *N Engl J Med* 1999; 340:101–107.

Baron JA, Cole BF, Sandler RS, Haile RW, Ahnen D, Bresalier R et al. A randomized trial of aspirin to prevent colorectal adenomas. *N Engl J Med* 2003; 348:891–899.

Bertagnolli MM, Eagle CJ, Zauber AG, Redston M, Solomon SD, Kim K et al. Celecoxib for the prevention of sporadic colorectal adenomas. *New Eng J Med* 2006; 355:873–884.

Bowen PE, Garg V, Stacewicz-Sapuntzakis M, Yelton L, Schreiner RS. Variability of serum carotenoids in response to controlled diets containing six servings of fruits and vegetables per day. *Ann N Y Acad Sci* 1993; 691:241–243.

Breslow N, Chan CW, Dhom G, Drury RAB, Franks LM, Gellei B et al. Latent carcinoma of praste at autopsy in seven areas collaborative study organized by the international agency for research on cancer, Lyons, France. *Int J Cancer* 1977; 20:680–688.

Burkitt DP. Epidemiology of cancer of the colon and rectum. *Cancer* 1971; 28:3–13.

Chlebowski RT, Blackburn GL, Thomson CA, Nixon DW, Shapiro A, Hoy MK et al. Dietary fat reduction and breast cancer outcome: Interim efficacy results from the women's intervention nutrition study. *J Natl Cancer Inst* 2006; 98:1767–1776.

Chlebowski RT, Johnson KC, Kooperberg C, Pettinger M, Wactawski-Wende J, Rohan T et al. Calcium plus vitamin D supplementation and the risk of breast cancer. *J Natl Cancer Inst* 2008; 100:1581–1591.

Clark LC, Combs GF, Turnbull BW, Slate EH, Chalker DK, Chow J et al. Effects of selenium supplementation for cancer prevention in patients with carcinoma of the skin: A randomized controlled trial. *JAMA* 1996; 276:1957–1963.

Cohen YC, Liu KS, Heyden NL, Carides AD, Anderson KM. Detection bias due to the effect of finasteride on prostate volume: A modeling approach for analysis of the prostate cancer prevention trial. *J Natl Cancer Inst* 2007; 99:1366–1374.

Cole BF, Baron JA, Sandler RS, Haile RW, Ahnen DJ, Bresalier RS et al. Folic acid for the prevention of colorectal adenomas a randomized clinical trial. *JAMA* 2007; 297:2351–2359.

Cole BF, Logan RF, Halabi S, Benamouzig B, Sandler RS, Grainge MJ et al. Aspirin for the chemoprevention of colorectal adenomas: Meta-analysis of the randomized trials. *J Natl Cancer Inst* 2009; 101:256–266.

Collin SM, Metcalfe C, Refsum H, Lewis SL, Zuccolo L, Davey Smith G et al. Circulating folate, vitamin B12, homocysteine, vitamin B12 transport proteins, and risk of prostate cancer: A case-control study, systematic review, and meta-analysis. *Cancer Epidemiology Biomarkers & Prevention* 2010; 19:1632–1642.

Combs GF. Impact of selenium and cancer-prevention findings on the nutrition-health paradigm. *Nutr Cancer* 2001; 40:6–11.

Figueiredo JC, Grau MV, Haile RW, Sandler RS, Summers RW, Bresalier RS et al. Folic acid and risk of prostate cancer: Results from a randomized clinical trial. *J Natl Cancer Inst* 2009; 101:432–435.

Fisher B, Costantino JP, Wickerham DL, Cecchini RS, Cronin WM, Robidoux A et al. Tamoxifen for the prevention of breast cancer: Current status of the national surgical adjuvant breast and bowel project p-1 study. *J Natl Cancer Inst* 2005; 97:1652–1662.

Fleshner NE, Kapusta L, Donnelly B, Tanguay S, Chin J, Hersey K et al. Progression from high-grade prostatic intraepithelial neoplasia to cancer: A randomized trial of combination vitamin-E, soy, and selenium. *Journal of Clinical Oncology* 2011; 29:2386–2390.

Gann PH, Ma J, Giovannucci E, Willett W, Sacks FM, Hennekens CH et al. Lower prostate cancer risk in men with elevated plasma lycopene levels: Results of a prospective analysis. *Cancer Res* 1999; 59:1225–1230.

Giovannucci E, Clinton SK. Tomatoes, lycopene, and prostate cancer. *Proceedings of the Society for Experimental Biology & Medicine* 1998; 218:129–139.

Giovannucci E, Stampfer MJ, Colditz GA, Hunter DJ, Fuchs C, Rosner BA et al. Multivitamin use, folate and colon cancer in women in the nurses' health study. *Ann Intern Med* 1998; 129:517–524.

Giovannucci E. The epidemiology of vitamin D and cancer incidence and mortality: A review (United States). *Cancer Causes Control* 2005; 16:83–95.

Giovannucci E, Liu Y, Rimm EB, Hollis BW, Fuchs CS, Stampfer MJ et al. Prospective study of predictors of vitamin D status and cancer incidence and mortality in men. *J Natl Cancer Inst* 2006; 98:451–459.

Greenberg ER, Baron JA, Tosteson TD, Freeman DH, Beck GJ, Bond JH et al. A clinical trial of antioxidant vitamins to prevent colorectal adenoma. *N Engl J Med* 1994; 331:141–147.

Hennekens CH, Buring JE, Manson JE, Stampfer M, Rosner B, Cook NR et al. Lack of effect of long-term supplementation with beta carotene on the incidence of malignant neoplasms and cardiovascular disease. *N Engl J Med* 1996; 334:1145–1149.

Huggins C, Hodges CV. Studies on prostatic cancer: I. the effect of castration, estrogen, and androgen injection on serum phosphatases in metastatic carcinoma of the prostate. *Cancer Res* 1941; 1:293–297.

Karp DD, Lee SJ, Wright GLS, Johnson DH, Johnston MR, Goodman GE et al. A phase III, intergroup, randomized, double-blind, chemoprevention trial of selenium (se) supplementation in resected stage I non-small cell lung cancer (NSCLC). *Journal of Clinical Oncology* 2010; 28(18s) *ASCO MEETING ABSTRACTS*:CRA7004.

Keith RL, Blatchford PJ, Kittelson J, Minna JD, Kelly K, Massion PP et al. Oral iloprost improves endobronchial dysplasia in former smokers. *Cancer Prevention Research* 2011; 4:793–802.

Klein EA, Thompson IM, Tangen CM, Crowley JJ, Lucia MS, Goodman PJ et al. Vitamin E and the risk of prostate cancer: The selenium and vitamin E cancer prevention trial (SELECT). *JAMA* 2011; 306:1549–1556.

Kramer BS, Hagerty KL, Justman S, Somerfield MR, Albertsen PC, Blot WJ et al. Use of 5a-reductase inhibitors for prostate cancer chemoprevention: American society of clinical oncology/American urological association 2008 clinical practice guideline. *Journal of Urology* 2009; 181:1642–1657.

Küçük Ö, Churley M, Goodman MT, Franke A, Custer L, Wilkens LR et al. Increased plasma level of cholesterol-5β,6β-epoxide in endometrial cancer patients. *Cancer Epidemiology Biomarkers and Prevention* 1994; 3:571–574.

Kurie JM, Lee JS, Khuri FR, Mao L, Morice RC, Lee JJ et al. N-(4 hydroxyphennyl)retinamide in the chemoprevention of squamous metaphasia and dysplasia of the bronchial epithelium. *Clinical Cancer Research* 2000; 6:2973–2979.

Kurie JM, Lotan R, Lee JJ, Lee JS, Morice, RC Liu DD et al. Treatment of former smokers with 9-cis-retinonic acid reverses loss of retinoic acid receptor-B expression in the bronchial epithelium: Results from a randomized placebo-controlled trial. *J Natl Cancer Inst* 2003; 95:206–214.

Lam S, MacAulay C, Le Riche JC, Dyachkova Y, Coldman A, Guillaud M et al. A randomized phase IIb trial of anethole dithiolethione in smokers with bronchial dysplasia. *J Natl Cancer Inst* 2002; 94:1001–1009.

Lam S, LeRiche JC, McWilliams A, MacAulay C, Dyachkova Y, Szabo E et al. A randomized phase IIb trial of pulmicort turbuhaler (budesonide) in people with dysplasia of the bronchial epithelium. *Clinical Cancer Research* 2004; 10:6502–6511.

Lee JE, Baba Y, Ng K, Giovannucci E, Fuchs CS, Ogino S et al. Statin use and colorectal cancer risk according to molecular subtypes in two large prospective cohort studies. *Cancer Prevention Research* 2011; 4:1808–1815.

Lev R. *Adenomatous polyps of the colon: Pathobiological and clinical features*. New York, NY: Springer-Verlag; 1990.

Lippman SM, Lee JJ, Karp DD, Vokes EE, Benner SE, Goodman GE et al. Randomized phase III intergroup trial of isotretinoin to prevent second primary tumors in stage I non-small-cell lung cancer. *J Natl Cancer Inst* 2001; 93:605–618.

Lippman SM, Klein EA, Goodman PJ, Lucia MS, Thompson IM, Ford LG et al. Effect of selenium and vitamin E on risk of prostate cancer and other cancers: The selenium and vitamin E cancer prevention trial (SELECT). *JAMA* 2009; 301:39–51.

Marshall JR, Tangen CM, Sakr WA, Wood DP, Berry DL, Klein EA et al. Phase III trial of selenium to prevent prostate cancer in men with high-grade prostatic intraepithelial neoplasia: SWOG S9917. Cancer Prevention Research 2011; 4:1761–1769.

McKeown-Eyssen G, Holloway C, Jazmaji V, Bright-See E, Dion P, Bruce WR. A randomized trial of vitamins C and E in the prevention of recurrence of colorectal polyps. *Cancer Res* 1988; 48:4701–4705.

Mettlin C, Graham S, Swanson M. Vitamin A and lung cancer. *J Natl Cancer Inst* 1979; 62:1435–1438.

Meyskens FL, Mc Laren CE, Pelot D, Fujikawa-Brooks S, Carpenter PM, Hawk E et al. Disfluoromethylornithine plus sulindac for the prevention of sporadic colorectal adenomas: A randomized placebo-controlled, double-blind trial. *Cancer Prevention Research* 2008; 1:32–38.

Newman VA, Parsons JK, Mohler J, Pierce JP, Paskett E, Marshall JR. In: *The men's eating and living (MEAL) study: A multi-center pilot trial of dietary intervention for the treatment of prostate cancer. National cancer institute and society of urologic oncology*; Bethesda, MD; 2006. p. 42.

Omenn GS, Goodman GE, Thornquist MD, Balmes J, Cullen MR, Glass A et al. Effects of a combination of beta carotene and vitamin A on lung cancer and cardiovascular disease. *N Engl J Med* 1996; 334:1150–1155.

Parsons JK, Newman V, Mohler JL, Pierce JP, Paskett E, Marshall J. The men's eating and living (MEAL) study: A cancer and leukemia group B pilot trial of dietary intervention for the treatment of prostate cancer. *Urology* 2008a; 72:633–637.

Parsons JK, Newman VA, Mohler JL, Pierce JP, Flatt S, Marshall J. Dietary modification in patients with prostate cancer on active surveillance: A randomized, multicentre feasibility study. *British Journal of Urology International* 2008b; 101:1227–1231.

Pastorino U, Infante M, Maioli M, Chiesa G, Buyse M, Firket P et al. Adjuvant treatment of stage I lung cancer with high-dose vitamin A. *Journal of Clinical Oncology* 1993; 11:1216–1222.

Pierce JP, Natarajan L, Caan BJ, Parker BA, Greenberg ER, Flatt SW et al. Influence of a diet very high in vegetables, fruit, and fiber and low in fat on prognosis following treatment for breast cancer. the women's health eating and living (WHEL) randomized trial. *JAMA* 2007; 298:289–298.

Prentice RL, Caan B, Chlebowski RT, Patterson R, Kuller LH, Ockene JK et al. Low-fat dietary pattern and risk of invasive breast cancer the women's health initiative randomized controlled dietary modification trial. *JAMA* 2006; 295:629–642.

Reid ME, Duffield-Lillico AJ, Garland L, Turnbull BW, Clark LC, Marshall JR. Selenium supplementation and lung cancer incidence: An update of the nutritional prevention of cancer trial. *Cancer Epidemiology Biomarkers Prevention* 2002; 11:1285–1291.

Sandler RS, Halabi S, Baron JA, Budinger S, Paskett E, Keresztes R et al. A randomized trial of aspirin to prevent colorectal adenomas in patients with previous colorectal cancer. *N Engl J Med* 2003; 348:883–890.

Schatzkin A, Freedman LS, Schiffman MH, Dawsey SM. Validation of intermediate end points in cancer research. *J Natl Cancer Inst* 1990; 82:1746–1752.

Schatzkin A, Lanza E, Corle D, Lance P, Iber F, Caan B et al. Lack of effect of a low-fat, high-fiber diet on the recurrence of colorectal adenomas: The polyp prevention trial study group. *N Engl J Med* 2000; 342:1149–1155.

Shike M, Latkany L, Riedel E, Fleisher M, Schatzkin A, Lanza E et al. Lack of effect of a low-fat, high-fruit, - vegetable, and -fiber diet on serum prostate-specific antigen of men without prostate cancer: Results from a randomized trial. *Journal of Clinical Oncology* 2002; 20:3592–3598.

Sporn MB. Combination chemoprevention of cancer. *Nature* 1980; 287:107–108.

Sporn MB, Hong WK. Clinical prevention of recurrence of colorectal adenomas by the combination of difluoromethylornithine and sulindac: An important milestone. *Cancer Prevention Research* 2008; 1:9–11.

The Alpha-Tocopherol,Beta Carotene Cancer Prevention Study Group. The effect of vitamin E and beta carotene on the incidence of lung cancer and other cancers in male smokers. *N Engl J Med* 1994; 330:1029–1035.

Thompson IM, Goodman PJ, Tangen CM, Lucia MS, Miller GJ, Ford LG et al. The influence of finasteride on the development of prostate cancer. *N Engl J Med* 2003; 349:215–224.

Thompson IM, Pauler DK, Goodman PJ, Tangen CM, Lucia MS, Parnes HL et al. Prevalance of prostate cancer among men with a prostate-specific antigen level <4.0 ng per milliliter. *N Engl J Med* 2004; 350:2239–2246.

Thompson IM, Lucia MS, Redman MW, Darke A, La Rosa FG, Parnes HL et al. Finasteride decreases the risk of prostatic intraepithelial neoplasia. *Journal of Urology* 2007; 178:107–110.

Thun MJ, Calle EE, Namboodiri MM, Flanders WD, Coates RJ, Byers T et al. Risk factors for fatal colon cancer in a large prospective study. *J Natl Cancer Inst* 1992; 84:1491–1500.

Trump DL, Deeb KK, Johnson CS, Candace S. Vitamin D: Considerations in the continued development as an agent for cancer prevention and therapy. *The Cancer Journal* 2010; 16:1–9.

Vogel VG, Costantino JP, Wickerham DL, Cronin WM, Cecchini RS, Atkins JN et al. Effects of tamoxifen vs raloxifene on the risk of developing invasive breast cancer and other disease outcomes: The NSABP study of tamoxifene and raloxifene (STAR) P-2 trial. *JAMA* 2006; 295:2727–2741.

Wactawski-Wende J, Kotchen JM, Anderson GL, Assaf AR, Brunner RL, O'Sullivan MJ et al. Calcium plus vitamin D supplementation and the risk of colorectal cancer. *N Engl J Med* 2006; 354:684–696.

World Cancer Research Fund/American Institute for Cancer Research. *Food, nutrition, physical activity, and the prevention of cancer: A global perspective*. Washington, DC: American Institute for Cancer Research; 2007.

Wynder EL, Hyams L, Shigmatsu T. Correlations of international cancer death rates. *Cancer* 1967; 20:113–126.

Wynder EL, Reddy B. Studies of large-bowel cancer: Human leads to experimental application. *J Natl Cancer Inst* 1973; 50:1099–1106.

Zell JA, Pelot D, Chen WP, McLaren CE, Gerner EW, Meyskens FL. Risk of cardiovascular events in a randomized placebo-controlled, double-blind trial of difluoromethylornithine plus sulindac for the prevention sporadic colorectal adenomas. *Cancer Prevention Research* 2009; 2:209–212.

Chapter 10
The Role of Hormonal Factors in Cancer Prevention

David B. Thomas

10.1 Introduction

Hormonal factors included in this chapter include reproductive factors that alter risk by influencing endogenous hormone level and that are directly modifiable by changes in human behavior. These include parity, age at first birth, and breast-feeding. Other hormonal factors, such as ages at menarche and menopause, are not considered because they are not directly modifiable; they are likely influenced by a variety of other factors including diet and are thus covered elsewhere. Exogenous hormones that have a direct effect on risk of specific cancers, and to which large numbers of individuals are exposed for purposes other than cancer prevention, are also included in this chapter. These include hormonal contraceptives and both estrogens and estrogen–progestin combinations used to treat or prevent conditions associated with menopause. Compounds that are given specifically to prevent cancer are covered in the chapter on chemoprevention.

The epidemiologic literature on hormonal factors and cancer is voluminous and reviews by expert committees and meta-analyses of pooled data from multiple studies have greatly facilitated our understanding of the relationships between hormonal factors and specific cancers. Reports of these reviews and analyses have been used in the preparation of this chapter along with results of individual studies published since these reports.

D.B. Thomas (✉)
Fred Hutchinson Cancer Research Center,
1100 Fairview Ave. N., PO Box 19024, Seattle, WA 98109, USA
e-mail: dbthomas@fhcrc.org

A.B. Miller (ed.), *Epidemiologic Studies in Cancer Prevention and Screening*, Statistics for Biology and Health 79, DOI 10.1007/978-1-4614-5586-8_10,

10.2 Endogenous Hormonal Factors

10.2.1 Childbearing

10.2.1.1 Summary of the Evidence

It has been known for over 40 years that risk of breast cancer is inversely related to the number of children that a woman has had and that risk decreases with decreasing age at which she had her first child. A meta-analysis of data from 47 epidemiologic studies (Collaborative Group on Hormonal Factors in Breast Cancer 2002) yielded estimates of a 7.0 % decline in risk for each birth (in the absence of breast-feeding) and a 3 % decline in risk for each year of age younger at the time of a woman's first birth. Risks of endometrial cancer (Dossus et al. 2010; Zucchetto et al. 2009) and ovarian cancer (Braem et al. 2010; Moorman et al. 2008; Tsilidis et al. 2011a; Tung et al. 2003; Yang et al. 2007) also decrease with number of full-term pregnancies, although risk of neither has consistently been shown to decrease with age at first child. Risk of ovarian cancer is also inversely related to parity in women with mutations in the BRCA1 and BCRA2 genes (Antoniou et al. 2009; McLaughlin et al. 2007; Milne et al. 2010).

Conversely, risk of invasive, but not of in situ, cervical cancer was found to increase with number of full-term pregnancies in a meta-analysis of data from 25 epidemiological studies (International Collaboration of Epidemiological Studies of Cervical Cancer 2006), and this relationship was shown for both squamous cell cancer and adenocarcinomas in a pooled analysis of data from 12 of these studies (Gonzales and Green 2007). Increased risks were also related to young age at first child. However, these associations were weakened after controlling for indices of sexual behavior, suggesting that residual confounding by sexual behavior may at least partially account for these observed relationships.

A meta-analysis of data from 53 epidemiologic studies (Beral et al. 2004) clearly showed no association between induced abortions and breast cancer. Induced abortions have also not consistently been associated with risk any other neoplasm.

10.2.1.2 Implications for Cancer Prevention

In developed countries, risks of cancers of the breast, ovary, and endometrium far outweigh risk of cervical cancer, and the chances of dying from the latter are greatly reduced by screening and human papillomavirus vaccines. On the other hand, screening for breast cancer is far from 100 % efficacious, and screening for endometrial and ovarian cancers is not currently available, so any means of appreciably reducing the risk of acquiring these neoplasms would be of considerable benefit. Many women have difficulty balancing the demands of their jobs with the desire to have children, and they consequently often have their children late in life. Given the strong relationship of breast cancer risk to age at first birth, it seems reasonable that this information should be part of any message to the lay public about breast cancer prevention. It would also be reasonable to use knowledge of this relationship to advocate for policy changes that would facilitate early childbearing without jeopardizing women's professional education or careers. Advocating having many children to reduce risk of cancer would clearly be unwise, given the many societal and personal reasons to limit family size. In developing countries, which tend to have high rates of birth and of cervical cancer and low rates of other gynecologic and breast cancers, the benefits of preventing unwanted pregnancies, reducing family size, and delaying childbearing clearly outweigh any benefits high parity and early childbearing have on risks of cancers of the breast, ovary, and endometrium, and family planning efforts may have the added benefit of reducing the incidence of cervical cancer.

10.2.2 Breast-feeding

10.2.2.1 Summary of the Evidence

After tightly controlling for number of live births as well as for other factors related to childbearing, a meta-analysis of data from 47 epidemiologic studies clearly showed that risk of breast cancer decreased with the total number of years that a women breast-fed (Collaborative Group on Hormonal Factors in Breast Cancer 2002). Risk of breast cancer decreased by 4.3 % for every 12 months of breast-feeding. Women who lactated for at least 4.5 years had a risk of 0.73 relative to women who never breast-fed. The reduction in risk was seen in post- as well as pre-menopausal women, suggesting that the apparent protective effect may be long-lasting. Many studies that have reported no significant reduction in risk with lactation were conducted in developed countries where women breast-fed for short periods of time. Recent case–control studies conducted in areas in which prolonged lactation is frequent have consistently shown breast-feeding to be associated with a reduction in risk. These include studies in Korea (Kim et al. 2007), Israel (Shema et al. 2007), Nigeria (Huo et al. 2008), India (Gajalakshmi et al. 2009), Sri Lanka (De et al. 2010a), and Tunisia (Awatef et al. 2010).

A reduction in risk of ovarian cancer has also been associated with breast-feeding. Although a large multinational European cohort study did not show such an association (Tsilidis et al. 2011a), only risk in relation to short-term lactation could be evaluated, and a pooled analysis of data from two cohort studies conducted in the USA showed a decrease in risk with lifetime duration of breast-feeding (Danforth et al. 2007). Most recent case–control studies that controlled carefully for parity also have shown decreasing trends in risk with duration of lactation (Jordan et al. 2010; Moorman et al. 2008; Titus-Ernstoff et al. 2010; Tung et al. 2003), although a study in Italy did not (Chiaffarino et al. 2005). No clear and consistent evidence has emerged that the apparent protective effect of lactation is specific for any particular histologic type of ovarian cancer. Risk of ovarian cancer has been shown to decrease with duration of lactation in carriers of BRCA1 and BRCA2 mutations (Antoniou et al. 2009; McLaughlin et al. 2007). Studies have not shown risk of endometrial cancer to be related to short-term breast-feeding (Dossus et al. 2010; Zucchetto et al. 2009), but the effect of prolonged lactation on risk has not been well studied. Surprisingly, a meta-analysis of data from four case–control studies of adenocarcinomas of the esophagus and gastroesophageal junction found a decreasing trend in risk of these tumors with increasing duration of lactation (Cronin-Fenton et al. 2010).

10.2.2.2 Implications for Cancer Prevention

There are many good reasons for breast-feeding and virtually no health-related reasons not to. Although the impact of short-term breast-feeding on risk of breast and ovarian cancers is small, women should be informed of these anticarcinogenic effects. These effects are additional reasons for women who work outside the home to have a place for breast-feeding and for breast pumping and maternal milk storage at their place of employment, and public health officials and concerned women's groups should advocate for such facilities. In developing countries where women traditionally breast-feed, efforts to promote bottle-feeding have been discouraged for nutritional and other reasons, and reduction in risk of breast and ovarian cancers is an additional benefit of breast-feeding that can be used to argue against bottle-feeding.

10.3 Exogenous Hormonal Factors

10.3.1 Combined Oral Contraceptives

10.3.1.1 Summary of the Evidence

Since combined oral contraceptives, containing an estrogen and a progestogen, were initially introduced in the late 1950s, they have been used by over 100 million women in all parts of the world, and it has been estimated that these preparations are currently used by about 10 % of all women of childbearing age (IARC 2011). Therefore, even a relatively small alteration in risk of cancer in users of these products would impact large numbers of women. In October 2008, a working group for the International Agency for Research on Cancer (IARC) updated previous reviews of the relationship of oral contraceptives to risk of various cancers. The results of this review (IARC 2011), plus subsequent publications, are the predominant sources used in this section.

The doses and specific types of estrogens and progestogens in the multitude of different oral contraceptives that have been marketed have varied temporarily and among countries, with a trend toward lower doses over time. They have been classified by estrogen dose as high dose (≥50 μ), intermediate dose (30–35 μ) and low dose (15–20 μ). They have also been classified by the type and strength of the progestogen and its androgenic activity. In addition, preparations may vary within a monthly cycle of use, with some having a fixed dose of estrogen and a varying dose of progestogen and others having a fixed dose of progestogen and a varying dose of estrogen. Most epidemiologic studies have not distinguished exposures to different formulations. The most useful classifications that have been used are based on estrogen dose and the relative potency of the estrogen and progestogen in the preparation.

Oral contraceptives have clearly been shown to reduce risk of ovarian cancer. In a meta-analysis of data from 45 epidemiological studies (Beral et al. 2008), risk declined with duration of use. Although the apparent protective effect diminished with time since last use, a statistically significant reduction in risk was seen over 30 years after use, with the level of protection after use greatest for the longest-term users. Compared to nonusers, the risk in women who had ever used oral contraceptives was 0.73(0.70–0.76), the risk in women who used them for over 15 years was 0.42 (0.36–0.49), and the risk in ever-users after 30 years since use was 0.86 (0.76–0.97). They appear to protect against both malignant and borderline tumors and against all histologic types, although the reduction in risk may be less for mucinous than other types (IARC 2011). The level of protection may be greater for lean than obese women (Tsilidis et al. 2011b), although this has not been consistently observed. Paradoxically, most studies that have assessed risk in relation to the strength of the preparations used have found that risk is actually lower in users of low- than high-dose oral contraceptives. Risk was also shown to be reduced in relation to duration of use of oral contraceptives in women with BRCA1 or BRCA2 mutations in the IARC review, in a subsequent meta-analysis (Iodice et al. 2010), and in a large cohort of women with these mutations (Antoniou et al. 2009). Relative risks of dying from ovarian cancer of 0.53 (0.06–4.53) over 10 years after last use (Hannaford et al. 2010) and of 0.5 (0.3–0.8) over 20 years since exposure (Vessey et al. 2010) were observed in two cohort studies in the United Kingdom.

Risk of endometrial cancer has also been shown to decrease with increasing duration of oral contraceptive use in comprehensive reviews of the literature (IARC 2011; Mueck et al. 2010) and in subsequent cohort (Dossus et al. 2010) and case–control (Zucchetto et al. 2009) studies. The relative risk in women who ever used oral contraceptives is approximately 0.5, and studies have demonstrated reduced risks up to over 25 years since exposure. The level of protection thus appears to be about the same for ovarian and endometrial cancers. Risk of the latter has been shown in two studies (Maxwell et al. 2006; Rosenblatt and Thomas 1991) to be lower in women who used preparations with high doses of progestogens than in users of low progestogen-dose products. Relative risk of death from uterine cancer other than cervical (i.e., largely endometrial) of 0.4 (0.1–1.0) over 20 years since last use has been documented in one of the United Kingdom cohort studies (Vessey et al. 2010).

Most studies have shown a decrease in risk of colorectal cancer in users of oral contraceptives. The relative risk of colorectal cancer in women who ever used oral contraceptives was estimated to be 0.81 (0.70–0.92) in a meta-analysis of data from 11 case–control studies and 7 cohort studies (Bosetti et al. 2009). Comparable relative risks of 0.85 (0.79–0.93) and 0.80 (0.70–0.92) were estimated separately for cancers of the colon and rectum, respectively. However, no trends in risk with duration of use were observed. A subsequent multinational cohort study in Europe (Tsilidis et al. 2011c) also showed a small decrease in risk in users and no trend in risk with duration of use. One of the cohort studies in the United Kingdom found a reduced risk of dying of colorectal cancer in users of oral contraceptives and a modest decreasing trend in risk with duration of use (Hannaford et al. 2010), but this was not observed in the other cohort study in that country (Vessey et al. 2010). The IARC Working Group (IARC 2011) concluded that it is unlikely that oral contraceptives increase the risk of colorectal cancer and that they may reduce risk.

In order to assess the usefulness of oral contraceptives in cancer prevention, consideration must also be given to possible increases in risk of neoplasms associated with their use. A meta-analysis of data from 54 epidemiologic studies (Collaborative Group on Hormonal Factors in Breast Cancer 1996) found that risk of breast cancer increased with duration of use of oral contraceptives, but only in current users, in women who had last used them in the past 10 years, and in women who started using them before the age of 20. Since current and recent users tend to be young women at low risk of breast cancer, the increase in relative risk of only about 20 % (in women who ever used oral contraceptive) meant that a very small excess number of breast cancers was actually observed. Furthermore, the excess risk was greater for tumors confined to the breast than for more widely disseminated tumors, and no increase in mortality from breast cancer in relation to duration of use or time since last use was subsequently observed in the 2 United Kingdom cohorts (Hannaford et al. 2010; Vessey et al. 2010), suggesting the possibility of detection bias as an explanation for the observed risk increase. No long-term increase in risk of breast cancer in relation to oral contraceptive use was reported in the two cohorts in the United Kingdom or in a cohort in Shanghai after the meta-analysis (IARC 2011), but in a cohort study of US nurses (Hunter et al. 2010), an increase in risk in current users was observed. Case–control studies conducted after the meta-analysis generally provided inconsistent results, but most of the best designed population-based studies generally supported the conclusion that increased risk was confined to recent users and young women. Although based on small numbers and not statistically significant, the meta-analysis found that high-dose products were associated with a somewhat higher risk than the newer lower-dose products. The Working Group was unable to determine whether the possible increase in risk was greater for lobular than ductal carcinomas or differed by estrogen receptor status of the tumor. The Working Group and a subsequent meta-analysis (Iodice et al. 2010) have provided evidence that oral contraceptives use is associated with an increased risk of breast cancer in women with mutations in the BRCA1 and BRCA2 genes, and in the meta-analysis, this increase was confined to products marketed before 1975, suggesting that the newer, lower-dose products may not alter risk in carriers of these gene mutations. The Working Group noted that the increased risk in the carriers may at least in part account for the increase in risk in young women who began using oral contraceptives at an early age.

An increase in risk of both in situ and invasive cervical cancer with duration of oral contraceptive use was observed in a meta-analysis of data from 24 epidemiological studies (Appleby et al. 2007). Based on data from 12 of these studies, a similar increasing trend in risk was also observed for both invasive cervical squamous cell carcinoma and adenocarcinoma (Gonzales and Green 2007). Risk of invasive cancer did not increase until after about 5 years of use and was increased by about 56 % in users of over 10-year duration relative to nonusers. Risk in women who used them for over 5 years returned to base-line level by 10 years after cessation of use. Risk of in situ disease was increased even in women who used them for less than 5 years and persisted for over 10 years after last use both in these short-term users and in women who used them for over 5 years. Although based on small numbers, both cohort studies in the United Kingdom (Hannaford et al. 2010; Vessey et al. 2010) reported increased risks of mortality from cervical cancer with duration of use and also persistence of an increased risk up to over 9 and over 20 years since last use, respectively. Although bias due to preferentially screening users of oral contraceptives may, at least in part, be an explanation for the increase in risk of in situ disease, it is less likely to account for the increase in risk of invasive and fatal carcinomas. Users of oral contraceptive may be more likely than nonusers to engage in sexual behavior conducive to the acquisition of human papillomaviruses, the primary causal agent of cervical carcinomas, and less likely to use barrier contraceptives. It is extremely difficult to collect reliable data on such behavior, and the possibility that residual confounding by sexual variables is an explanation for at least part of the observed increases in risk cannot be confidently ruled out. However, the pattern of an increasing risk with duration of use and the decline in risk with time since exposure suggest that the observed associations may represent a true biological phenomenon. Reports from cohort studies that oral contraceptives apparently increase the likelihood of persistence of HPV infection (Marks et al. 2011; Nielsen et al. 2010) provide a possible mechanism.

In case–control studies conducted in countries not endemic for hepatitis B, a primary cause of hepatocellular carcinoma, risk in this neoplasm has been shown to increase with duration of oral contraceptive use (IARC 2011). However, this association has not been observed in cohort studies in non-hepatitis B endemic areas where the disease is rare and the expected numbers of cases are small or in studies in areas endemic for this virus, clearly indicating that this apparent complication of oral contraceptive use is rare and does not potentiate the carcinogenic effect of hepatitis B.

10.3.1.2 Implications for Cancer Prevention

Use of oral contraceptives clearly protects against ovarian and endometrial cancers. The longer the use, the greater the protection, and protection can last for over a quarter of a century after last use. Risk of colorectal cancer may also be reduced in users of oral contraceptives. These benefits clearly outweigh the small increase in risks of cancers of the breast and liver. The increase in risk of the former is a rare phenomenon confined to young women who are current or recent users, may at least in part be a spurious observation due to preferential screening in users of oral contraceptives, and may be lower for the newer low-dose preparations than for the older products, suggesting that any adverse effect on breast cancer occurrence may be even smaller in the future than in the past. Liver cancer is an extremely rare consequence of oral contraceptive use and has not been observed in hepatitis B endemic areas or in carriers of this virus. Like breast cancer, the increase in risk of invasive cervical cancer in users of oral contraceptives seems to be confined to the decade after cessation of use, is therefore observed primarily in young women, and hence is a relatively rare event. Although the observed increase in risk of in situ disease may be longer lasting, it may in part be due to preferential screening in users of oral contraceptives, and the observed increase in both in situ and invasive diseases may be partly due to residual confounding by sexual variables and differences in use of barrier methods of contraception in users and nonusers of oral contraceptives. Nonetheless women who use oral contraceptives constitute a group at increased risk of cervical cancer, and provision of oral contraceptives provides an opportunity for screening and thus secondary cervical cancer prevention.

Although use of oral contraceptives clearly reduces the risk of ovarian cancer in women with mutations in the BRCA genes, the apparent increase in risk of the more common breast cancer in these women probably outweighs this protective effect. However, future quantification of risks of these two neoplasms in oral contraceptive users with these mutations may alter this conclusion.

10.3.2 Progestational Contraceptives

10.3.2.1 Summary of the Evidence

The results of epidemiologic studies of cancer risks in relation to progestogen-only oral contraceptives and to the long-acting injectable contraceptive, depot medroxyprogesterone acetate (DMPA), were reviewed by the IARC Working Group in 1998 (IARC 1999). Too few women had used progestogen-only oral contraceptives to allow an adequate evaluation of their possible carcinogenic effects in humans. Since these products are seldom used today, any effects they may exert on risks of cancer in women are now of little public health importance or applicability. However, DMPA has been used by many millions of women and is currently a commonly used method of birth control in some countries. Its impact on cancer risk is therefore of considerable interest. Few epidemiologic studies of DMPA and cancer in humans have been conducted since the IARC review, and the conclusions of the Working Group are largely valid today.

Although based on small numbers, a case–control study in Thailand showed risk of endometrial cancer to be reduced in users of DMPA. In a joint analysis of data from case–control studies in Thailand and Mexico, no significant association between DMPA use and ovarian cancer was observed. Based on a combined analysis of data from a multinational hospital-based case–control study by the World Health Organization (WHO) and a population-based case–control study in New Zealand, no significant association between use of DMPA and breast cancer was found. Two studies in hepatitis B endemic areas found no increase in risk of liver cancer in DMPA users. In a meta-analysis of data from most studies of cervical cancer and DMPA (International Collaboration of Epidemiological Studies of Cervical Cancer 2006), a 22 % increase in risk of invasive cervical cancer was observed in women who used this product for over 5 years. There was no significant trend in risk with time since last use and no significant association with carcinoma in situ. In a cohort study in the United States (Harris et al. 2009), users of DMPA were at increased risk of acquiring an HPV infection, but at reduced risk of subsequent cervical intraepithelial neoplasia 1, 2, and 3. As with oral contraceptives, the possibility that the increase in risk of cervical cancer is a spurious result of confounding by sexual variables, or preferential screening in users, cannot be ruled out.

10.3.2.2 Implications for Cancer Prevention

DMPA protects against endometrial cancer. Women who use DMPA may be at increased risk of cervical cancer and should be screened for this condition; and the provision of DMPA provides an opportunity for secondary prevention of this neoplasm. There is no strong evidence that risks of other cancer are altered in users of DMPA.

10.3.3 Estrogen-Only and Combined Estrogen–Progestogen Menopausal Therapy

10.3.3.1 Summary of the Evidence

Estrogens alone were initially used as hormonal therapy for symptoms associated with the menopause, such as hot flashes, and for prevention of chronic conditions such as osteoporosis and ischemic heart disease that occur primarily in the postmenopausal period. Progestogens were added to the regimens beginning in 1975, after it was discovered that estrogen therapy increased the risk of endometrial cancer. Estrogens alone are currently given almost exclusively to hysterectomized women. Use of estrogen–progestogen combinations peaked in 2002 and then declined, and duration of therapy was shortened in response to a report from a randomized trial that showed an increased incidence of breast cancer in users of estrogen–progestogen combinations (Rossouw et al. 2002). Estrogens alone and estrogen–progestogen combinations are considered together in this section to facilitate comparisons of their relative carcinogenic and anticarcinogenic effects on various organs. Conjugated estrogens have been the most frequently used estrogens in the United States and some other countries, whereas various synthetic estrogens are more commonly used in some European countries and elsewhere. Estrogens alone have been given in various doses, and estrogen–progestogen combinations vary in the types of estrogens and progestogens used, their doses, and the numbers of days in a month during which the progestogen is given with the estrogen. Because of the large number of different products and regimens that have been used, information on the risks and benefits of specific products and patterns of use is limited, and specific regimens have generally not been distinguished in reviews of studies in humans and assessments by expert committees. The evidence for the carcinogenic and anticarcinogenic effects of these products was reviewed by the US Preventive Services Task force in 2004–2005 (U.S. Preventive Services Task Force 2005) and in 2008 by an IARC Working Group (IARC 2011).

Based on results from 7 cohort studies and over 35 case–control studies, the IARC Working Group concluded that risk of endometrial cancer increases with duration of estrogen therapy. Risk decreases with time since cessation of use but risk remains elevated for at least 10 years after cessation of use (International Agency for Research on Cancer 2011). This iatrogenic tumor production can be reduced or prevented by addition of a progestogen to the estrogen regimen. Risk decreases with the number of days during a monthly cycle that the progestogen is given, but results of studies vary as to the number of days per month that it must be taken in order to reduce the risk to that of nonusers of any hormones or to further reduce risk to provide a true protective effect. Continuous use of a progestogen reduced risk below that of non-hormone users in some studies (Allen et al. 2010; Jaakkola et al. 2009, 2011), but not in others (Karageorgi et al. 2010; Razavi et al. 2010).

In a meta-analysis of data from 51 epidemiological studies performed when most menopausal hormone therapy was estrogen-only (Collaborative Group on Hormonal Factors in Breast Cancer 1997), risk of breast cancer was found to increase with duration of use and to decrease with time since cessation use, with no statistically significant increase in risk after 5 years since last exposure. Risk specifically in users of only estrogens has subsequently been reported in multiple studies, with somewhat inconsistent results (IARC 2011). Some studies have shown clear increases in risk with duration of use, some have shown risk to be confined primarily to current users irrespective of duration of use suggesting a screening bias, and others have shown no increase in risk in users. In the Women's Health Initiative (WHI) trial, risk was actually somewhat lower in women who were given 0.625 mg of conjugated equine estrogen daily than in women who received a placebo, although the difference was only of borderline statistical significance (Rossouw et al. 2002). Risk of breast cancer has more consistently, and more strongly, been associated with use of estrogen–progestogen combinations than with estrogen alone. The WHI trial was stopped, after a mean of 5.6 years of treatment and an average of 7.9 years of follow-up, in part because of an increased risk of breast cancer in women who received O.625 mg of conjugated equine estrogens and 2.5 mg medroxyprogesterone acetate daily (Rossouw et al. 2002). Subsequent analyses after an average of 11 years of follow-up showed a 25 % increase in risk of invasive breast cancer, an excess particularly of tumors that had spread to the lymph nodes, and an increased risk of deaths from breast cancer (Chlebowski et al. 2010). Risk began to decline within a year of cessation of use and was near that of the placebo group within 2 years (Chlebowski et al. 2009). A large number of cohort and case–control studies have also consistently shown increased risks in users of combined products with duration of use, as well as a decline in risk with cessation of use (IARC 2011). Recent cohort studies, in which risks of breast cancer in users of estrogens alone and in users of combined products can be directly compared, have shown risks to be higher in women who used the latter preparations than in users of estrogens alone (Bakken et al. 2011; Saxena et al. 2010). The WHI trial (Prentice et al. 2009a) and a cohort study in Europe (Fournier et al. 2009) also showed use of combined products within 5 and 3 years of menopause to be associated with an increase in risk of breast cancer after 2 years since initial use and after 5 years of use, respectively, suggesting that even relatively short-term use may increase risk of breast cancer if given near menopause (Bernstein 2009). Use of these combined regimens increased following realization in about 1979 that estrogens alone increased risk of endometrial cancer and then declined following the WHI trial report in 2002 of an increased risk of breast cancer in users of these products. Commensurate with these changes in prescribing practices, the incidence rates of breast cancer in general populations in North America and Europe increased from the 1980s to 2002, and then declined, particularly in the age and ethnic groups in which hormone replacement therapy is most commonly used (De et al. 2010b; Farhat et al. 2010; IARC 2011). It has been estimated that about half of the decline in rates of breast cancer in the United States since 2002 in the relevant age groups can be explained by changes in exposure to postmenopausal hormones (Sprague et al. 2011). The demonstration that estrogen–progestogen combinations, and probably also estrogens alone, cause breast cancer has clearly resulted in changes in prescribing practices that have prevented large numbers of iatrogenic breast cancers.

A large number of cohort and case–control studies and 3 meta-analyses reviewed by the latest IARC Working Group (IARC 2011) have, in the aggregate, provided fairly consistent evidence that risk of ovarian cancer increases with duration of exposure to menopausal estrogen-only therapy and declines with time since cessation of use, and the Working Group concluded that these products can cause ovarian cancer. In a subsequent analysis of published data from 15 studies (Pearce et al. 2009), the relative risk (and 95 % confidence interval) of ovarian cancers was estimated to be 1.22 (1.18–1.27) per 5 years of use of estrogen-only products and 1.10 (1.04–1.16) per 5 years of use of estrogen–progestogen combinations. This difference was unlikely due to chance. The estimates for individual studies were quite consistent for estrogen-only users, but there was considerable heterogeneity of results for users of combined products, with many showing no increase in risk. Among studies in which risk in users of both products could be compared, risk was uniformly higher in users of estrogens alone, and this has also been observed in most subsequent studies (Hildebrand et al. 2010; Tsilidis et al. 2011a; Wernli et al. 2008), although not in all (Morch et al. 2009). The IARC Working Group concluded that it is unlikely that estrogen–progestogen menopausal therapy alters the risk of ovarian cancer. Thus, the addition of progestogens to estrogen therapy has likely prevented iatrogenic ovarian cancers.

The IARC Working Group noted that results of 14 case–control studies and 7 cohort studies of colorectal cancer were inconsistent, with about half showing a decreased risk and half showing no significant alteration in risk in users of estrogen-only preparations (IARC 2011). The observed reductions in risk were observed primarily in current and recent users, and trends in risk with duration of use were generally not seen. Subsequent reports from four additional cohort studies similarly reveal either no alterations in risk in users of estrogens alone (Tsilidis et al. 2011c) or a decrease in risk (Delellis et al. 2010; Hildebrand et al. 2009; Johnson et al. 2009), with inconsistencies among studies with respect to duration of use and time since last use. The results of 12 studies of estrogen–progestogen combinations reviewed by the Working Group were more consistent, with most showing a reduction in risk of colorectal cancers primarily in current users and some showing a decreasing trend in risk with duration of use. The results of the WHI randomized trials are consistent with these observations: the hazard ratios for colorectal cancer were estimated to be 1.12 (0.77–1.63) and 0.56 (0.38–0.81) in women assigned to receive conjugated estrogens alone and conjugated estrogens plus medroxyprogesterone acetate, respectively. However, more recent reports do not fully support the contention that estrogen–progestogen combinations protect against colorectal cancer. In the observational cohort portion of the WHI, hazard ratios of 0.80 (0.55–1.20) and 1.15 (0.74–1.79) were observed in users of estrogen alone and estrogen plus progestogen, respectively (Prentice et al. 2009b); and no alteration in risk was observed in two recent cohort studies (Hildebrand et al. 2009, Tsilidis et al. 2011c), although a decrease in risk, but no trend in risk with duration of use, was observed in the other two others (Delellis et al. 2010; Johnson et al. 2009). It can confidently be concluded that risk of colorectal cancer is not increased in users of either estrogens alone or estrogens plus a progestogen. These products may offer some protection against these neoplasms, but the evidence is inconsistent.

In a combined analysis of data from the WHI trials and observational study, risk of squamous cell esophageal carcinomas, but not of adenocarcinomas, was significantly reduced in users of estrogens plus a progestogen, but not in users of estrogens alone (Bodelon et al. 2011). This unexpected result requires independent confirmation. Risks of no other neoplasms have been convincingly associated with menopausal hormonal therapy.

10.3.3.2 Implications for Cancer Prevention

The iatrogenic production of cancers of the endometrium and ovary by menopausal estrogen therapy was reduced by addition of a progestogen to the regimen, but this increased the risk of breast cancer. In the 2005 Preventive Services Task Force recommendation statement on hormonal therapy for the prevention of chronic conditions (U.S. Preventive Services Task Force 2005), it was noted that menopausal therapy with both estrogen alone and with estrogen plus progestogen has also been associated with increased risks of stroke, venous thromboembolism, cholecystitis, dementia, and cognitive dysfunction; that the combined regimen has also been related to increased risk of coronary heart disease; and that estrogen alone does not reduce risk of this condition. Although both regimens have been shown to increase bone density and reduce risk of fractures, it was judged that these benefits, plus the reduced risks in users of combined products of iatrogenic endometrial and ovarian cancers, and the possible reduction in risk of colorectal cancers were outweighed by the noncancerous adverse effects and the increased risk of breast cancer. The Task Force recommended against the long-term use of both estrogens alone and estrogen–progestogen combinations for prevention of chronic conditions in the postmenopausal years. Results of subsequent studies of risks of various neoplasms and a report from the WHI on risks of multiple endpoints (Prentice et al. 2009a) are consistent with the results of studies considered by the Task Force and do not provide evidence that these recommendations should be revised. Although use of estrogens and progestogens for less than a year for treatment of acute symptoms of the menopause is unlikely to appreciably alter risks of any cancers, except possibly breast cancer, alternative treatments should be generally given first, and if hormones are used, they should be given only for a short period of time and in the lowest doses needed to achieve the desired results. The reduction in use of postmenopausal hormonal therapeutic agents has prevented iatrogenic cancers of the endometrium and breast and probably also of the ovary that otherwise would occur in users of these products.

References

Allen NE, Tsilidis KK, Key TJ, Dossus L, Kaaks R, Lund E, et al. Menopausal hormone therapy and risk of endometrial carcinoma among postmenopausal women in the European Prospective Investigation into Cancer and Nutrition. *Am J Epidemiol* 2010; 172:1394–1403.

Antoniou AC, Rookus M, Andrieu N, Brohet R, Chang-Claude J, Peock S, et al. Reproductive and hormonal factors, and ovarian cancer risk for BRCA1 and BRCA2 mutation carriers: results from the International BRCA1/2 Carrier Cohort Study. *Cancer Epidemiol Biomarkers Prev* 2009; 18:601–610.

Appleby P, Beral V, Berrington de GA, Colin D, Franceschi S, Goodhill A, et al. Cervical cancer and hormonal contraceptives: collaborative reanalysis of individual data for 16,573 women with cervical cancer and 35,509 women without cervical cancer from 24 epidemiological studies. *Lancet* 2007; 370:1609–1621.

Awatef M, Olfa G, Imed H, Kacem M, Imen C, Rim C, et al. Breastfeeding reduces breast cancer risk: a case-control study in Tunisia. *Cancer Causes Control* 2010; 21:393–397.

Bakken K, Fournier A, Lund E, Waaseth M, Dumeaux V, Clavel-Chapelon F, et al. Menopausal hormone therapy and breast cancer risk: impact of different treatments. The European Prospective Investigation into Cancer and Nutrition. *Int J Cancer* 2011; 128:144–156.

Beral V, Bull D, Doll R, Peto R, Reeves G. Breast cancer and abortion: collaborative reanalysis of data from 53 epidemiological studies, including 83,000 women with breast cancer from 16 countries. *Lancet* 2004; 363:1007–1016.

Beral V, Doll R, Hermon C, Peto R, Reeves G. Ovarian cancer and oral contraceptives: collaborative reanalysis of data from 45 epidemiological studies including 23,257 women with ovarian cancer and 87,303 controls. *Lancet* 2008; 371:303–314.

Bernstein L. Combined hormone therapy at menopause and breast cancer: a warning--short-term use increases risk. *J Clin Oncol* 2009; 27:5116–5119.

Bodelon C, Anderson GL, Rossing MA, Chlebowski RT, Ochs-Balcom HM, Vaughan TL. Hormonal factors and risks of esophageal squamous cell carcinoma and adenocarcinoma in postmenopausal women. *Cancer Prev Res* 2011; 4:840–850.

Bosetti C, Bravi F, Negri E, La VC. Oral contraceptives and colorectal cancer risk: a systematic review and meta-analysis. *Hum Reprod Update* 2009; 15:489–498.

Braem MG, Onland-Moret NC, van den Brandt PA, Goldbohm RA, Peeters PH, Kruitwagen RF, et al. Reproductive and hormonal factors in association with ovarian cancer in the Netherlands cohort study. *Am J Epidemiol* 2010; 172:1181–1189.

Chiaffarino F, Pelucchi C, Negri E, Parazzini F, Franceschi S, Talamini R, et al. Breastfeeding and the risk of epithelial ovarian cancer in an Italian population. *Gynecol Oncol* 2005; 98:304–308.

Chlebowski RT, Anderson GL, Gass M, Lane DS, Aragaki AK, Kuller LH, et al. Estrogen plus progestin and breast cancer incidence and mortality in postmenopausal women. *JAMA* 2010; 304:1684–1692.

Chlebowski RT, Kuller LH, Prentice RL, Stefanick ML, Manson JE, Gass M, et al. Breast cancer after use of estrogen plus progestin in postmenopausal women. *N Engl J Med* 2009; 360:573–587.

Collaborative Group on Hormonal Factors in Breast Cancer. Breast cancer and hormonal contraceptives: collaborative reanalysis of individual data on 53 297 women with breast cancer and 100 239 women without breast cancer from 54 epidemiological studies. *Lancet* 1996; 347:1713–1727.

Collaborative Group on Hormonal Factors in Breast Cancer. Breast cancer and hormone replacement therapy: collaborative reanalysis of data from 51 epidemiological studies of 52,705 women with breast cancer and 108,411 women without breast cancer. *Lancet* 1997; 350:1047–1059.

Collaborative Group on Hormonal Factors in Breast Cancer. Breast cancer and breastfeeding: collaborative reanalysis of individual data from 47 epidemiological studies in 30 countries, including 50302 women with breast cancer and 96973 women without the disease. *Lancet* 2002; 360:187–195.

Cronin-Fenton DP, Murray LJ, Whiteman DC, Cardwell C, Webb PM, Jordan SJ, et al. Reproductive and sex hormonal factors and oesophageal and gastric junction adenocarcinoma: a pooled analysis. *Eur J Cancer* 2010; 46:2067–2076.

Danforth KN, Tworoger SS, Hecht JL, Rosner BA, Colditz GA, Hankinson SE. Breastfeeding and risk of ovarian cancer in two prospective cohorts. *Cancer Causes Control* 2007; 18:517–523.

De SM, Senarath U, Gunatilake M, Lokuhetty D. Prolonged breastfeeding reduces risk of breast cancer in Sri Lankan women: a case-control study. *Cancer Epidemiol* 2010a; 34:267–273.

De P, Neutel CI, Olivotto I, Morrison H. Breast cancer incidence and hormone replacement therapy in Canada. *J Natl Cancer Inst* 2010b; 102:1489–1495.

Delellis HK, Duan L, Sullivan-Halley J, Ma H, Clarke CA, Neuhausen SL, et al. Menopausal hormone therapy use and risk of invasive colon cancer: the California Teachers Study. *Am J Epidemiol* 2010; 171:415–425.

Dossus L, Allen N, Kaaks R, Bakken K, Lund E, Tjonneland A, et al. Reproductive risk factors and endometrial cancer: the European Prospective Investigation into Cancer and Nutrition. *Int J Cancer* 2010; 127:442–451.

Farhat GN, Walker R, Buist DS, Onega T, Kerlikowske K. Changes in invasive breast cancer and ductal carcinoma in situ rates in relation to the decline in hormone therapy use. *J Clin Oncol* 2010; 28:5140–5146.

Fournier A, Mesrine S, Boutron-Ruault MC, Clavel-Chapelon F. Estrogen-progestagen menopausal hormone therapy and breast cancer: does delay from menopause onset to treatment initiation influence risks? *J Clin Oncol* 2009; 27:5138–5143.

Gajalakshmi V, Mathew A, Brennan P, Rajan B, Kanimozhi VC, Mathews A, et al. Breastfeeding and breast cancer risk in India: a multicenter case-control study. *Int J Cancer* 2009; 125:662–665.

Gonzales A, Green J. Comparison of risk factors for invasive squamous cell carcinoma and adenocarcinoma of the cervix: collaborative reanalysis of individual data on 8,097 women with squamous cell carcinoma and 1,374 women with adenocarcinoma from 12 epidemiological studies. *Int J Cancer* 2007; 120:885–891.

Hannaford PC, Iversen L, Macfarlane TV, Elliott AM, Angus V, Lee AJ. Mortality among contraceptive pill users: cohort evidence from Royal College of General Practitioners' Oral Contraception Study. *BMJ* 2010; 340:c927.

Harris TG, Miller L, Kulasingam SL, Feng Q, Kiviat NB, Schwartz SM, et al. Depot-medroxyprogesterone acetate and combined oral contraceptive use and cervical neoplasia among women with oncogenic human papillomavirus infection. *Am J Obstet Gynecol* 2009; 200:489e1–498e8.

Hildebrand JS, Gapstur SM, Feigelson HS, Teras LR, Thun MJ, Patel AV. Postmenopausal hormone use and incident ovarian cancer: Associations differ by regimen. *Int J Cancer* 2010; 127:2928–2935.

Hildebrand JS, Jacobs EJ, Campbell PT, McCullough ML, Teras LR, Thun MJ, et al. Colorectal cancer incidence and postmenopausal hormone use by type, recency, and duration in cancer prevention study II. *Cancer Epidemiol Biomarkers Prev* 2009; 18:2835–2841.

Hunter DJ, Colditz GA, Hankinson SE, Malspeis S, Spiegelman D, Chen W, et al. Oral contraceptive use and breast cancer: a prospective study of young women. *Cancer Epidemiol Biomarkers Prev* 2010; 19:2496–2502.

Huo D, Adebamowo CA, Ogundiran TO, Akang EE, Campbell O, Adenipekun A, et al. Parity and breastfeeding are protective against breast cancer in Nigerian women. *Br J Cancer* 2008; 98:992–996.

IARC. *Hormonal Contraception and Post-Menopausal Hormonal Therapy*. IARC Monographs on the Evaluation of Carcinogenic Risks to Humans Vol 72. Lyon, International Agency for Research on Cancer 1999;72.

IARC. A Review of Human Carcinogens. IARC Monographs on the Evaluation of Carcinogenic Risks to Humans. *Part A: Pharmaceuticals*. Vol 100. Lyon, International Agency for Research on Cancer 2011;100.

International Collaboration of Epidemiological Studies of Cervical Cancer. Cervical carcinoma and reproductive factors: collaborative reanalysis of individual data on 16,563 women with cervical carcinoma and 33,542 women without cervical carcinoma from 25 epidemiological studies. *Int J Cancer* 2006; 119:1108–1124.

Iodice S, Barile M, Rotmensz N, Feroce I, Bonanni B, Radice P, et al. Oral contraceptive use and breast or ovarian cancer risk in BRCA1/2 carriers: a meta-analysis. *Eur J Cancer* 2010; 46:2275–2284.

Jaakkola S, Lyytinen H, Pukkala E, Ylikorkala O. Endometrial cancer in postmenopausal women using estradiol-progestin therapy. *Obstet Gynecol* 2009; 114:1197–1204.

Jaakkola S, Lyytinen HK, Dyba T, Ylikorkala O, Pukkala E. Endometrial cancer associated with various forms of postmenopausal hormone therapy: a case control study. *Int J Cancer* 2011; 128:1644–1651.

Johnson JR, Lacey JV, Jr., Lazovich D, Geller MA, Schairer C, Schatzkin A, et al. Menopausal hormone therapy and risk of colorectal cancer. *Cancer Epidemiol Biomarkers Prev* 2009; 18:196–203.

Jordan SJ, Siskind V, Green C, Whiteman DC, Webb PM. Breastfeeding and risk of epithelial ovarian cancer. *Cancer Causes Control* 2010; 21:109–116.

Karageorgi S, Hankinson SE, Kraft P, De VI (2010) Reproductive factors and postmenopausal hormone use in relation to endometrial cancer risk in the Nurses' Health Study cohort 1976–2004. Int J Cancer 126:208–216.

Kim Y, Choi JY, Lee KM, Park SK, Ahn SH, Noh DY, et al. Dose-dependent protective effect of breast-feeding against breast cancer among ever-lactated women in Korea. *Eur J Cancer Prev* 2007; 16:124–129.

Marks M, Gravitt PE, Gupta SB, Liaw KL, Tadesse A, Kim E, et al. Combined oral contraceptive use increases HPV persistence but not new HPV detection in a cohort of women from Thailand. *J Infect Dis* 2011; 204:1505–1513.

Maxwell GL, Schildkraut JM, Calingaert B, Risinger JI, Dainty L, Marchbanks PA, et al. Progestin and estrogen potency of combination oral contraceptives and endometrial cancer risk. *Gynecol Oncol* 2006; 103:535–540.

McLaughlin JR, Risch HA, Lubinski J, Moller P, Ghadirian P, Lynch H, et al. Reproductive risk factors for ovarian cancer in carriers of BRCA1 or BRCA2 mutations: a case-control study. *Lancet Oncol* 2007; 8:26–34.

Milne RL, Osorio A, Cajal T, Baiget M, Lasa A, Diaz-Rubio E, et al. Parity and the risk of breast and ovarian cancer in BRCA1 and BRCA2 mutation carriers. *Breast Cancer Res Treat* 2010; 119:221–232.

Moorman PG, Calingaert B, Palmieri RT, Iversen ES, Bentley RC, Halabi S, et al. Hormonal risk factors for ovarian cancer in premenopausal and postmenopausal women. *Am J Epidemiol* 2008; 167:1059–1069.

Morch LS, Lokkegaard E, Andreasen AH, Kruger-Kjaer S, Lidegaard O. Hormone therapy and ovarian cancer. *JAMA* 2009; 302:298–305.

Mueck AO, Seeger H, Rabe T. Hormonal contraception and risk of endometrial cancer: a systematic review. *Endocr Relat Cancer* 2010; 17:R263–R271.

Nielsen A, Kjaer SK, Munk C, Osler M, Iftner T. Persistence of high-risk human papillomavirus infection in a population-based cohort of Danish women. *J Med Virol* 2010; 82:616–623.

Pearce CL, Chung K, Pike MC, Wu AH. Increased ovarian cancer risk associated with menopausal estrogen therapy is reduced by adding a progestin. *Cancer* 2009; 115:531–539.

Prentice RL, Manson JE, Langer RD, Anderson GL, Pettinger M, Jackson RD, et al. Benefits and risks of postmenopausal hormone therapy when it is initiated soon after menopause. *Am J Epidemiol* 2009a; 170:12–23.

Prentice RL, Pettinger M, Beresford SA, Wactawski-Wende J, Hubbell FA, Stefanick ML, et al. Colorectal cancer in relation to postmenopausal estrogen and estrogen plus progestin in the Women's Health Initiative clinical trial and observational study. *Cancer Epidemiol Biomarkers Prev* 2009b; 18:1531–1537.

Razavi P, Pike MC, Horn-Ross PL, Templeman C, Bernstein L, Ursin G. Long-term postmenopausal hormone therapy and endometrial cancer. *Cancer Epidemiol Biomarkers Prev* 2010; 19:475–483.

Rosenblatt KA, Thomas DB. Hormonal content of combined oral contraceptives in relation to the reduced risk of endometrial carcinoma. The WHO Collaborative Study of Neoplasia and Steroid Contraceptives. *Int J Cancer* 1991; 49:870–874.

Rossouw JE, Anderson GL, Prentice RL, LaCroix AZ, Kooperberg C, Stefanick ML, et al. Risks and benefits of estrogen plus progestin in healthy postmenopausal women: principal results From the Women's Health Initiative randomized controlled trial. *JAMA* 2002; 288:321–333.

Saxena T, Lee E, Henderson KD, Clarke CA, West D, Marshall SF, et al. Menopausal hormone therapy and subsequent risk of specific invasive breast cancer subtypes in the California Teachers Study. *Cancer Epidemiol Biomarkers Prev* 2010; 19:2366–2378.

Shema L, Ore L, Ben-Shachar M, Haj M, Linn S. The association between breastfeeding and breast cancer occurrence among Israeli Jewish women: a case control study. *J Cancer Res Clin Oncol* 2007; 133:539–546.

Sprague BL, Trentham-Dietz A, Remington PL. The contribution of postmenopausal hormone use cessation to the declining incidence of breast cancer. *Cancer Causes Control* 2011; 22:125–134.

Titus-Ernstoff L, Rees JR, Terry KL, Cramer DW. Breast-feeding the last born child and risk of ovarian cancer. *Cancer Causes Control* 2010; 21:201–207.

Tsilidis KK, Allen NE, Key TJ, Dossus L, Kaaks R, Bakken K, et al. Menopausal hormone therapy and risk of ovarian cancer in the European prospective investigation into cancer and nutrition. *Cancer Causes Control* 2011a; 22:1075–1084.

Tsilidis KK, Allen NE, Key TJ, Dossus L, Lukanova A, Bakken K, et al. Oral contraceptive use and reproductive factors and risk of ovarian cancer in the European Prospective Investigation into Cancer and Nutrition. *Br J Cancer* 2011b; 105:1436–1442.

Tsilidis KK, Allen NE, Key TJ, Sanjoaquin MA, Bakken K, Berrino F, et al. Menopausal hormone therapy and risk of colorectal cancer in the European Prospective Investigation into Cancer and Nutrition. *Int J Cancer* 2011c; 128:1881–1889.

Tung KH, Goodman MT, Wu AH, McDuffie K, Wilkens LR, Kolonel LN, et al. Reproductive factors and epithelial ovarian cancer risk by histologic type: a multiethnic case-control study. *Am J Epidemiol* 2003; 158:629–638.

U.S.Preventive Services Task Force. Summaries for patients. Hormone therapy to prevent chronic conditions in postmenopausal women: recommendations from the U.S. Preventive Services Task Force. *Ann Intern Med* 2005; 142:I59.

Vessey M, Yeates D, Flynn S. Factors affecting mortality in a large cohort study with special reference to oral contraceptive use. *Contraception* 2010; 82:221–229.

Wernli KJ, Newcomb PA, Hampton JM, Trentham-Dietz A, Egan KM. Hormone therapy and ovarian cancer: incidence and survival. *Cancer Causes Control* 2008; 19:605–613.

Yang CY, Kuo HW, Chiu HF. Age at first birth, parity, and risk of death from ovarian cancer in Taiwan: a country of low incidence of ovarian cancer. *Int J Gynecol Cancer* 2007; 17:32–36.

Zucchetto A, Serraino D, Polesel J, Negri E, De PA, Dal ML, et al. Hormone-related factors and gynecological conditions in relation to endometrial cancer risk. *Eur J Cancer Prev* 2009; 18:316–321.

Chapter 11
Controlling Environmental Causes of Cancer

Paolo Vineis

11.1 Introduction

The generally long life expectancy experienced by Western populations owes much to the advent of large-scale public health measures in sanitation during the nineteenth century. This led to a dramatic decrease in infectious diseases and marked gain in population health. Can such a dramatic improvement be achievable for today's predominant diseases on a global scale and specifically for cancer? In overviews concerning 'environmental cancers' (see, e.g. Boffetta 2006; Boffetta et al. 2007; Doll and Peto 1981; Prüss-Üstün and Corvalan 2006; Vineis and Xun 2009; World Health Organization 2002), the definition of 'environmental' can vary considerably in terms of the list of exposures considered due to differences in inclusion criteria. The methodological difficulties encountered in the investigation of environmental causes of disease are often neglected in these publications, which in addition tend to focus mainly or exclusively on Western populations. In this chapter, I will summarize some of the evidence concerning environmental risks of cancer in both low-income and high-income countries and discuss methodological issues with particular emphasis on policy and control.

P. Vineis (✉)
Centre for Environment and Health,
School of Public Health, Imperial College,
511 5th Floor, Medical School, St Mary's Campus, London, UK
e-mail: p.vineis@imperial.ac.uk

A.B. Miller (ed.), *Epidemiologic Studies in Cancer Prevention and Screening*, Statistics for Biology and Health 79, DOI 10.1007/978-1-4614-5586-8_11,

11.2 Estimates for Environmentally Related Cancer Burden in Low-Income Countries

For a long time, it has been claimed that most chronic diseases have an environmental origin (using the term 'environment' in a broad sense). This claim was based on descriptive data showing the broad range of incidence rates in different parts of the world, the rapid temporal changes—such as those currently occurring in China and India—and the crucial observation of incidence rates in migrant populations. The latter unequivocally showed that migrants rapidly acquire—sometimes already in the first generation after migration—the risk of disease that is typical of the population where they move.

The interpretations of the word 'environment' differ between researchers: for example, in the 'gene–environment interaction' field, by environment researchers just mean nongenetic (inherited) determinants.

A recent document released by WHO (Prüss-Üstün and Corvalan 2006) has estimated the worldwide risk for different diseases attributable to environmental exposures. The proposed value for cancer was 19 % on the basis of previously published results and expert opinions. Conversely, Boffetta et al. (2007), from the International Agency for Research on Cancer (a WHO agency), proposed a much more conservative figure of ~ 1–3 %. What is surprising is not only the large discrepancy between the two estimates but also the general lack of sound information behind the figures, especially for developing countries. In fact, Boffetta et al. (2007) extrapolated their global estimate from a figure that was originally proposed by Doll and Peto (1981) for the United States in the late 1970s.

With a colleague we have published an overview of the cancer burden due to environmental exposures in low-income countries (Vineis and Xun 2009). This topic is usually neglected and it offers room for methodological considerations. For the sake of clarity, I will use here the term environment in a restricted way, meaning 'pollutants' of air, food, water and soil. I am thus excluding many nongenetic external causes, like tobacco smoking, alcohol and dietary habits. I will also exclude occupational exposures for which considerable work has already been done (Pearce et al. 1994). For the same reason, I exclude infectious or parasitic causes of cancer, which explain ~ 15 % of all cancers (a figure that is based on sound evidence Pisani et al. 1997).

In our chapter, we focused on prospective cohort studies whenever possible. Controversial exposures with limited evidence were also exempt from our overview; such examples include electromagnetic fields (Wakeford 2004), nonoccupational exposure to pesticides (Alavanja and Bonner 2005; Alavanja et al. 2007), disinfection by-products (Villanueva et al. 2007) and exposure to solvents (except benzene) (Lynge et al. 1997). Although considerable evidence does exist for some of these exposures, it often comes predominantly from case–control studies and is therefore less persuasive than prospective cohort studies. We have also excluded UV light, although it is a well-established carcinogen, and focused on chemical exposures.

The conclusion of our work was that the burden of cancers due to environmental exposures in developing countries is unknown, but it can sum up to several hundred thousands of cases if we just limit our estimates to the main known carcinogenic exposures (arsenic, air pollution, aflatoxin, PCB, asbestos) (Vineis and Xun 2009). The effects of additional exposures such as metals (chromium, cadmium, nickel, beryllium) and other known human carcinogens are difficult to quantify because virtually no information is available on the number of exposed people.

The development of an effective strategy to prevent environmental cancer, particularly in low-income countries, goes beyond the scope of this chapter. However, it is clear that such a strategy involves (1) a survey of the number of people potentially exposed in developing countries, (2) a strict international policy about transfer of hazardous contaminants from developed to developing countries and (3) an international programme for early detection of potential carcinogens through in vitro tests and animal experiments.

11.3 Low Doses and Acquired Susceptibility to Disease

Most environmental exposures in high-income countries (with significant exceptions) are at low or very low doses, in contrast with low-income countries. In the 1970s and 1980s, many researchers thought it was impossible to detect plausible causal associations with such low-level exposures. The underlying idea was that 'noise' (bias, confounding) was larger than the signal. However, a large number of well-conducted studies have been published since: in the case of second-hand tobacco smoke, more than 60 studies show (with few exceptions) increased risks of lung cancer in the order of 1.25, that is, the same magnitude as the gene for the nicotine acetylcholine receptor (Lynge et al. 1997; Vineis et al. 2007). For air pollution, an association with lung cancer has been reported in six cohort studies. One of these studies is sufficiently large as to show the association in non-smokers (Vineis et al. 2007). Again, the relative risk is around 1.25. In both cases, biomarkers for second-hand smoke, such as cotinine or nicotine-derived nitrosamine ketone (NNK), and DNA adducts as a marker for air pollution have contributed to make the association more plausibly causal.

In recent studies, it has also been possible to identify clear associations between second-hand smoke, air pollution and cardiovascular disease. Again, these are well-conducted cohort studies, and biomarkers have substantiated the epidemiological observations. We have thus to acknowledge that second-hand smoke and air pollution (mainly due to traffic exhaust) are able to induce, after long-term exposure, chronic diseases such as cancer and coronary artery disease. The interesting observation is that this happens at dose levels that are much lower than those of mainstream tobacco smoke or 'classical' carcinogens. For example, exposure to second-hand smoke occurs at levels that are 1/100 compared to active smoking.

One potential explanation for the effects of extremely low doses and the absence of a threshold is based on acquired susceptibility and the cumulative effects of different exposures. As defined by Rothman and Greenland (1998), 'the cause of a disease event is an antecedent event, condition or characteristic that was necessary (given that all other conditions are fixed) for the occurrence of the disease at the moment it occurred'. Said in other words, a cause can also be viewed as something that 'completes an incomplete causal chain'(Vineis and Kriebel 2006) or precipitates a chain of events which creates a state of vulnerability. Exposure to low levels of, for example, second-hand smoke or air pollution is not a 'cause' of cancer in itself (like an accident is the cause of a death), but possibly because it occurs on top of pre-existing vulnerability. This could well explain why small changes in environmental exposures can have big effects, if they occur in a population of vulnerable subjects.

Vulnerability can be acquired or genetically based. The concept of acquired 'clinical vulnerability' is related to previous insults/pathophysiological changes that predispose to disease. An example is the finding of a greater effect of second-hand smoke among ex-smokers compared to never smokers in a large prospective investigation (Vineis et al. 2005a). It is plausible that ex-smokers have a greater vulnerability because of already existing mutations or epigenetic changes, so that further exposure to second-hand smoke leads to selection and clonal expansion of mutated cells.

Another type of vulnerability (more often called susceptibility) is genetically determined. Many years ago we showed that subjects with the genetically based NAT2 slow acetylator genotype could have greater susceptibility to being damaged by tobacco smoke-related arylamines at lower levels of exposure rather than at higher levels (Vineis et al. 1994). Our reasoning was that on very rare occasions, for example, among people exposed to extremely high doses of potent carcinogens, the whole population or a vast majority develops cancer. This is what happened among British chemical workers exposed to 2-naphthylamine in the 1950s and before. For example, all 15 workers exposed to 2-naphthylamine in a plant developed bladder cancer, probably the only known example of a 'sufficient' exposure in the history of carcinogenesis (Case et al. 1954). It is clear that in that case genetic susceptibility was totally irrelevant. In the vast majority of situations, however, people are exposed to moderate/low doses of carcinogens, and—as we have suggested—individual susceptibility can then become relevant. How genetic information on individual susceptibility can be included into public health practice is still contentious and raises ethical issues (Vineis et al. 2005b), as the recent lively debate in the Journal of Public Health, stimulated by a paper by Zimmern (2011), clearly suggests.

11.4 Methodological Issues

Most epidemiological estimates are based on surrogate markers of exposure, such as through questionnaire interviews. It is not surprising that such measures can lead to inaccurate estimates. Although bias can occur in both directions (i.e. overestimations as well as underestimations are possible), the most likely implication of inaccuracy is underestimation of the risks.

When methods of biomarker measurements become available to improve accuracy in exposure assessments, estimates of risk for the same risk factors can increase substantially. For example, when sexual habits were used as a surrogate to investigate the relationships between human papilloma virus (HPV) infection and sexual habits, the relative risks for cervical cancer were estimated to be in between 2 and 8. This increased to up to 500 when specific strains of HPV were considered (Schiffman et al. 2007).

Some human cancers may take 20–30 years or longer from the time of first exposure to clinical manifestation. Waiting for high incidence of such cancers is not an ethically acceptable method for identifying human carcinogens.

11.5 Alternatives to Epidemiology: Research in Animals, Biomarkers and Omics

For the reasons described above, Lorenzo Tomatis, former director of the International Agency for Research on Cancer (IARC), proposed in the 1970s that prevention of human cancer could not rely on epidemiology alone and promoted research in animals as a surrogate for research in humans. The IARC Monographs are the most prestigious instrument for cancer prevention, thanks to their sound scientific methodology, and besides human epidemiological evidence rely heavily on research in animals for the categorization of carcinogens. This is illustrated in the case of 1,3-butadiene, whose carcinogenicity was confirmed by a review of the Working Group of the IARC Monographs in 2007 (Grosse et al. 2007). More than 20 years ago, experiments in rodents showed that this widely used chemical induced cancers at multiple organ sites, including a very high incidence of otherwise extremely rare cancers (e.g. heart hemangiosarcomas). Also an excess of lymphopoietic cancers was found in animals. There was no doubt that the chemical was a potent animal carcinogen, given the consistency of the observations, the presence of a dose–response relationship, the unusual type of tumours induced and the very high incidence. Even today, we still lack a satisfactory number of sound epidemiological studies capable of confirming these observations in humans. The results from the available studies, however, are remarkably consistent with animal studies, at least for lymphopoietic tumours, given the considerable difficulties encountered in such investigations.

11.6 The Strategies of Public Health

As has been brilliantly suggested by Nancy Cartwright, there are three equally important elements in the decisional process: *quality of the evidence, relevance and evaluation* (Cartwright N, Personal Communication, 2010). This applies also to public health. It is well known that sometimes extremely sophisticated and accurate knowledge is totally irrelevant for the population's health, while at least as often we lack essential knowledge in crucial areas of public's protection.

Geoffrey Rose (Rose 1985, 1992) set out the main advantages and disadvantages of a 'high-risk group' preventive strategy. In Rose's words, this is a strategy with some clear and important advantages: the 'high-risk' strategy produces interventions that are appropriate to the particular individuals identified and consequently has the advantage of enhanced subject motivation; it also offers a more cost-effective use of limited resources and a more favourable ratio of benefits to risks. When the outcome we want to prevent (i.e. an environmentally caused disease) is frequent (e.g. in a high-risk group) the number needed to treat (in fact, the number needed to prevent, see below) is particularly low, a well-known property of public health interventions. Also, the frequency of harm tends to be constant irrespective of the frequency of the outcome, though harm is uncommon with primary prevention. Therefore, the benefit/risk ratio is particularly favourable for high-risk groups.

Despite these advantages, the 'high-risk' strategy of prevention has some serious disadvantages and limitations. Firstly, one is likely to meet problems with compliance, and the tendency is for the response to be greatest among those who are often least at risk of the disease; this, however, may be true for voluntary exposures but not necessarily for environmental exposures. There is another related reason why the effectiveness of the 'high-risk' strategy of prevention could be weak. This is well illustrated by data which relate breast cancer to parity and other reproductive factors. High-risk women generate a relatively small proportion of the cases, too few to justify pre-screening for the identification of selected women to whom to offer mammography. The lesson from this example—and many others—is that a large number of people at smaller risk may give rise to more cases of disease than the small number who are at a high risk. This situation seems to be common, and it limits the utility of the 'high-risk' approach to prevention. Combined with the first disadvantage mentioned—that is, the fact that those who are most likely to change their behaviour or seek treatment are often those at least risk—implies that the effectiveness of the high-risk strategy as a public health measure may be significantly lower than expected.

11.7 Number Needed to Prevent

One important property of prevention is that the NNP (number needed to prevent one case of disease) can be lower than 1. This situation does not occur with therapies (number needed to treat) or with screening (number needed to screen), for which the relevant measures are always greater than 1. It occurs in primary prevention when a relatively limited preventive action has an impact that goes beyond those who are directly affected by it, for example, by an indirect fallout. The typical example is *herd immunity*: vaccinating a relatively limited number of subjects prevents the disease in many more, for example, by vaccinating 10 we save 100. Similarly, banning smoking in public places has a positive effect not only on those potentially exposed to second-hand smoke (the target population) but also on smokers, who will smoke less. Even more extreme is the case of a limitation of CO_2 emissions in developed countries that would lead to big advantages (avoidance of the consequences of climate change) in the large populations of developing countries. Zulman et al. (2008) have considered how the NNT helps disentangle the efficacies of different public health strategies, including focused strategies aimed at high-risk groups vs. unfocused strategies aimed at the general population. They notice that a population-based intervention is a good option (in terms of NNT, though it should be more adequately called NNP) if there are no adverse effects, while a targeted approach may prevent more deaths while treating fewer people if adverse effects are present.

11.8 Conclusions

To be able to estimate the 'cancer burden' due to environmental carcinogens and to implement complete and effective preventive strategies for environmental carcinogens, we need better and larger studies that overcome the serious problem of misclassification of exposures. However, this is not the main point. What we dramatically lack is a detailed and updated knowledge of exposure to known carcinogens (who, where and to what concentrations there is exposure), particularly in low-income countries; a systematic plan for action; and huge investments in both occupational settings and the general environment to get rid of carcinogens according to a precautionary philosophy.

References

Alavanja MC, Bonner MR. Pesticides and human cancers. *Cancer Invest* 2005; 23:700–711.

Alavanja MC, Ward MH, Reynolds P. Carcinogenicity of agricultural pesticides in adults and children. *J Agromedicine* 2007; 12:39–56.

Boffetta P. Human cancer from environmental pollutants: the epidemiological evidence. *Mutat Res* 2006; 608:157–162

Boffetta P, McLaughlin JK, la Vecchia C, Autier P, Boyle P. 'Environment' in cancer causation and etiological fraction: limitations and ambiguities. *Carcinogenesis* 2007; 28:913–915.

Case RA, Hosker ME, Mc DD, Pearson JT. Tumours of the urinary bladder in workmen engaged in the manufacture and use of certain dyestuff intermediates in the British chemical industry. I. The role of aniline, benzidine, alpha-naphthylamine, and beta-naphthylamine. *Br J Ind Med* 1954; 11:75–104.

Doll R, Peto R. *The Causes of Cancer. Quantitative Estimates of Avoidable Risks of Cancer in the United States Today*. 1981. Oxford: Oxford University Press

Grosse Y, Baan R, Straif K, Secretan B, El Ghissassi F, Bouvard V et al. Carcinogenicity of 1,3-butadiene, ethylene oxide, vinyl chloride, vinyl fluoride, and vinyl bromide. *Lancet Oncol* 2007; 8:679–680.

Lynge E, Anttila A, Hemminki K. Organic solvents and cancer. *Cancer Causes Control* 1997; 8:406–419.

Pearce N, Matos E, Boffetta P, Kogevinas M, Vainio H. Occupational exposures to carcinogens in developing countries. *Ann Acad Med Singapore* 1994; 23:684–689.

Pisani P, Parkin DM, Munoz N, Ferlay J. Cancer and infection: estimates of the attributable fraction in 1990. *Cancer Epidemiol Biomarkers Prev* 1997; 6:387–400.

Prüss-Üstün A, Corvalan C. *Preventing Disease through Health Environments. Towards an Estimate of the Environmental Burden of Disease.* 2006. Geneva: World Health Organization.
Rose G. Sick individuals and sick populations. *Int J Epidemiol* 1985; 14:32–38.
Rose G. *The strategy of preventive medicine.* 1992; Oxford: Oxford University Press
Rothman K, Greenland S. *Modern Epidemiology*, 3rd edition 1998; Lippincott Williams & Wilkins
Schiffman M, Castle PE, Jeronimo J, Rodriguez AC, Wacholder S. Human papillomavirus and cervical cancer. *Lancet* 2007; 370:890–907.
Villanueva CM, Cantor KP, Grimalt JO, Malats N, Silverman D, Tardon A et al. Bladder cancer and exposure to water disinfection by-products through ingestion, bathing, showering, and swimming in pools. *Am J Epidemiol* 2007; 165:148–156.
Vineis P, Airoldi L, Veglia F, Olgiati L, Pastorelli R, Autrup H et al. Environmental tobacco smoke and risk of respiratory cancer and chronic obstructive pulmonary disease in former smokers and never smokers in the EPIC prospective study. *BMJ* 2005a; 330:277–280.
Vineis P, Ahsan H, Parker M. Genetic screening and occupational and environmental exposures. *Occup Environ Med.* 2005b; 62:657–662.
Vineis P, Bartsch H, Caporaso N, Harrington AM, Kadlubar FF, Landi MT et al. Genetically based N-acetyltransferase metabolic polymorphism and low-level environmental exposure to carcinogens. *Nature* 1994; 369:154–156.
Vineis P, Hoek G, Krzyzanowski M, Vigna-Taglianti F, Veglia F, Airoldi L et al. Lung cancers attributable to environmental tobacco smoke and air pollution in non-smokers in different European countries: a prospective study. *Environ Health* 2007;6: 7.
Vineis P, Kriebel D. Causal models in epidemiology: past inheritance and genetic future. *Environ Health* 2006; 5:21.
Vineis P, Xun W. The emerging epidemic of environmental cancers in developing countries. *Ann Oncol* 2009; 20:205–212.
Wakeford R. The cancer epidemiology of radiation. *Oncogene* 2004; 23:6404–6428.
World Health Organization. *The World Health Report 2002: Reducing Risks, Promoting Healthy Life.* 2002; Geneva.
Zimmern RL. Genomics and individuals in public health practice: are we luddites or can we meet the challenge? *J Publ Health* 2011; 33:477–482.
Zulman DM, Vijan S, Omenn GS, Hayward RA. The relative merits of population-based and targeted prevention strategies. *Milbank Q* 2008; 86:557–580.

Chapter 12
A Historical Moment: Cancer Prevention on the Global Health Agenda

Andreas Ullrich

12.1 Introduction

Primary prevention of cancer includes comprehensive cancer risk-reduction strategies which cover a broad variety of exposures from lifestyle factors such as tobacco use, some viral infections such as HBV and HPV and environmental and occupational carcinogens. Reducing these risks requires a large variety of interventions which only in part can be delivered by health systems with regard to some specific interventions for cancer prevention such as vaccination or tobacco cessation. Changing lifestyles requires individual and collective changes in societies which can only be achieved by involving a large variety of stakeholders, governmental, non-governmental and the private sector. Governmental engagement and commitment beyond the health sector and across mostly all sectors is required so that cancer prevention is effective.

The World Health Organization's (WHO) non-communicable disease (NCD) framework and action plan groups the four major chronic conditions cardiovascular disease, diabetes, chronic obstructive pulmonary disease and cancers and their risk factors in order to bundle global risk-reduction strategies. The starting point for any WHO guidance is the evidence about what causes diseases and which strategies are proven to be effective to control them. This applies also to WHO's cancer prevention strategies. By creating the WHO specialized research agency, the International Agency for Research on Cancer (IARC) four decades ago, the World Health Assembly was visionary in its endeavour to increase knowledge about cancer prevention, which now with the steady increase of the cancer burden all over the

Based on a speech at the occasion of the international cancer control congress Marrakesh/Morocco in January 2012. http://www.contrelecancer.ma/fr/marrakech-call

A. Ullrich, MD MPH (✉)
Department of Chronic Diseases and Health Promotion (CHP),
World Health Organization Cancer Control Programme,
Avenue Appia 20, CH – 1211 Geneva 27, Switzerland
e-mail: ullricha@who.int

A.B. Miller (ed.), *Epidemiologic Studies in Cancer Prevention and Screening*, Statistics for Biology and Health 79, DOI 10.1007/978-1-4614-5586-8_12,

world is so much needed. IARC has set international standards in identifying cancer risks and strategies to prevent and detect cancers early. Much of the knowledge generated by IARC was the foundation for strategies, for example, to prevent tobacco use.

12.2 Cancer Prevention in the Context of National Cancer Control Plans and the WHO NCD Action Plan

Nearly two decades ago, WHO developed a policy framework known as the National Cancer Control Programme (NCCP) concept (WHO 1995). Crucially, this framework addresses the full continuum of care from primary prevention, early detection including screening, diagnosis and treatment, through to palliative care. In terms of public health actions, NCCPs encompass population interventions for prevention/screening as well as healthcare system-strengthening aspects, so that cancer patients get optimal care. In accordance with this framework, national cancer control planners need to work from both ends of the health system, taking in a healthcare system perspective as well as a population-based social medicine perspective. All the known causes of cancer such as tobacco, infectious carcinogens or radiation require national policies and strategies to reduce population exposure. By these means, the burden of cancer could be substantially reduced. Tobacco control is advocated as an integral part of national cancer plans, so that professional organizations involved in cancer control (e.g. oncologists, radiotherapists and surgeons) might consider it as part of their role and in their interaction with patients and their families. Encouragingly, many countries have started to develop national cancer plans. These plans are greatly dependent upon national health priorities, background cancer risks and available resources. However, WHO recommends that even in very low-resource settings, prevention should be part of national cancer plans.

NCCPs are embedded in a broader overall NCD action plan developed through several steps of consultations with WHO Member States and stakeholders and was endorsed by the World Health Assembly (WHO 2008a). The WHO NCD action plan is the result of a broad consensus among governmental and non-governmental stakeholders. The action plan defines the roles WHO Member States and non-governmental organizations will play in reducing the NCD burden. It also gives an overview of the technical areas which need to be tackled so that risk-reduction strategies and service delivery for NCD cure and care are both addressed. From the cancer prevention perspective, the generic NCD framework needs to be translated into the specificities of what causes cancers and what are the strategies to reduce population and individual exposure to those cancer risks which go beyond the shared behavioural risks with other NCDs. This NCD action plan encompasses a set of six objectives which are aimed at halting the NCD epidemic. The development of national NCD plans (Objective 2) and implementing NCD prevention strategies (Objective3) are central elements of the NCD framework. The action plan 2008 has a timeframe for implementation until 2013. A follow-up action plan is under development by following the same principles of stakeholder involvement as in the first period.

12.3 The WHO Behavioural Risk-Reduction Policies and Strategies and Related Tools

Over the last decade and starting from a first generic NCD framework in 2000, WHO has accomplished a series of milestones in population-based risk-reduction strategies for NCDs. The WHO secretariat put forward and obtained endorsement by the World Health Assembly in 2003 for the tobacco control strategy as the WHO Framework Convention on Tobacco Control (FCTC), in 2004 for the global strategy on diet and physical activity and in 2010 the global alcohol control strategy.

The FCTC is the first global health treaty. This legally binding convention came into force in 2005 and its implementation is coordinated by the FCTC secretariat hosted by WHO headquarters. As of April 2012, national parliaments of 174 WHO Member States have ratified the FCTC becoming contracting parties to the treaty.[1] The FCTC provides new legal dimensions for tobacco control. It is a comprehensive approach since it includes mechanisms for demand and supply reduction of tobacco products. Price and tax policies, labelling of tobacco products and protection from exposure to second-hand smoke, that is, promoting smoke-free environments, are evidence-based strategies to reduce demand which are included in the FCTC. Central elements of demand and cancer risk reduction are smoking cessation programmes for current smokers (quit lines, treatment of nicotine dependency). Supply reduction policies include measures to reduce illicit trade in tobacco products (smuggling), banning sales to minors and encouraging alternatives to tobacco growing in the agriculture sector. Although in force for several years, the implementation of the FCTC has still a long way to go. According to the most recent report, only 5 % of the world population was covered by smoke-free environments, 8 % by cessation programmes, 8 % by tobacco health warnings, 9 % by advertising bans and 6 % by taxation on tobacco products (WHO 2008b).

The WHO Global Strategy on Diet, Physical Activity and Health (DPAS) is a prevention-based strategy that aims to significantly reduce the prevalence of common risk factors, primarily unhealthy diet and physical inactivity for NCDs (WHO 2003).

Its overall objectives are to increase awareness and understanding of the relationships between diet, physical activity and NCDs including cancer. DPAS provides the framework to develop, strengthen and implement global, regional, national policies and action with the intent to reduce obesity, unhealthy diet and physical inactivity in populations through public health actions. DPAS is underpinned

[1] Updates of the implementation of the FCTC are online. (http://www.who.int/fctc/signatories_parties/en/index.html)

by a series of WHO guidelines which have a specific focus on the prevention of childhood obesity since this is linked closely to future obesity levels in adulthood.

The WHO global strategy to reduce harmful use of alcohol focuses on a series of ten key areas of policy options and interventions at the national level and four priority areas for global action WHO (2011a). These include drink-driving policies and countermeasures, policies on the availability of alcohol and the marketing of alcoholic beverages. The four priority areas for global action are public health advocacy and partnership, technical support and capacity building, production and dissemination of knowledge.

12.4 The WHO Specific Cancer Risk-Reduction Policies and Strategies and Related Tools: Infections and Environmental Causes

A series of risk factors are not shared with other NCDs and are less determined by individual choices (see Tanaka, this volume). These are infectious causes of cancer such as HBV and HPV both causally related to specific cancer types, HBV to hepatocellular carcinoma (HCC) and HPV to cervical cancer. Vaccination against HBV is part of the WHO expanded programme of immunization (EPI). A more comprehensive approach to prevent hepatitis has been requested by the World Health Assembly. WHO is in the process of developing a hepatitis prevention and control strategy which, further to immunization, encompasses measures to prevent HBV infections through patient safety measures.[2]

With the recent progress in development and availability of HPV vaccines (see Bosch, this volume), WHO has taken the firm position to recommend the introduction of HPV vaccines as part of comprehensive cervical cancer prevention and control plans which also should include cervical screening. A series of technical documents provide hands-on guidance for national decision-makers to rationally plan and implement HPV vaccine programmes.[3]

Preventing HIV infections can also be subsumed among cancer prevention interventions as HIV and cancer are closely related. HIV-positive populations are at increased risk of developing a large variety of cancers. WHO's guidance on sexual education and the prevention of sexually transmitted diseases is therefore an important component in comprehensive cancer prevention and opens up cross-links and options for integration between programmes.

Exposure to carcinogenic chemicals in the environment can occur through drinking water or pollution of indoor and ambient air. Exposure to carcinogens also occurs via the contamination of food by chemicals, including aflatoxins or dioxins. Aflatoxin is a cofactor together with HBV infection in the carcinogenesis of HCC.

[2] http://www.who.int/csr/disease/hepatitis/en/

[3] http://www.who.int/nuvi/hpv/resources/en/

Indoor air pollution from coal fires increases the risk of lung cancer, particularly among women.

With regard to occupational exposure, a great variety of agents, mixtures and exposure circumstances in the working environment are classified by IARC as carcinogenic (and see Blair et al., this volume). Occupational cancers are concentrated among specific groups of the working population, for whom the risk of developing a particular form of cancer may be much higher than for the general population. For example, mesothelioma is to a large extent caused by work-related exposure to asbestos.

It is well known that ionizing radiation due to environmental or medical diagnostic and therapeutic exposure is carcinogenic to humans. Ionizing radiation can induce leukaemia and a number of solid tumours, with higher risks at young age of exposure. Residential exposure to radon gas from soil and building materials can cause lung cancers, making it the second cause of lung cancer after tobacco smoke.[4]

Ultraviolet (UV) radiation, and in particular solar radiation, is carcinogenic to humans, causing all major types of skin cancer, such as basal cell carcinoma (BCC), squamous cell carcinoma (SCC) and melanoma. Avoiding excessive exposure, use of sunscreen and protective clothing are effective preventive measures. UV-emitting tanning devices are now also classified as carcinogenic to humans based on their association with skin and ocular melanoma cancers (IARC 2012).

WHO is promoting evidence-based exposure reduction strategies to reduce environmental and occupational cancer risks such as guidance in improving ventilation and sealing of floors to reduce radon levels in homes. Reducing exposure is effective if food safety systems (i.e. legislation and monitoring) are implemented focusing on key contaminants of food which can cause cancers. The reduction of the use of biomass and coal for heating and cooking at home and promotion of the use of clean burning and efficient stoves is a powerful tool to reduce the burden of lung cancer burden in particular among women.

12.5 The UN Political Declaration on Non-communicable Diseases (NCDs) and Implications for Cancer Prevention

One of the many factors which contributed to put NCDs including cancer on the agenda of the UN General Assembly in September 2011 was the increased awareness and knowledge about the current and projected future burden of NCDs as well as their economic impact. Driven by population ageing, unplanned urbanization, globalization of trade and marketing, the unhealthy lifestyles that fuel the NCD epidemic are spreading rapidly. At the microeconomic level, there is a spiral of poverty caused by NCDs/cancer which affects more and more families which ends up in catastrophic expenditures for NCD cure and care because of insufficient insurance coverage. At the macroeconomic level, NCD care requires an increasing proportion of health budgets in low- and middle-income countries. The productivity

[4] http://www.who.int/ionizing_radiation/en/

loss due to NCD-related mortality and impairments affects economies in low- and middle-income countries in particular where 16 % of the overall mortality is due to NCDs below the age of 60. With WHO providing the global picture on NCD burden and trends, the political will to tackle NCDs became a momentum. The political determination of a group of UN Member States lead by the Caribbean Community of countries (CARICOM) finally reached its objective in 2011 to discuss the problem of NCDs at the highest political level as was the case for HIV a decade earlier.

In preparing the background documents for the UN General Assembly High-level Meeting (HLM) on NCDs, WHO focused on the cost-effectiveness of the interventions to be proposed as solutions for controlling NCDs. The concept of 'best buys'—defined as the interventions with the most extensive health impact by monetary unit invested—was highly promoted and condensed in one of the key publications available to the event (WHO 2011b).

Among the selected interventions included in the 'best buys', two of them are specifically relevant for cancer prevention: screening for cervical cancer and immunization against HBV infection to prevent liver cancer.

The UN HLM resulted in a political declaration[5] which expresses the firm commitment of the signing UN Member States to develop national NCD strategies along the lines of WHO's technical advice. Fundamental to the declaration was the World Health Assembly resolutions on risk-reduction strategies (tobacco, diet, physical inactivity and alcohol) and well as the NCD action plan framework. Cancer prevention is covered by the UN resolution with regard to these behavioural factors. However, there are several entry points in the resolution which are providing bridges to infectious and environmental causes and related health systems delivering preventive interventions. Operative paragraph 43/j makes reference to the infectious cause of cancer and the call for increase in vaccination against HBV. In operative 43/k, the declaration mentions screening as an important intervention to control NCDs. Among all NCDs, cancer screening is the most established intervention which in the case of cervical cancer is also preventive since it is focusing on precancer (see the chapters of Hakama and Broutet). The cross-link between cancer prevention and reproductive health is specifically mentioned in operative paragraphs 45/r and 45/o. To translate these intentions as expressed in the declaration into practice, cancer prevention programmes in settings where infectious causes are of major importance such as in high HIV prevalence countries will need to build upon existing systems with focus at the primary care level or equivalent (reproductive health, anti-HIV programmes).

12.6 Conclusion

The UN HLM declaration provides a historical opportunity for improved agenda setting for cancer control. In the past, high-income countries have reacted to the increasing NCD burden through massive investment in healthcare systems.

[5] http://www.who.int/nmh/events/un_ncd_summit2011/en/index.html

This applies in particular to cancer. Nevertheless, by prioritizing heath care, high-income countries have paid less attention to dealing with the underlying causes. This 'model' is apparently a solution neither for high- nor low- and middle-income countries. Due to the WHO's continuous efforts over the last decade, it is now well accepted that NCD prevention needs to be an integral part of controlling NCDs. It is also more and more recognized that NCDs including cancers are also a problem in low- and middle-income countries. The globalization of markets has the consequence that NCD risks are spreading worldwide. The WHO has a key role to play in the NCD agenda because of its technical expertise and the credibility afforded to it by its UN mandate. WHO is the independent broker able to catalyze the necessary changes in societies through national and international decision-making and priority setting. These key turning points are related to tobacco control, halting the epidemic of overweight/obesity, increasing physical activity and limiting alcohol use.

To tackle NCDs and their underlying causes is complex and difficult because of the close relationship between risk factors, market forces, social and economic development and health outcomes. NCDs appear on the global health agenda to many as still less menacing compared to communicable diseases, as countries may experience acute outbreaks of conditions due to contagious agents. As a consequence, for decades NCDs were considered as a problem restricted to affluent societies and were therefore 'invisible' as a development issue. The agreement of all UN Member States on a joint political declaration would not have been possible if developing countries had not already perceived the NCD burden as a major threat to their public health and economies. The historical window for setting the pace to address NCDs needs now to be used so that the necessary changes at the global, regional and national health agendas are implemented.

References

IARC *A Review of Human Carcinogens: Radiation.* IARC Monographs on the Evaluation of Carcinogenic Risks to Humans, Volume 100D 2012. Lyon, International Agency for Research on Cancer.

WHO *National cancer control programmes. Policies and managerial guidelines.* Miller AB, Stjernsward J (eds). 1995. Geneva, World Health Organization.

WHO *Diet, nutrition and the prevention of chronic diseases.* Report of a Joint WHO/FAO Expert Consultation. WHO Technical Report Series No. 916, 2003. Geneva, World Health Organization. http://www.who.int/dietphysicalactivity/en/index.html

WHO *2008–2013 action plan for the global strategy for the prevention and control of noncommunicable diseases: prevent and control cardiovascular diseases, cancers, chronic respiratory diseases and diabetes.* 2008a. Geneva, World Health Organization.

WHO *Status of the Framework Convention on Tobacco Control.* 2008b. Geneva, World Health Organization. http://www.who.int/tobacco/en/

WHO *Global Status Report on Alcohol and Health* 2011a Geneva, World Health Organization. http://www.who.int/topics/alcohol_drinking/en/

WHO *Scaling up action against noncommunicable diseases: How much will it cost?* 2011b. Geneva, World Health Organization. http://www.who.int/nmh/publications/cost_of_inaction/en/index.html

Part II
Screening for Cancer

Chapter 13
Evidence-Based Cancer Screening

Anthony B. Miller

13.1 Introduction

Screening of asymptomatic people is one component of early detection of cancer, in the expectation that it will change the incurable patient into one that is curable by effective therapy, resulting in a reduction in the death rate from the disease and thus reduction in health-care costs. The other component of early detection is encouraging the early diagnosis of people with symptomatic cancer. Neither should be promoted unless there are adequate facilities for diagnosing people with suspicious findings and treating those who are found to have cancer. Effective therapy is essential and adequate compliance of the target population is the key to impact at the population level.

Early diagnosis is obtained through education of the target population and health-care professionals, especially at the primary care level. Education programs should be culturally sensitive, designed to dispel myths that cancer is an incurable, inevitably fatal disease; these are important in many low- and middle-income countries and even in some segments of the population in high-income countries. Education of primary care practitioners should facilitate their recognition of the signs of early cancer, which are often subtle, very different from the signs of advanced cancer. Education programs should precede the introduction of screening programs and should be an integral part of such programs.

Screening was defined by the US Commission on Chronic Illness (1957) as "the presumptive identification of unrecognized disease or defect by the application of tests, examinations or other procedures that can be applied rapidly." Although more recent definitions have been adopted (Wald 2001), this one is still probably the most useful.

A.B. Miller (✉)
Dalla Lana School of Public Health, University of Toronto,
155 College Street, Toronto, ON M5T 3M7, Canada
e-mail: ab.miller@sympatico.ca

A.B. Miller (ed.), *Epidemiologic Studies in Cancer Prevention and Screening*,
Statistics for Biology and Health 79, DOI 10.1007/978-1-4614-5586-8_13,

In screening for cancer too often the right people are not screened, many false-positive screening tests occur, the death rate from the cancer is reduced by a negligible amount, and health-care costs increased.

Part of the difficulty is that for far too many cancers, an effective screening test, acceptable to the population at risk, has not yet been developed, and even if cancer is detected "early," treatment is not as effective as hoped. However, another major difficulty is that screening is advocated under circumstances where there is no evidence that it works, and very often, the natural history of the disease is not sufficiently understood to apply screening effectively, yet such a requirement is a prerequisite for screening (Wilson and Junger 1968).

Screening is a process, and there are many components of that process that need attention if screening is to be effective (Miller 2010). In the chapters that follow in this part of the book, screening is considered for the major cancer sites in America and Europe and, increasingly, in other parts of the world. In this chapter, I shall consider some of the issues that are becoming increasingly of interest in evaluating screening at the present time.

13.2 Evaluation of Screening

Elsewhere, I and others have described the biases that can affect the evaluation of screening, especially if survival is considered (Miller 1996, 2010; Hakama this volume). The only design that eliminates the effect of these biases is the randomized screening trial (Prorok et al. 1984), but only if mortality from the disease (i.e., deaths related to the person-years of observation) is used as the endpoint rather than survival (Miller 2006). Survival could be used in a randomized screening trial only under special circumstances. These are that there is good evidence because of the equivalence in cumulative numbers of cases during the relevant period of observation that there is no overdiagnosis bias; and providing that the start of the period of observation of the cases is taken as the date of randomization, as that will eliminate differential lead time. Length bias and selection bias are not issues, the latter having been equally distributed by the randomization and the former by having started at the same point in time and by including all cases that occur during follow-up in the evaluation.

It has been suggested that because of potential biases in death attribution, all cause mortality should be used as the preferable endpoint (Black et al. 2002). Unfortunately, the sample size required to demonstrate reduction in all cause mortality as distinct from cancer site-specific mortality would be prohibitive. All cause mortality should be compared in a randomized screening trial; however, if it is identical in the screening and control arms and cancer-specific mortality is reduced in the screening arm; this suggests that there is an issue with cause of death attribution, or an adverse consequence of screening, which should be evaluated.

Outside a randomized trial, if the screening test detects a precursor, reduction in incidence of the clinically detected disease can be expected and evaluated.

This effect has been well demonstrated in the Nordic countries in relation to screening for cancer of the cervix (Hakama this volume). If the screening test does not detect a precursor, or even if it does but the main yield is invasive cancer, then the incidence can be expected to increase initially following the introduction of screening, and remain elevated while screening continues, though there may be some reduction toward the baseline after continued screening, if the application of the test results in most at risk subjects being included, and the subsequent screening tests are largely used for rescreening. Under such circumstances, when further reduction in incidence cannot be anticipated and improvement in survival cannot be relied upon because of the biases already discussed, the only valid outcome for assessment of results of a screening program is mortality from the disease in the total population offered screening.

A randomized screening trial can either be an efficacy trial or an effectiveness trial. Efficacy trials are based on randomization of the screening test, which answers the biologically relevant question as to whether mortality is reduced in those screened. An effectiveness trial is based on the randomization of invitations to attend for screening, and more nearly replicates the circumstances that may eventually pertain in practice in a population. Both those who accept the invitation as well as those who refuse will have to be included in the assessment of outcome. Thus, it tests the impact of introducing screening in a population. Some trials of this type involve randomization by cluster. However, cluster randomization can lead to difficulties in determining whether the trial results are valid, especially if it cannot be confirmed that the randomized groups were balanced or if there is evidence that they were not.

If for some reason randomization is believed inappropriate, a second-best method is the quasi-experimental study in which screening is offered in some areas and unscreened areas as comparable as possible are used for comparison purposes. However, this design is not a cheap and easy way out but demands the same methodological accuracy as required for randomized trials. Further, in view of the substantially larger populations that may have to be studied than in randomized trials, it may prove to be more expensive than the preferred design. Critically, difficulties in analysis may ensue if the baseline mortality in the comparison areas differ.

Nevertheless, ethical issues may preclude the utilization of randomized trials, particularly for programs that were introduced before the necessity of utilizing trials as far as possible for evaluation was appreciated as for screening for cancer of the cervix (Hakama this volume). One approach under these circumstances is to compare the mortality in defined populations before and after the introduction of screening programs, preferably with data available on the trends in acceptance of screening so that changes in mortality can be correlated with the mortality trends. Such a correlation study will be strengthened if other data that could be related to changes in the outcome variable are entered into a multivariate analysis (Miller et al. 1976).

A case-control study of screening is another approach that has been used to evaluate programs that were introduced sufficiently long before the study that an effect could be expected to have occurred. Case-control studies depend on comparing the screen histories of the cases with the histories of comparable controls drawn from the population from which the cases arose. Individuals with early stage disease if sampled would be eligible as a control, providing the date of diagnosis was not earlier than that of the case, as diagnosis of disease truncates the screening history. However, a bias would arise if advanced disease is compared only with early stage disease, as the latter is likely to be screen detected, though this is just a function of the screening process, not its efficacy (Weiss 1983). Cases have to reflect the end points used to evaluate screening, that is, those that would be expected to be reduced by screening. Thus, cases are often deaths from the disease or advanced disease as a surrogate for deaths, or if a precursor of the disease is detected through screening, incident cases in the population. If incident cases are screen detected, the controls should be drawn from those screened in the same program; if the cases are not screen detected, the controls should be population based (Sasco et al. 1986).

One difficulty with case-control studies of screening is that they may be affected by selection bias as the health conscious may select themselves for screening. This may be difficult to correct in the analysis, though such a correction should be attempted if the relevant data on risk factors for the disease (confounders) are available. Such a bias may not be a problem, however, in other circumstances, if it can be demonstrated that the incidence of cancer in those who declined the invitation to the screening program is similar to that expected in an unscreened population.

However, even if data are available on risk factors for disease, adjusting for them may not result in avoiding the effect of selection bias. For breast cancer, for example, experience in studies in Sweden and the UK, where case-control studies were performed within trials, shows that although those who refused invitations for screening had similar breast cancer incidence to the unscreened controls in the trial, their breast cancer mortality experience was worse than that of those controls. This meant that the estimate of the effect of screening in such case-control studies was greater than could have been expected in the total population (Miller et al. 1990; Moss 1991).

In addition to assessing effectiveness of screening, case-control studies may also be of use to assess other aspects of screening programs. For example, a method has been proposed for estimation of the natural history of preclinical disease from screening data based on case-control methodology (Brookmeyer et al. 1986). The cohort study design may also provide an estimate of the effect of screening, an approach in which the mortality from the cancer of interest in an individually identified and followed screened group (the cohort) is compared to the mortality experience in a control population, often derived from the general population. In these studies it has to be recognized that those recruited into a screening program are initially free of the disease of interest so that it is not appropriate to apply population mortality rates for the disease to the person-years experience of the study cohort. Rather, as is required in estimating the sample size required for a controlled trial of screening, it is first necessary to determine the expected incidence of the cases of interest, then apply to that expectation the expected case-fatality rate from the disease to derive the expectation for the deaths (Moss et al. 1987). In practice, a cohort study of screening suffers from the same problem of selection bias as for case-control studies, so the results have to be interpreted with caution.

Indirect indicators of effectiveness are often desired in evaluating screening programs, especially one that would predict subsequent mortality. Compliance with screening, and rate of screen detection, as well as the ratio of prevalence and incidence can be indicators of potentially effective screens (Day et al. 1989). The cumulative prevalence (not the percentage distribution) of advanced disease is one such measure (Prorok et al. 1984, and see Autier, this volume). However, case detection frequency, numbers of small tumors, and stage shift in percentages of the total should not be used as indicators of effectiveness as they potentially reflect all four screening biases.

In evaluating whether screening programs are effective in a population, different methods are generally to be used. Evaluation is an intermittent activity. It is essential for all programs to ensure that the resources used achieve the benefit expected. Process measures such as the numbers of screens performed, the numbers of positive tests reported, the number (and proportion) of those screened referred for diagnosis and therapy, the numbers of cases of disease diagnosed, and the numbers of precursor and benign lesions detected should be derivable, providing the data are collected from the screening centers and the treating institutions and collated. Such data must be analyzed by age to confirm that those in the target age group are being screened and receive appropriate subsequent management. However, such data cannot evaluate the effectiveness in terms of the likely prevention of occurrence of disease or of deaths from the disease, unless the data can be related to that derived from the total population on an ongoing basis, which requires linkage to a preexisting disease register or vital statistics system or to a register of cases of the relevant disease established for this purpose.

Depending on the endpoint that should be affected by screening, for example, deaths from the cancer of interest, the simplest form of surveillance and evaluation that will provide measures of the effectiveness of the program in the population is to be able to demonstrate a change in the slope of the trend in mortality from the disease in the population. More detailed evaluation requires the identification of all who develop the disease and die from it in the target population and documentation of their screening history. Such documentation could be done by comparing incident cases of disease in the target population with a register of those from the same population who have been screened. This will permit an estimate of the risk in those who have been screened and in those who failed to attend screening, and the combined effect can then be compared with the prescreening period. Where such registers have not been established, a screening history should be obtained from subjects with the disease, though this may not be reliable as many are unable to recall whether a screening test has been taken in the past. Efficient surveillance requires a system of linked records. A population register (or available substitute) allows periodic callback for rescreening at appropriate intervals. The screening program register, when linked with a disease register, permits the active surveillance of those detected with abnormalities, to ensure recall for diagnosis and therapy. Evaluation of the program can then be performed with regard to assessment of management of those screened with positive tests, disease diagnosed between the screening interval, and groups missed in the target population.

However, the main issue that has arisen is determining whether the program as introduced in a population has achieved the reduction in mortality from the disease in question. This is especially difficult if treatment for the disease has improved during the same period that the program was being introduced. Theoretically, this will not reduce the relative benefit of screening, but it could have a major impact on the absolute benefit derived from screening until the effect may become almost negligible (Glasziou and Houssami 2011). This situation is considered for breast screening by Autier (this volume).

13.3 Evaluating a New Screening Test for Cancer

The question this section of the chapter is seeking to address is "What is required to permit the introduction of a new screening test for a cancer for which previous research has established efficacy for another screening test for that cancer?" In other words, do we have to go through the expense and delay of a large randomized screening trial each time a new promising test becomes available? It is important to recognize that just because a test detects an early cancer, this does not necessarily mean that the individual has received benefit, that is, *case detection is not equivalent to efficacy,* for the reasons more fully set out in Miller (2010). For cancers where no efficacy has yet been established for any screening test, a new test which is introduced will have to be evaluated by means of a carefully designed randomized screening trial where the prime comparison will be between screening and no screening (Miller 2006). However, in this section I address whether demonstration of improved sensitivity of the new test compared to the old is sufficient to replace the old test by the new.

Lord et al (2006) have addressed this issue for diagnostic tests. They concluded that accuracy studies suffice if a new diagnostic test is safer or more specific than, but of similar sensitivity to, an old test. They pointed out that if a new test is more sensitive than an old test, it leads to the detection of extra cases of disease and that results from treatment trials that enrolled only patients detected by the old test may not apply to these extra cases.

Among the requirements for medical screening, Strong et al. (2005) noted these characteristics desired of an ideal screening test:

- Simple and safe
- Distributions of test values in affected and unaffected individuals known
- Cost-effective
- Acceptable to those screened

If a new screening test were to be simpler and safer than the existing test, or less costly, or shown to be more acceptable, and the distributions of test values in affected and unaffected individuals identical, as demonstrated in appropriate circumstances, it would be justifiable to substitute the new test for the old, though subsequent outcomes should be monitored to make sure there were no unintended consequences of the change. However, it is the circumstances whereby the distributions of test values in affected and unaffected individuals are determined which are of concern and which need further consideration. In practice, these distributions result in the determination of the sensitivity and specificity of the screening test. Improved specificity if sensitivity remains the same will reduce costs and could justify adopting a new test where the efficacy of the old had been demonstrated. However, the same is not necessarily true of sensitivity.

13.3.1 Determining the Sensitivity of a Screening Test

Sensitivity is defined as the proportion of those who have the disease who are positive to the test. The sensitivity of a test to be used for screening should be done within screening circumstances, not, as for a diagnostic test, among those who have already been diagnosed by other means as having the disease. In practice, the term sensitivity can have a number of connotations, as discussed by Hakama (this volume). Sometimes, an attempt is made to determine the sensitivity of a new test by applying it simultaneously with the old test in the same people, obtaining an estimate of the *relative* sensitivity of the two tests. However, this approach has a number of fundamental disadvantages. If one of the tests has the disadvantage of detecting nonprogressive lesions (overdiagnosis), a test that failed to detect these lesions might be inappropriately judged adversely. Further, it would normally be regarded as ethically indefensible to fail to act on the positive finding of any of the tests. This would mean that although the tests could be compared in terms of counts of the cases detected and the characteristic of those cases, only relative sensitivity based on screen-detected cases could be determined and an assumption that the test that detected more cases was superior could be false (Miller 2010).

Instead of such an approach, a method is needed to estimate the efficacy of the test in detecting cancers that would otherwise progress within a relatively short interval, say a year. A test with high efficiency in doing so is in fact detecting rapidly progressive cancers, cancers that are more likely to result in death than the majority of cancers detected by screening which tend to be slow growing (length bias). The method recommended is the incidence method, that is, the determination of the rate of interval cancers in comparison with the expected incidence (Day 1985). Rules will have to be developed and applied equally to identify and exclude as interval cancers those who were detected as a result of a diagnostic process initiated at the previous screen, when they should be labeled screen detected. Then the other cancers that present within the defined period before the next screen is due will be the interval cancers. The test that results in fewer such cancers is the most sensitive in detecting progressive cancers. Day (1985) described the incidence method under the circumstances when the sensitivity of a single test was being determined within the context of a randomized screening trial, as the unscreened control group provided the expected incidence in the absence of screening. However, when two screening tests are compared in a randomized screening trial, it is not necessary to know the expected incidence; the relative sensitivity of the two tests can be determined for *progressive* disease by comparing the interval cancer rates directly; the fact that we do not obtain a measure of the absolute sensitivity of the two tests is immaterial for our purpose. If the interval cancer rate following the new test is significantly less than the interval cancer rate following the old test, it can be concluded that the new test is more sensitive for progressive disease than the old. Some have objected to this method because of the need for randomization, and implicitly, twice as many subjects as when you apply the two tests in the same person. However, we should be prepared to pay this price to obtain the answer without the result being confounded by overdiagnosis.

13.3.2 The Problem of Overdiagnosis

If a randomized screening trial is performed with the immediate objective of determining the relative sensitivity of the new test compared with the old for progressive disease as just described and the sensitivity of the new test for progressive disease is demonstrated to be superior to the old, is that sufficient to justify substituting the new test for the old in routine screening programs? Unfortunately not, as there is at least one other feature of the test to estimate in order to be able to compare the cost of the management of the abnormalities detected by the two tests and especially the extent the new test results in more overdiagnosis than the old, defining overdiagnosis as the detection of disease in an individual that was not destined to progress and cause symptoms in that individual's lifetime. Although it may be possible to use some indicators of the probability of progression to obtain some indication of the probability of overdiagnosis, such as the Gleason score for prostate cancer, an overdiagnosed case may be histologically and biochemically indistinguishable from a case that is destined to progress, because of the effect of competing causes of mortality.

Overdiagnosis is probably universal for all cancer screening, even when there may be no efficacy demonstrable for the screening. If, in a randomized trial performed to assess the sensitivity for progressive disease, the cancer detection rate from screening is significantly greater for the new test than the old, the increase in detection could be due to greater lead time from the new test or increased overdiagnosis or both. If screening stops in both arms, further follow-up without screening which exceeds the lead time gained by the two tests will indicate whether all the increase is due to lead time, when the cumulative incidence becomes equal. But if the cumulative incidence in the two arms never equalize, the difference between the two cumulative incidence rates will indicate the contribution of additional overdiagnosis from the new test.

Determining the extent or even the presence of overdiagnosis of cancer when the screening test detects a presumed precursor of the cancer as well as any cancers present is very difficult. For example, incidence is reduced following screening for colorectal cancer because some of the adenomas are destined to progress to invasive cancer, and their detection and removal prevents this. The incidence gap between screened and control groups will continue to widen until the effect of such removal is spent. In this instance because of the effect of the removal of precursors, incidence of invasive cancers will be less in the screened group than the control. Nevertheless, it is still likely that some overdiagnosis of cancer is occurring; it is being masked by the removal of precursor lesions. It is also likely, by analogy with other sites, that the greater the sensitivity of the test the greater the extent of overdiagnosis. So it is likely that overdiagnosis will be greater with new tests than with the old.

13.4 Conclusions

There is no substitute for the randomized screening trial in evaluating the efficacy of screening for a cancer where, so far, efficacy of screening has not been established. Unfortunately, for a cancer where screening has already been determined to be effective, there is no definitive set of rules to decide if a new screening test should be substituted for the old. Practical issues, including acceptability to the target group and better quality control in laboratories, will tend to trump apparent improved sensitivity.

However, very careful assessment is required under these circumstances, especially in deciding whether indeed the test is more sensitive for progressive and therefore potentially fatal disease. Fortunately, a method to use is available, and hopefully this will receive much wider recognition in the future.

References

Black WC, Haggstrom DA, Welch HG. All-cause mortality in randomized trials of cancer screening. J Natl Cancer Inst. 2002;94:167–73.

Brookmeyer R, Day NE, Moss S. Case-control studies for estimation of the natural history of preclinical disease from screening data. Stat Med. 1986;5:127–38.

Commission on Chronic Illness. Chronic illness in the United States: prevention of chronic illness. Cambridge, MA: Harvard University Press; 1957.

Day NE. Evaluating the sensitivity of a screening test. J Epidemiol Community Health. 1985;39:364–6.

Day NE, Williams DRR, Khaw KT. Breast cancer screening programmes: the development of a monitoring and evaluation system. Br J Cancer. 1989;59:954–8.

Glasziou P, Houssami N. The evidence base for breast screening. Prev Med. 2011;53:100–2.

Lord SJ, Irwig L, Simes RJ. When is measuring sensitivity and specificity sufficient to evaluate a diagnostic test, and when do we need randomized trials? Ann Intern Med. 2006;144:850–5.

Miller AB. Fundamental issues in screening for cancer. In: Schottenfeld D, Fraumeni Jr JF, editors. Cancer epidemiology and prevention. 2nd ed. New York: Oxford, Oxford University Press; 1996. p. 1433–52.

Miller AB. Design of cancer screening trials/randomized trials for evaluation of cancer screening. World J Surg. 2006;30:1152–62.

Miller AB. Conundrums in screening for cancer. Mini review. Int J Cancer. 2010;126:1039–46.

Miller AB, Lindsay J, Hill GB. Mortality from cancer of the uterus in Canada and its relationship to screening for cancer of the cervix. Int J Cancer. 1976;17:602–12.

Miller AB, Chamberlain J, Day NE, Hakama M, Prorok PC. Report on a workshop of the UICC project on evaluation of screening for cancer. Int J Cancer. 1990;46:761–9.

Moss SM. Case-control studies of screening. Int J Epidemiol. 1991;20:1–6.

Moss S, Draper GJ, Hardcastle JD, Chamberlain J. Calculation of sample size in trials of screening for early diagnosis of disease. Int J Epidemiol. 1987;16:104–10.

Prorok PC, Chamberlain J, Day NE, Hakama M, Miller AB. UICC Workshop on the evaluation of screening programmes for cancer. Int J Cancer. 1984;34:1–4.

Sasco AJ, Day NE, Walter SD. Case-control studies for the evaluation of screening. J Chronic Dis. 1986;39:399–405.

Strong K, Wald N, Miller A, Alwan A, on behalf of the WHO Consultation Group. Current concepts in screening for noncommunicable disease: World Health Organization Consultation Group Report on methodology of noncommunicable disease Screening. J Med Screen. 2005;12:12–9.

Wald NJ. Guidance on terminology. J Med Screen. 2001;8:56.

Weiss NS. Control definition in case-control studies of the efficacy of screening and diagnostic testing. Am J Epidemiol. 1983;116:457–60.

Wilson JMG, Junger G. Principles and Practice of Screening for Disease. Public Health Paper # 34, WHO 1968. Geneva Switzerland.

Chapter 14
Comprehensive Cervical Cancer Control: Strategies and Guidelines

Nathalie Broutet

14.1 Introduction

Cancer of the uterine cervix is the second most important cancer among women in the world, in nearly all low- and middle-income (LMI) countries; it is number one in importance. In comparison with other cancers, the number of deaths from cancer of the cervix among women 25–64 years old each year in LMI countries was estimated at 133,200, compared to 128,000 for breast cancer, 54,900 for lung cancer and 57,900 for cancer of the stomach; in high-income countries the corresponding numbers were 18,300, 82,200, 40,000 and 20,800, respectively (Ferlay et al. 2010).

It is estimated that over a million women worldwide currently have cervical cancer. Most of these women have not been diagnosed, nor do they have access to treatment that could cure them or prolong their lives. In 2005, almost 260,000 women died of the disease, nearly 95 % of them in low-income countries, making cervical cancer one of the gravest threats to women's lives Yang et al. (2004). Without urgent attention, deaths due to cervical cancer are projected to rise by almost 25 % over the next 10 years.

Most women who die from cervical cancer, particularly in LMI countries, are in the prime of their life. They may be raising children, caring for their family and contributing to the social and economic life of their town or village. Their death is both a personal tragedy and a sad and unnecessary loss to their family and their community with enormous repercussions for the welfare of both. These deaths are unnecessary because there is compelling evidence that cervical cancer is one of the most preventable and treatable forms of cancer as long as it is detected early and managed effectively (see Hakama this volume).

N. Broutet (✉)
Department of Reproductive Health and Research,
World Health Organization, 1211, Geneva 27, Switzerland
e-mail: broutetn@who.int

A.B. Miller (ed.), *Epidemiologic Studies in Cancer Prevention and Screening*, Statistics for Biology and Health 79, DOI 10.1007/978-1-4614-5586-8_14,

Therefore, it is important for the World Health Organization (WHO) to assume a leadership role over control of cancer of the cervix.

14.2 WHO Recommended Strategies for Cervical Cancer Control

The major issue over cervical cancer control is, as expressed by Madon et al. (2007), *'we face a formidable gap between innovations in health (vaccines, tests, drugs and strategies for care) and their delivery to communities'*, especially in the countries that need them most.

So why do these stark inequalities in health status exist?

In addition to the obvious answer regarding the lack of effective health systems and financial resources in developing countries, it is important to underscore one of the most often overlooked but influential drivers of health inequities, the position of women in a given society. Gender inequality in many developing countries underlies some key risk factors, as well as the availability and access to women's health services. Gender inequality interacts with other social hierarchies, such as class, caste, race and other social markers, to worsen vulnerability, risks, access to care and outcomes for the most marginalized women.

The WHO programme on Comprehensive Cervical Cancer Control incorporates primary, secondary and tertiary prevention components.

For primary prevention, an important emphasis is on education to reduce high-risk sexual behaviour and thus limit transmission or acquisition of infection by oncogenic types of the human papillomavirus (HPV). Important components of these programmes are messages to promote delay in age of first sexual intercourse, condom use, limits in the number of sexual partners and change to less risky sexual behaviour for both male and female adolescents. Gender inequality underlies important risk factors for STIs, HPV infection and cervical cancer, such as early age at first sexual intercourse, childbearing and parity and number of sexual partners. For instance, girl's lack of knowledge, inability to negotiate sex or safe sex, sexual coercion and cultural demands for marriage at a young age result in high incidence of sexually transmitted infections. Gender inequality and norms related to masculinity encourage men to have more sexual partners and older men to have sexual relations with much younger women. In some settings, this contributes to far greater sexually transmitted infection rates among young women (15–24 years) compared to young men.

At the community level, many women and men have not heard of cervical cancer and do not recognize early signs and symptoms when they occur. Women at risk may not be aware of the need to be tested, even when they have any symptoms. New is the availability of HPV vaccines, creating for the first time the potential for providing complete protection against the HPV types included in the vaccine, as well as some cross protection against those related types not in the vaccine (see Bosch, this volume).

For secondary prevention, the WHO promotes programmes of early detection of the disease to facilitate effective treatment (WHO Guide for Effective Programmes 2007). Early detection has two components: early diagnosis, that is, identify and treat early cancer while the chance of cure is still good (will reduce cervical cancer mortality if effective) and screening, that is, identify and treat precancerous lesions of the cervix before they progress to cervical cancer (will reduce cervical cancer incidence and mortality if effective).

Beyond risk, gender inequality also affects women's access to and interaction with health services. To address gender-based inequities in access to vaccines and screening, it is crucial to consider the different needs and constraints of women and men when accessing services in different settings – and design interventions accordingly. For example, women's access is more likely to be affected by restricted mobility, difficulties in accessing transport and childcare and lack of treatment literacy, as compared to men's. As gender intersects with age, ethnicity, social and economic status and other social categories, these barriers can vary across settings and within populations, often creating different sets of issues for adolescent girls and boys and for women and men in different situations (e.g. migrant workers, sex workers, housewives, others).

Further, stigmatization of women's bodies may prevent women from seeking care. In many cultures, the female genital tract is considered private, polluted or profane, and women may be hesitant to discuss symptoms related to it. This is especially true in settings where the health-care provider is a man or is from a different culture. Destigmatizing discussion of the female genital tract may be an important strategy in encouraging women to be screened and to seek care if they have symptoms suggestive of cervical cancer. Gender norms discourage women from displaying knowledge and communicating about sex and related topics with partners and even with health professionals.

For tertiary prevention, the WHO promotes adequate treatment of invasive cancer, but if treatment is not possible, palliative care.

14.3 Strengthening Health Systems

In nearly all LMI countries, for cervical cancer control programmes to succeed, a major requirement is the strengthening of health systems. Unless governments are able to make the necessary investments, the advances in cervical cancer control that are possible will not be realized.

The need for adequate resources and improved health care for women in developing countries has to be addressed. It is also crucial to better understand and take into account gender inequality in the design of health policies and programmes and work alongside other sectors to change unequal gender power relations at the heart of gender inequality and other important social determinants of health.

At the present time, there are many opportunities for the advancement of cervical cancer control. As already emphasized, the new HPV vaccines offer a completely

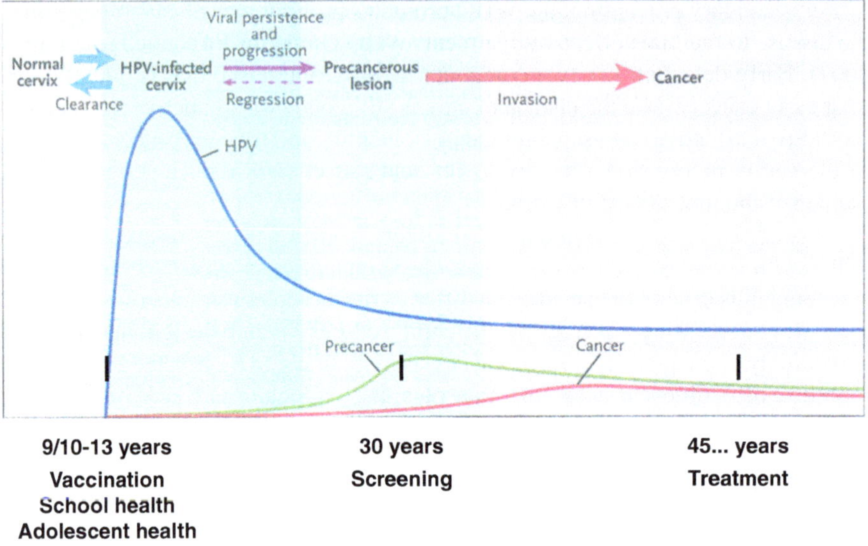

Fig. 14.1 Integration of health programmes: target age groups of different interventions and links with cervical cancer prevention

new strategy for primary prevention. But in addition, there are new assays and new algorithms for improved cervical cancer screening, which may permit the identification of precancerous and cancerous lesions with greater accuracy, less complexity and with fewer barriers to access. These new technologies offer new possibilities for widespread access to effective prevention that in itself has the ability to reduce inequity. These opportunities are resulting in new advocates, with new interest and new energy.

While WHO continues to advocate for greater attention and resources for women's health beyond maternal care and family planning, WHO is also actively involved in strengthening health systems in general and in developing, testing and implementing appropriate technologies to make comprehensive cervical cancer care feasible and affordable in low- and middle-income countries.

However, to achieve the advances possible, we need to envisage the integration of health programmes which will target different age groups for different interventions with links to cervical cancer prevention.

Figure 14.1 is illustrative. With the peak in acquisition of HPV infection at late adolescence, the target group for vaccination has principally to be girls ages 9–13 who have not yet had their sexual debut. This means that vaccination programmes have to be linked to existing school health and especially adolescent health programmes, or such programmes especially created for the purpose. The peak for development of cervical intraepithelial neoplasia is around age 30, though the peak for development of high-grade lesions (CIN3) in some countries may be 5 years later. Given that the peak in development of invasive cervical cancer is some 15 years later, the target group for initiation of screening will be women ages 30–35 or even later (for further discussion of these issues, please see Hakama this volume). In terms of the target group for treatment of invasive cervical cancer, this will be extremely rare in women in their twenties and will reach a maximum at about age 45.

Interdisciplinary approaches are required to span cervical control interventions. This is commonplace in high-income countries but may be very difficult to achieve in many LMI countries. It is important that Ministries of Health recognize the need; the recent UN Declaration on Non-communicable Disease Prevention and Control will hopefully encourage leaders of cancer control to ensure the necessary expertise is available or, if not, train people to meet the needs (see Ullrich, this volume). In that respect primary care services will be critical to ensure women do not fall through the cracks in the system. It may be necessary to ensure the availability of trained nurses in primary health settings to ensure girls and women attend the appropriate facility and do not miss critical appointments for diagnosis or treatment.

14.4 The Role of HPV Vaccination Programmes

To amplify further on the new opportunities for primary prevention, it is important to recognize that the HPV vaccine is an effective new tool that targets adolescent girls.

HPV vaccination is designed for a new target population, not one previously served routinely by immunization programmes (World Health Organization 2006). HPV vaccination programmes can now become an entry point for integrated services to adolescents, who are often largely ignored by health services in LMI countries though adolescents represent 1 in 5 of the world's population. Adolescent girls are particularly vulnerable and deserve special attention, and the HPV vaccine provides an opportunity to reach adolescents with a wider range of proven health information and services, for which tools are available.

In order to effectively deliver HPV vaccines, in many countries it will be necessary to strengthen the health system. HPV vaccination raises issues of cost and financing and programme delivery to adolescents. But it may strengthen or support adolescent immunization programmes, through schools or other delivery systems, according to country-specific needs and within their sociocultural context. It may also link immunization with other public health interventions for adolescents, especially sexual health and other health interventions. Further, by creating partnerships between mothers and daughters over these issues, it could increase cervical cancer screening rates among mothers.

In order to achieve high HPV vaccination rates, it will be necessary to improve education of patients, parents and communities. Messages and patient or parental notification, approval or consent methods, should be tailored to local cultural context and the information needs of various audiences (e.g. candidates for vaccination, parents and clinicians). These messages should stress that vaccines do not cure cancer, they prevent some HPV-related cancers, and they are most effective when given before the onset of sexual activity. It is also important that girls and their parents are warned that for fully effective vaccination, three vaccine doses are required. Also, because of the lack of information, it is wise to emphasize that vaccination is not recommended for pregnant females. Further, vaccination is not a cancer or a universal infectious disease preventive agent; for example, it will not prevent HIV infection, other sexually transmitted diseases or pregnancy. If it has been decided to use the quadrivalent vaccine in the programme, it will be appropriate to note that an additional benefit will be wart prevention.

Thus, educational campaigns are recommended to improve knowledge about cervical cancer and HPV and to increase vaccine acceptance, and these will have to be sustained to ensure adequate vaccination coverage.

14.5 The Role of Screening

Even if a decision has been taken to initiate a vaccination programme, secondary prevention is still needed at adult ages. This is because up to 30 % of all cervical cancer cases are caused by HPV types other than 16 and 18; for their control, there will be a continuing need for future cervical cancer screening, and screening of the non-vaccinated older and eventually young population, who are likely to be at high risk, will still be required. There is also the concern that as yet, the existing vaccines have an unknown effect on invasive cervix cancer, and it will be important to maintain screening programmes pending resolution of this issue.

An important consideration in planning for screening as an integral part of cervical cancer control will be to decide which screening test will be selected for which population and where will it be used. The options are the conventional Pap smear, the DNA-based tests, visual inspection with acetic acid (VIA) or with Lugol's iodine (VILI) or, when it becomes available, the HPV rapid DNA test. In making the decision, it is important to understand why new approaches are needed for secondary prevention in LMI countries. This is because clinical expertise is often limited, there is very limited capacity for confirmatory or diagnostic testing, there is poor infrastructure with limited reporting and opportunity for monitoring, while it is often difficult to contact patients. Available and accepted screening methods (particularly the Pap smear) are not practical or accessible to the majority of women living in many countries, while in addition, the predictive value of applied screening tests will change with the implementation of HPV vaccination.

The choice of a screening test should be based upon the effectiveness of the test (i.e. its sensitivity and specificity) in the target women. There needs to be capacity to reach (coverage) a significant proportion (at least 80 %) of target women and adequate local infrastructure where the test will be used, and it must be possible to meet the cost of the test and the infrastructure to ensure its effectiveness. Table 14.1 summarizes the characteristics of the available screening tests for secondary prevention.

Table 14.1 Characteristics of the available cervical screening tests

Characteristics	Conventional cytology	HPV DNA tests	Visual inspection tests VIA	VILI
Sensitivity	47–62 %	66–100 %	67–79 %	78–98 %
Specificity[a]	60–95 %	62–92 %	49–86 %	73–91 %
Comments	Assessed over the last 50 years in a wide range of settings in developed and developing countries	Assessed over the last decade in many settings in developed and relatively few in developing countries	Assessed over the last decade in many settings in developing countries	Assessed by IARC over the last 4 years in India and 3 countries in Africa. Need further evaluation for reproducibility
Number of visits required for screening and treatment	2 or more visits	2 or more visits	Can be used in single-visit or 'see and treat' approach where outpatient treatment is available	

[a]For high-grade lesions and invasive cancer

To ensure adequate coverage requires increase in availability and access to quality services: tests should be easy to perform and acceptable at the level of the health system where they are intended to be used; and information and knowledge in the community about the existence of quality services to ensure women do go to the services.

There are alternative programmatic approaches for cervical cancer screening. The conventional approach, as in most high-income countries, is to screen, diagnose, confirm and treat in progressive steps, a strategy that involves multiple visits for those who test positive. Such a strategy is likely to fail in many LMI countries, as return visits for diagnosis and treatment create many opportunities for women to fail to attend.

The new paradigms involve, as far as possible, 'screen and treat approaches' (as pioneered by the Alliance for Cervical Cancer Prevention – ACCP). These screen and treat strategies involve one or at most two visits and losses are minimized. They are dependent on a test that can be read almost instantaneously and are particularly suited to visual methods with treatment on the spot. Cryotherapy is acceptable, but procurement is an issue, as well as maintenance of liquid nitrogen for freezing.

WHO is supporting Ministries of Health to strengthen evidence-based cervical cancer screening programmes – with advice on appropriate use of screening tests: cytology, visual methods, HPV DNA assays; different combinations may be used in different countries and even in a given country, depending on the level of infrastructure (Blumenthal et al. 2007; Denny et al. 2005; RTCOG/JHPIEGO 2003; Sankaranarayanan et al. 2004).

Figure 14.2 illustrates how screening has to be integrated at the different levels of health care, from VIA offered at the primary care level through VIA and cryotherapy at the secondary care level to treatment for extensive lesions or invasive cancer at the tertiary care level. Control of cervical cancer can be strengthened if there is integration of these levels and monitoring of performance.

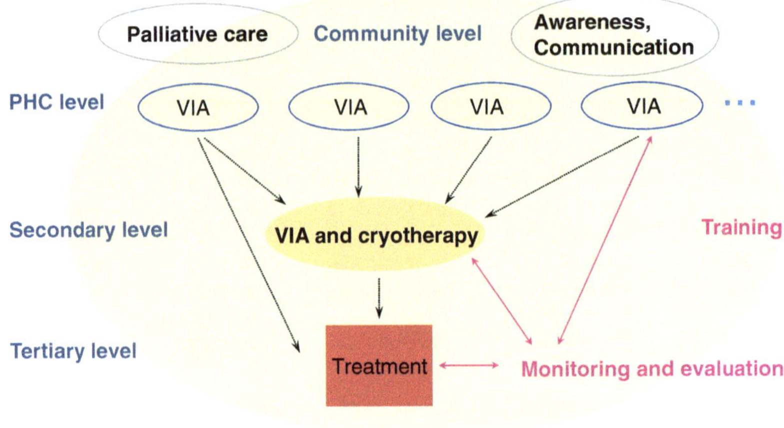

Fig. 14.2 Strengthening cervical cancer screening programmes – operational framework

Different situations arise with different screening tests. Cytology detects precancerous lesions (e.g. CIN 1/2/3 and worse). However, for diagnosis, colposcopy with biopsy is required and adequate treatment. As nearly all CIN 1 and much of CIN 2 and 3 regress, especially in younger women, there is risk of substantial overtreatment, especially if women are screened at too young an age or too frequently.

The HPV test identifies infection with oncogenic types of HPV, but cannot determine whether this is likely to be persistent or results in high-grade CIN. Again there is risk of substantial overtreatment, and it is generally agreed the test should not be used on women under the age of 30 as the vast majority of infections in younger women are transitory. Diagnosis requires application of a triage test, if available cytology, but if not VIA. Treatment has to be decided based on the results of the triage test. HPV tests raise the question of the diagnosis of a sexually transmitted infection (STI), and according to WHO best practice, other STIs should be looked for and the partner treated also.

The VIA test will identify a cervical lesion, but it cannot determine if it is CIN or something else. It provides the option for immediate treatment with cryotherapy or referral of those non-eligible for treatment elsewhere if the lesion is extensive. Because of relatively low specificity, there is likely to be overtreatment, though this does not seem to result in harm.

14.6 Key Issues for Programmes

From the WHO pilot programmes to strengthen cervical cancer control conducted in several African countries (Madagascar, Malawi, Nigeria, Tanzania, Uganda, Zambia), several important lessons have been learnt for scaling up VIA followed by

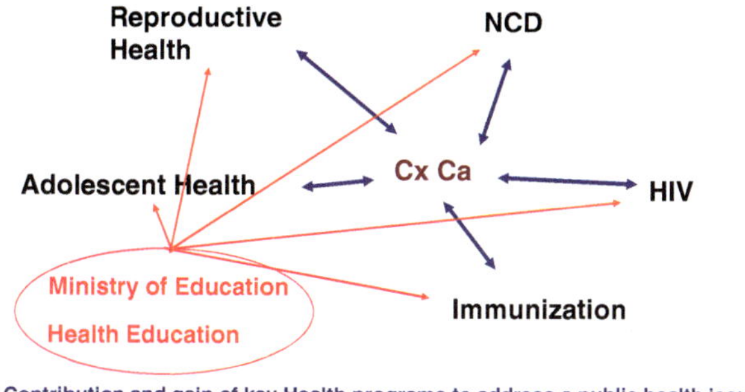

Fig. 14.3 Health system approach to address cervical cancer control

cryotherapy to increase screening and treatment coverage. These include the importance of supervision, organization of the necessary training, monitoring and evaluation of the programme (a cancer registry, or failing that a special register of cervical cancers should be in place), feedback of attendance for referral and means to procure and maintain cryotherapy equipment.

Access to treatment for high-grade lesions and cervical cancer has to be in place. The implementation of the policy should include linkages with HIV and sexual and reproductive health as well as other related programmes. Figure 14.3 illustrates the health system approach to address cervical cancer control, emphasizing the need for integration.

In summary, good secondary and tertiary cervical control programmes must be able to effectively test (with high sensitivity and specificity) the target women. They should reach a significant proportion of at-risk women (coverage), treat and manage women who test positive and ensure effective follow-up and be able to monitor and evaluate programme impact. It is not one size fits all.

New stakeholders and partners are needed for cervical cancer control. They include various departments within Ministries of Health; such as those responsible for immunization, sexual and reproductive health, adolescent health, cancer control and HIV prevention. Ministries of Education also have a role, especially departments responsible for school health. Women's groups can be partnered to facilitate education and adequate coverage, and community-based groups who can help to reach girls out of school. Interdisciplinary coordination will be needed.

14.7 The WHO Guides

The first-ever comprehensive guide from WHO on cervical cancer control was published in 2006 (WHO 2006). This has been translated into the six official WHO languages and adopted and adapted in many countries, for example, China, Sri Lanka, Vietnam, Cambodia, Thailand, Nigeria, Malawi, Zambia, Tanzania, Uganda, some Latin American countries and others.

The key technical messages are:

- Health education is integral to cervical cancer control.
- If sufficient resources exist, cytology is recommended but not under the age of 25 year nor annually.
- Visual screening methods followed by cryotherapy should be offered in piloted or closely monitored settings.
- HPV DNA-based methods should not be used in women before 30 years of age.
- Women should be offered the same cervical cancer screening and treatment options regardless of their HIV status.

WHO will shortly be offering an update of this guide. The purpose of the update is to expand the health education section, to include the role of HPV vaccines and to provide new data on use of screening tests and algorithms and new data on HIV and cervical cancer.

WHO offers guidelines in several other publications (Table 14.2).

Table 14.2 Recommendations on cervical cancer control in WHO guides

Context	Recommendation		Quality of evidence	Strength
Use of cryotherapy for prevention of CIN	1a	The expert panel recommends cryotherapy over no treatment	⊕OOO	Strong
	1b	In settings where LEEP is available and accessible, the expert panel suggests treatment with LEEP over cryotherapy	⊕⊕OO	Conditional
Lesion Size	2.	Among women with CIN Lesions covering more than 75% of the ectocervix, or with lesions extending beyond the cryo tip being used, the expert panel suggests performing or referring for excisional therapy	⊕⊕OO	Conditional
Lesions extending into the endocervical canal	3a.	In settings where LEEP is available and accessible, and women present with CIN lesions extending into the cervical canal, the expert panel suggests treatment with LEEP over cryotherapy	⊕⊕OO	Conditional
	3b.	In settings where excisional procedures (e.g. LEEP, laser or CKC) or referral to additional treatment are not available, the expert panel suggests that women with lesions extending into the endocervical canal be treated with cryotherapy	⊕OOO	Conditional

(continued)

Table 14.2 (continued)

Context	Recommendation		Quality of evidence	Strength
Cryotherapy technique and procedure	4.	The expert panel suggests double freeze using a 3 minute freeze, 5 minute thaw, 3 minute freeze cycle over single-freeze cryotherapy	⊕⊕OO	Conditional
	5.	The expert panel recommends cryotherapy using either carbondioxide (CO_2) or nitrous oxide (N_2O) gas	⊕⊕OO	Strong
		In settings where both gases are available, the expert panel suggests cryotherapy with CO_2 rather than with N_2O	⊕OOO	Conditional
	6.	The expert panel recommends that the "cough technique" *should not be used* during cryotherapy	⊕OOO	Strong
	7.	The expert panel suggests that prophylactic antibiotics *should not be used.* when providing cryotherapy	⊕OOO	Conditional
Providers	8.	The expert panel recommends that health-care workers (including non-physicians) trained in cryotherapy perform the procedure for women when it is indicated	⊕⊕OO	Strong
		The expert panel also suggests that trained nurses or trained midwives rather than physicians may perform cryotherapy	⊕OOO	Conditional
Use of cryotherapy during pregnancy	9a.	In pregnant women, the expert panel suggests deferring cryotherapy until after pregnancy	⊕OOO	Conditional
	9b.	In women whose pregnancy status is unknown (or there is no clinical evidence of pregnancy), the expert panel suggests using cryotherapy	⊕OOO	Conditional
Retreatment of CIN lesions with cryotherapy	10a.	The expert panel recommends cryotherapy over no treatment for women who screen positive after prior cryotherapy treatment	⊕OOO	Strong
	10b.	In settings where LEEP is available and accessible, the expert panel suggests treatment with LEEP over cryotherapy for women who screen positive after prior cryotherapy treatment	⊕⊕OO	Conditional

14.8 Challenges

There are many challenges for cervical cancer control programmes. They include the availability of human resources because of a shortage of trained health workers for vaccinating, screening and treating. An adequate organization is essential to ensure effective programmes. Coordination is needed between partners who are not used to working together over immunization, sexual and reproductive health, cancer control, child and adolescent health, school health and health system strengthening. It is necessary to identify the best affordable programmatic practices for a given country, vaccine delivery, the appropriate, screening-treatment algorithms and accessibility to a cancer treatment centre. Establishing monitoring and evaluation will not be easy but essential in order to ensure that relative failures are identified and rectified, and successes built upon. Financial resources will have to be secured because of the high costs of many new technologies, the requirements for new delivery systems and concerns over economic downturn so that government and donor resources may be limited.

14.9 Conclusions

Cancer is an increasing public health threat, in particular in low- and middle-income countries. WHO recommends a comprehensive and integrated approach to cervical cancer control of which HPV vaccination is one element. Gender inequality not only influences health inequities with respect to cervical cancer but in many other ways damages the physical and mental health of millions of girls and women across the globe and also of boys and men despite the many tangible benefits it gives men through resources, power, authority and control. Because of the numbers of people involved and the magnitude of the problems, taking action to improve gender equity in health and to address women's rights to health is one of the most direct and potent ways to reduce health inequities and ensure effective use of health resources.

Acknowledgments *Acknowledgments to my colleagues on the WHO working group on Cervix Cancer Prevention.*

Venkataram Chandra-Mouli, Tracey Goodman, Silvana Luciani, Gabrielle Ross, Andreas Ullrich, Susan Wang

IARC: Rengaswamy Sankaranarayanan, Eric Lucas

References

Blumenthal PD, Gaffikin L, Deganus S, Lewis R, Emerson M, Adadevoh S et al. Cervical cancer prevention: safety, acceptability, and feasibility of a single-visit approach in Accra, Ghana. *Am J Obstet Gynecol* 2007; 196:407.e1–407.e9.

Denny L, Kuhn L, De Souza M, Pollack AE, Dupree W, Wright TC, Jr. Screen-and-Treat Approaches for Cervical Cancer Prevention in Low-Resource Settings: A Randomized Controlled Trial. *JAMA* 2005; 294:2173–2181.

Ferlay J, Shin HR, Bray F, Forman D, Mathers C, Parkin DM. Estimates of worldwide burden of cancer in 2008: GLOBOCAN 2008. *Int J Cancer* 2010; 127:2893–2917.

Madon T, Hofman KJ, Kupfer L, Glass RI. Policy forum: Public Health. Implementation Science. *Science* 2007; 318:1728–1729.

Royal Thai College of Obstetricians and Gynaecologists (RTCOG) and the JHPIEGO Corporation Cervical Cancer Prevention Group. Safety, acceptability, and feasibility of a single-visit approach to cervical-cancer prevention in rural Thailand: a demonstration project. *Lancet* 2003; 361:814–820.

Sankaranarayanan R, Rajikumar R, Theresa R, Esmy PO, Mahe C, Begyalakshmi KR et al. Initial results from a randomized trial of cervical visual screening in rural south India. *Int J Cancer* 2004; 109:461–467.

Yang BH, Bray FI, Parkin DM, Sellors JW, Zhang Z-F. Cervical cancer as a priority for prevention in different world regions: an evaluation using years of life lost. *Int J Cancer* 2004; 109:418–424.

WHO. *Comprehensive cervical cancer control – A guide to essential practice*. 2006 Geneva, World health Organization.

WHO Guide for Effective Programmes. *Cancer Control. Knowledge into Action: Early Detection.* 2007. Geneva, World Health Organization.

World Health Organization. Department of Reproductive Health and Research. Preparing for the introduction of HPV vaccines. Policy and programme guidance for countries. 2006. Geneva, World Health Organization. http://www.who.int/reproductivehealth/publications/cancers/RHR_06.11/en/index.html

Chapter 15
Screening for Cervical Cancer

Matti Hakama

15.1 Benefits and Harms of Screening

Screening for cancer involves the identification of preclinical disease by a relatively simple test. The objective of screening is to reduce the risk of death, i.e., mortality from cancer among those subjected to screening. For cervical cancer, the screening test is aimed at detection of preinvasive lesions. Therefore, reduction in the incidence of invasive disease results from screening, and a valid indicator for the effect is also a change of incidence.

Screening may have benefits other than an effect on incidence and mortality. If the treatment of disease detected at screening is less invasive or less radical, or results in less morbidity than that of clinically detected disease, then the quality of life of the screened population is possibly improved. This is an obvious benefit in screening for cervical cancer because the identification of preinvasive lesions allows conservative operation. Correct negative results also have a beneficial effect in that they reassure women without the disease. This is another relevant aspect as a positive test results in no conclusion on whether to regard the woman as a patient or as healthy. The woman probably experiences anxiety and stress if the diagnosis is postponed.

Because the aim of cervical screening is to provide a diagnosis of preinvasive disease, there is a prolonged period of morbidity – from the time of diagnosis at screening to the hypothetical time at which a clinical diagnosis would have been made had the patient not been screened. This lead time, while a prerequisite of effective screening, is an adverse effect because of the prolongation of anxiety and morbidity due to diagnosis and treatment of the lesion.

M. Hakama (✉)
Tampere School of Public Health, Cancer Registry of Finland,
University of Tampere, Fl-33014 Helsinki, Finland
e-mail: marita.hallila@uta.fi; matti.hakama@uta.fi

A.B. Miller (ed.), *Epidemiologic Studies in Cancer Prevention and Screening*,
Statistics for Biology and Health 79, DOI 10.1007/978-1-4614-5586-8_15,

Cases detected at screening are confirmed by standard clinical diagnostic methods. Many such cases are borderline abnormalities, some of which would progress to clinical disease and some of which would not, even if left untreated. The diagnosis of carcinoma in situ and severe dysplasia results in an invasive treatment. A proportion of these lesions would not have progressed to clinical disease during the woman's life span. These are indistinguishable from the truly abnormal cases that will progress into the clinical phase in the absence of early treatment. One of the adverse effects of screening is therefore the consequent treatment of screenees with such lesions. This results in anxiety and morbidity. Conversely, a false-negative result is falsely reassuring. If it results in postponement of clinical diagnosis and worsens the outcome of treatment, screening is disadvantageous.

Many screening programs involve expensive techniques and are applied to large populations. The total budget required for health services is thus likely to increase if a screening program is adopted.

A decision about whether to screen requires weighing the beneficial and harmful effects. As is general in medicine, value judgments are involved in such weighting, so also ethical issues are closely related to screening.

15.2 Sensitivity

Sensitivity is in general defined as the ability of the test to identify an unrecognized disease. In screening for cervical cancer, sensitivity is the ability of the screening test to identify the cancer when still in the detectable preinvasive phase (DPIP).

Sensitivity is an essential indicator in the comparison of several competing tests. In screening for cervix cancer, this is especially timely because several tests have been proposed for routine use. While most of the evidence is on the Pap test, other competing technologies exist. The most important of them is the application of computer automation, of visual inspection, and especially of the etiology-based human papillomavirus (HPV) test.

Another extension of sensitivity is the concept itself. Traditionally, sensitivity in screening is the characteristic of the test. Also the diagnostic confirmation and the target population are included in the screening process from the point of view of clinical practice and public health. Therefore, it is useful to define episode and program sensitivities. Some of the test positives may be erroneously classified at diagnostic confirmation as healthy. Therefore, the sensitivity of the test may be better than the sensitivity of the total process from the test to the final diagnostic conclusion. We call the corresponding time as episode and the corresponding sensitivity as the episode sensitivity. Further, we define the program sensitivity as the ability of the screening program to identify cancer in the DPIP among all the women in the target population (Hakama et al. 2007).

The sensitivity of the screening test for cervix cancer is usually given at the preinvasive stage level as CIN2 or worse or CIN3 or worse and estimated on the basis of detection rates at screen (IARC 2005). Such cases include nonprogressive lesions as well, and one will not know whether an estimate of high sensitivity is describing true sensitivity or high overdiagnosis. Therefore, the proper sensitivity estimate is based on interval cancers between two successive screens, i.e., on failures of the screen, and the method of estimation is called the incidence method.

Most published results do not distinguish between the test and the episode, and most of them erroneously include also preinvasive lesions in the data. In a review analysis, Fahey et al. (1995) found that the sensitivity of the Pap test was from 40 % to 80 %. Early studies corresponding to the incidence method at the threshold level of invasive cancer implied substantially better sensitivity. The largest of those studies was the collaborative study coordinated by the International Agency for Research on Cancer (Hakama et al. 1986). It showed that eradication of the disease is an unrealistic goal and that maximal protection after a negative smear is about 90 %, which remains roughly the same during several years after the test. In other words, the sensitivity of the Pap test to detect a lesion in the DPIP was about 90 %. This conclusion is in accordance with the results of studies on the natural history of the disease, which have shown that most preinvasive lesions progress to frankly invasive cancer only over several years. Variation in the estimates of sensitivity from 40 % to 90 % stems from conceptual differences, from the methods used, and from the programs reported.

Automation-assisted cytology was proposed in the 1980s. Two basic methods formed the basis of the screening algorithm. One with neural networks is no more under commercial production. Another with discriminant function application is no longer in wide use. Both sensitivity and specificity were quite similar with the automation-assisted and the traditional Pap test (IARC 2005; Nieminen et al. 2007).

The first attempts based on visual inspection were known as downstaging (Stjernswärd 1990; Sankaranarayanan et al. 2007). The experience is largest with visual inspection with acetic acid (VIA). Visual inspection with Lugol's iodine (VILI) was shown to be comparable with the Pap smear in a developing country setting. VIA and VILI are simple tests, and they allow a see-and-treat policy, essential in a developing country. Their problem is poor specificity that results in overtreatment, and most of the studies show a modest benefit only. However, the results seem to depend on the effort made in training, and with extensive training, better results were observed (Sankaranarayanan et al. 2005, 2007).

The etiology-based HPV test has repeatedly yielded higher detection rates of preinvasive lesions than the traditional Pap test, which was interpreted as higher sensitivity. Therefore, it is widely recommended and has gained popularity in recent years. The high detection rates were found at the risk of lower specificity (IARC 2005). However, studies on invasive cancer are few (Malila et al. 2012; Naucler et al. 2007; Ronco et al. 2010). Based on a randomized health services study design and within a well-organized screening program, there was no difference in the sensitivity between traditional Pap test and HPV test (Malila et al. 2012). Therefore, it may be that recommendations to use the HPV test need to be reconsidered.

For the time being, the convincing evidence on sensitivity of screening for cervix cancer is with the Pap test. The HPV test is likely to have similar sensitivity as the

Pap smear but at the risk of more overdiagnosis. In a developing country, it is likely that visual inspection works (Sankaranarayanan et al. 2007).

15.3 Effectiveness

Effectiveness of screening for cervix cancer can be measured as the reduction in the incidence of cancer in the total target population. If based on mortality, one would expect somewhat smaller estimates of effectiveness because the fast growing cancers with poor prognosis are less likely to be detected when in the DPIP than the slow growing ones. In practice, the difference is small in reduction of mortality or in incidence (Miller et al. 1991). Therefore, screening as a public health policy is assessed by means of effectiveness based on incidence of cancer. The ultimate effect of the program depends on the screening test used, attendance, the screening interval, and the success of referral for diagnostic confirmation of cases found at screening (Table 15.1). In principle, screening for cervical cancer reduces the incidence of invasive disease and is applicable as public health policy. However, a wide variation is seen, from highly effective programs to relatively poor ones (IARC 2005).

The effectiveness of screening for cervical cancer was not demonstrated with a randomized screening trial before the large-scale application of the Pap test in routine screening. Canada was a pioneer in screening for cervical cancer (Miller et al. 1976). Large screening programs started in the 1960s. Only in the 2000s were the first results based on randomized trials published on the effectiveness of

Table 15.1 Essential elements of an organized screening program (Hakama et al 1986)

1.	The target population has been identified
2.	Individual women are identifiable
3.	Measures are available to guarantee high coverage and attendance, such as personal letter of invitation
4.	There are adequate field facilities to take the smear and adequate laboratory facilities to examine them
5.	There is an organized program for quality control of the taking of smears and of interpreting them
6	Adequate facilities exist for diagnosis and for appropriate treatment of confirmed neoplastic lesions and for the follow-up of treated women
7.	There is a carefully designed and agreed referral system, an agreed link between the women, the laboratory, and the clinical facility for diagnosis of an abnormal screening test, for management of any abnormality found, and for providing information about normal screening tests
8.	Evaluation and monitoring of the total program is organized in terms of incidence and mortality rates among those attending, and among those not attending, at the level of the total target population. Quality control of these epidemiological data should be established

screening with the Pap test (Sankaranarayanan et al. 2005). By that time, practically in all high and in many medium-resource countries, routine screening was a well-established activity (IARC 2005).

Much of the information on the applicability of screening for cervix cancer as a public health policy originated from the organized programs practiced in the Nordic countries since the mid-1960s (Laara et al. 1987). Most of the Nordic countries have nationwide screening programs that fulfill the general prerequisites of an organized program and make it possible to follow up each woman for the occurrence of intraepithelial cervical neoplasia and for cervical cancer. The programs define the ages and the frequencies of screening, use personal invitations with times and places for screening, and give personal information about the results of screening even when the smear is negative.

Within the organized programs, there have been differences in cervical cancer screening policies between the Nordic countries. In Finland, Iceland, and Sweden, nationwide population-based organized programs were in operation at least since the early 1970s, whereas only a few counties in Denmark, including the most populous ones, had organized screening programs. The programs were run by voluntary cancer organizations in Finland and Iceland and by the counties in Denmark and Sweden. The recommended age groups to be covered are 30–60 years in Finland, 25–69 years in Iceland, and 30–49 years in Sweden. The screening intervals recommended are 2–3 years in Iceland, 4 years in Sweden, and 5 years in Finland. In Denmark, the practice varies by county, but the National Board of Health recommendation is to have a smear every 3 years from the age of 23–59 and every 5 years from 60 to 75. In Norway, only 5 % of the population was covered by an organized program. Since early 1990s, an organized program was designed to substitute the spontaneous one in case the woman had not attended screening in the last 3 years. In most of the Nordic countries, cytological smears are, however, frequently taken outside the organized system by private gynecologists and elsewhere.

There was a strong correlation between the extent of the organized screening program and changes in the incidence of invasive cervical cancer (Fig. 15.1). The relative reduction in the risk was steepest in Finland and Sweden and intermediate in Denmark. In Norway the incidence rates of cervical cancer increased up to the 1970s. During the 25-year period from the 1960s to 1990s, the incidence rates fell by 70 % in Finland and 20 % in Norway. The substantial decrease in incidence from the 1960s to the 1970s in Iceland is partly because prevalent microinvasive lesions were diagnosed during the first round of screening in the late 1960s more frequently than in the other Nordic countries. The rates in Iceland are subject to large random variation owing to the small population and relatively few cases of cancer.

The most substantial reduction in the risk of cervical cancer occurred in the age group 40–49 years of age, which probably came under the most intensive screening by the organized program. Again, the reduction was highest in Finland (80 %) and lowest in Norway (50 %). By calendar time, the rates somewhat increased at young ages, sharply decreased for the middle aged, and were relatively stable in the elderly. The trends since 1990 are considered under the section on equity.

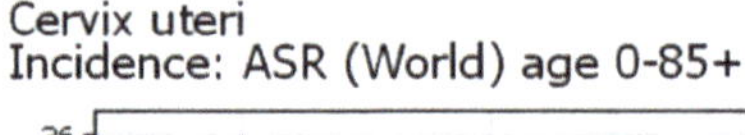

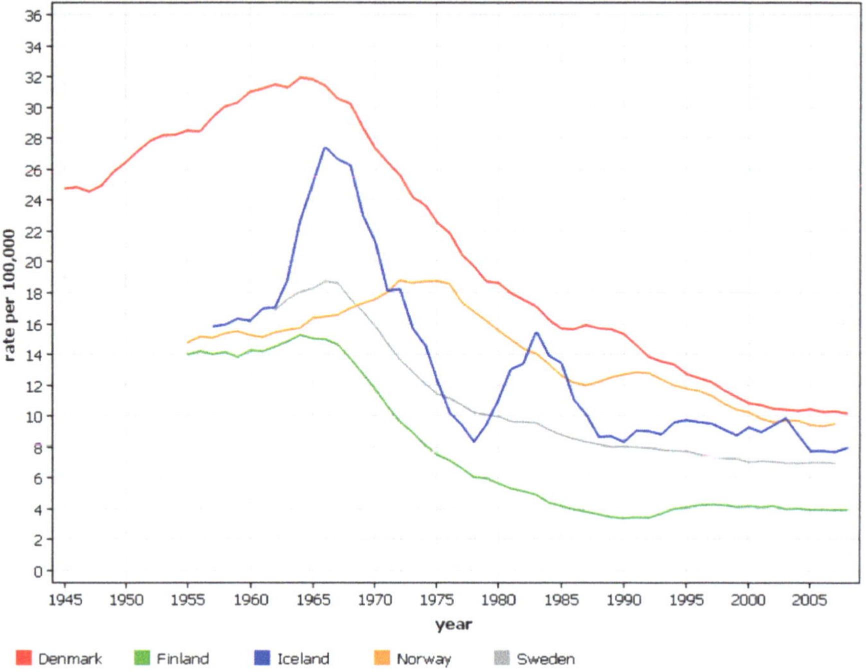

Fig. 15.1 Annual age-adjusted incidence rates in the Nordic countries in 1945–2008 (5-year moving averages)

The most significant determinant of risk reduction is how well the program is organized. A comparison of the Nordic countries shows very little relation between the interval between the screening rounds and reduction of risk, or very little relation between the target age range and reduction of risk. An IARC working group concluded on the basis of several large-scale programs that the protective effect of screening is high for screening intervals up to 5 years and for a lower age limit up to 30 years (Hakama et al. 1986). Organized programs, as contrasted to opportunistic ones, promote adequate quality control and high attendance (e.g., by personal letters of invitation and of response) and have control to prevent breaks in the screening path. High coverage and attendance seem to be the single most important determinants of a successful screening. Opportunistic screening has problems in catching those who would benefit most from screening, and it has less responsibility to maintain linkages in the screening path from population to treatment.

In Finland it was confirmed by a case-control study at the individual level that effectiveness was better for the organized screening than for the spontaneous smear-taking activity (Nieminen et al. 1999).

15.4 Efficiency

In spite of the coverage of the total target population, screening for cervical cancer can be relatively inexpensive; those programs with the largest effect have been low in cost. It seems that screening starting at the age of 25 or even at the age of 30, repeating the smears at 5-year intervals, and having an upper age limit of 60 years will provide practically maximal reduction in the risk of cervical cancer. The program assumes 7 or 8 smears during the woman's lifetime. Such a program compares favorably with those that start at age 20 with annual smears, which result in a total of 40 or more tests during the woman's lifespan.

Screening for cervical cancer is relatively inexpensive compared also to the economic costs of screening for cancers of other primary sites. In fact, the costs of an organized screening program can be compensated by savings due to more frequent treatment of the disease at preinvasive stage compared to the treatment costs of invasive cancers detected through normal practice without screening (Hristova and Hakama 1997). However, poor specificity and high rate of overdiagnosis will increase the cost of screening.

15.5 Equity

Equity is the third dimension, in addition to effect and cost, in health services activities. Often there is a trade-off between effectiveness, efficiency, and equity. Screening for cervical cancer is an exception. As pointed out above, the effect in terms of reduction in risk is in practice inversely related to cost: programs with a large reduction in risk are based on relatively few smears. The Finnish program is also an example of an effective program with improvement in equity, measured by the outcome (reduction in risk) in different population groups. In the mid-1960s, the risk was high in remote areas and in lower social classes. Some of the remote areas had benefited most, and at the same time, the social class differences were reduced (Fig. 15.2). In the early 1970s, the relative risk between the lowest and highest social class was 2.6, as compared to 1.7 in the 1980s. The difference in risk between social classes had disappeared, except that the lowest class was still at a higher risk than the other classes.

Gradually from the 1990s, there appeared changes in both the society and the screening program. The objective of these changes was to provide more choices for the subjects using the health services and to have more competition between the providers of health services. The highly organized screening program was based on the Cancer Society of Finland's Mass Screening Registry and cytological laboratories in different parts of the country. The screening laboratories were mainly replaced by private ones. This resulted in more demands on the coordination and sometimes in breaks in the screening path on referral system of the woman from target population to the eventual treatment (cf. the essential elements in Table 15.1).

It is likely that changes in society resulted in changes in the risk of invasive cervical cancer. The downward trend did not continue, and, in fact, there was a

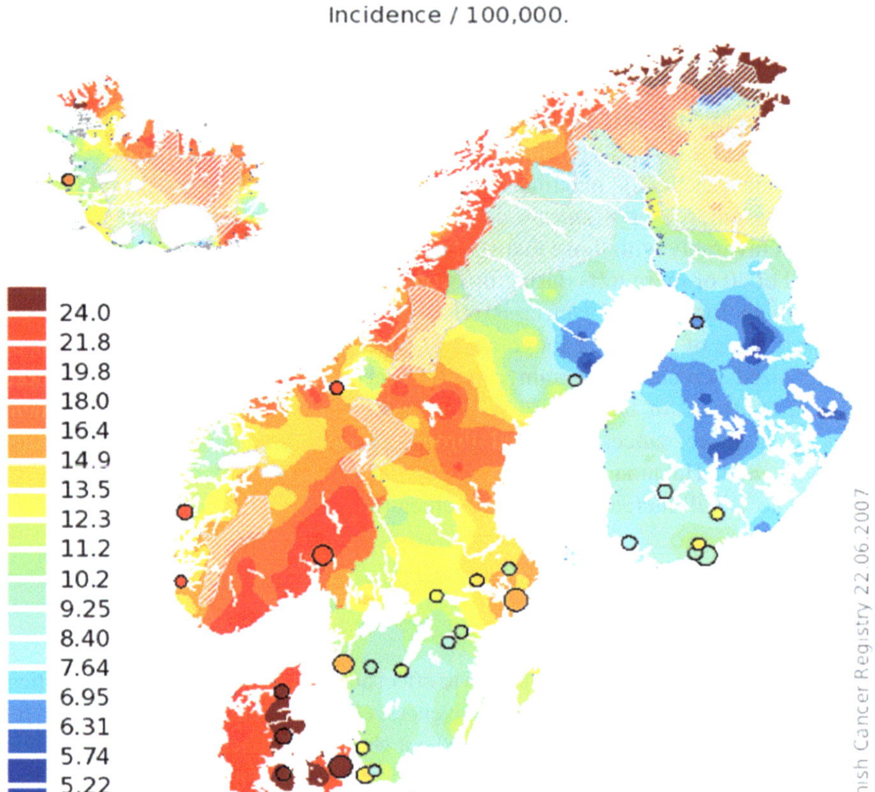

Fig. 15.2 Cervix cancer incidence (per 100,000 person-years, age 35–39) in the Nordic countries in 1971–1976

small overall increase in the incidence of cervix cancer in 1990s. It was, however, especially large in young women and detrimental for the efforts to improve equity. While the risk in the highest social class went down by calendar time, the reduction was much smaller in the other SES classes (Fig. 15.3). The difference between the social classes was in the early 2000s proportionally larger than in the early years of screening in Finland (Pukkala et al. 2010).

15.6 The Future with Vaccination

An important determinant of screening for cervix cancer will be vaccination against HPV infection. Many countries have incorporated HPV vaccination in their national vaccination programs. Such decisions are based on the causal chain from efficacy of

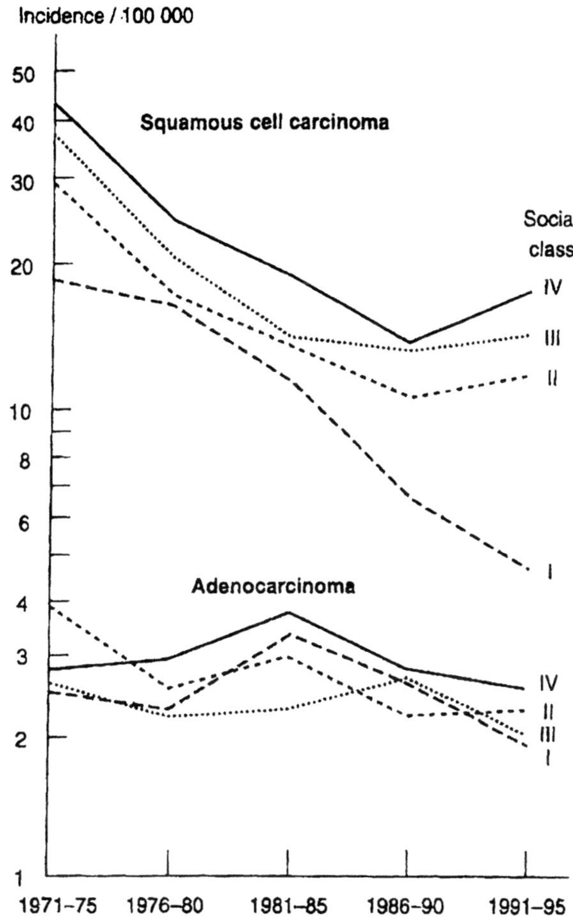

Fig. 15.3 Age-adjusted incidence of adenocarcinoma and squamous cell carcinoma of cervix uteri by socioeconomic status (SES) among Finnish women aged 45–64 at the beginning of each 5-year period between 1971 and 1995

the vaccine to prevent infection to the role of oncogenic HPV viruses in the etiology of cervix cancer. For the time being, there is no direct evidence on prevention of invasive cervix cancer by HPV vaccination, and such evidence may take decennia to emerge. Especially, it would not be an evidence-based policy to replace screening by vaccination against cervix cancer in the target age group for screening. On the other hand, present routine screening policies and pressure to change them to a vaccination policy provide an opportunity to find the evidence. This is best done by randomizing the women in the target population into a vaccination and a screening arm. The evidence needed will be found within one screening round if a sufficiently large target population is randomized. Meanwhile, screening for cervix cancer will continue to have its role in cancer control (Rebolj and Lynge 2011). At present the best evidence is for an organized program with the Pap test in high-resource countries, whereas visual inspection with a see-and-treat policy may the best option in low- and medium-resource countries.

References

Fahey MT, Irwig L, Macaskill P. Meta-analysis of Pap test accuracy. *Am J Epidemiol* 1995;141:-680-689.

Hakama M, Auvinen A, Day NE, Miller AB. Sensitivity in cancer screening. *J Med Screen* 2007;14:174-177.

Hakama M, Miller AB, Day NE, editors. *Screening for cancer of the uterine cervix* (IARC Scientific Publications No. 76). Lyon: International Agency for Research on Cancer, 1986.

Hristova L, Hakama M. Effect of screening for cancer in the Nordic countries on deaths, cost and quality of life up to the year 2017. *Acta Oncol* 1997;36 Suppl 9:1-60.

IARC Handbooks of cancer prevention Cervix Cancer Screening. Lyon: IARC Press, 2005.

Laara E, Day NE, Hakama M. Trends in mortality from cervical cancer in the Nordic countries: association with organised screening programmes. *Lancet* 1987:1:1247-1249.

Malila N, Leinonen M, Kotaniemi-Talonen L, Tarkkanen J, Laurila P, Hakama M. The HPV test has similar benefit but more harm than the Pap test – A randomised health services study on cervical cancer screening in Finland. Submitted for publication in Int J Cancer 2012.

Miller AB, Chamberlain J, Day NE, Hakama M, Prorok PC, editors. *Cancer screening* (Published on behalf of International Union Against Cancer). Cambridge: Cambridge University Press, 1991.

Miller AB, Lindsay J, Hill GB. Mortality from cancer of the uterus in Canada and its relationship to screening for cancer of the cervix. *Int J Cancer* 1976;17:602-612.

Naucler P, Ryd W, Tornberg S, Strand A, Wadell G, Hansson BG, et al. HPV type-specific risks of high-grade CIN during 4 years of follow-up: a population-based prospective study. *Br J Cancer* 2007;97:129-132.

Nieminen P, Kallio M, Anttila A, Hakama M. Organised vs. spontaneous Pap-smear screening for cervical cancer: A case-control study. *Int J Cancer* 1999;83:55-58.

Nieminen P, Kotaniemi-Talonen L, Hakama M, Tarkkanen J, Martikainen J, Toivonen T et al. Randomised evaluation trial on automation assisted screening for cervical cancer: Results after 770000 invitations. *J Med Screen* 2007;14:23-28.

Pukkala E, Malila N, Hakama N. Socioeconomic differences in incidence of cervical cancer in Finland by cell type. *Acta Oncologica* 2010;49:180-184.

Rebolj M, Lynge E. Has cytology become obsolete as a primary test in screening for cervical cancer? *J Med Screen* 2011;17:1-2.

Ronco G, Giorgi-Rossi P, Carozzi F, Confortini M, Dalla Palma P, Del Mistro A, et al. Efficacy of human papillomavirus testing for the detection of invasive cervical cancers and cervical intraepithelial neoplasia: a randomised controlled trial. *Lancet Oncol* 2010;11;249-257.

Sankaranarayanan R, Esmy PO, Rajkumar R, Muwonge R, Swaminathan R, Shanthakumari S, et al. Effect of visual screening on cervical cancer incidence and mortality in Tamil Nadu, India: a cluster-randomised trial. *Lancet* 2007:370:398-406.

Sankaranarayanan R, Nene BM, Dinshaw KA, Mahe C, Jayant K, Shastri SS, et al. A cluster randomized controlled trial of visual, cytology and human papillomavirus screening for cancer of the cervix in rural India. *Int J Cancer* 2005;116:617-623.

Stjernswärd J. National training of radiotherapists in Sri Lanka and Zimbabwe: priorities and strategies for cancer control in developing countries. *International journal of radiation oncology, biology, physics* 1990;19:1275-1278.

Chapter 16
Screening for Colon Polyps and Cancer

Swati G. Patel and Dennis J. Ahnen

16.1 Introduction

Colorectal cancer (CRC) is a major cause of morbidity and mortality in the world. In 2008, there were over 1.2 million new cases and about 610,000 deaths from CRC worldwide, making CRC the third most common cancer and the fourth most common cause of cancer death in the world (Center et al. 2009). Similarly, in the USA, CRC is the fourth most common malignancy and the second leading cause of cancer-related death; in 2011 it was estimated that there were 141,210 new cases and 49,380 deaths due to CRC (NCI 2011). An average-risk individual in the USA has an approximately 5% lifetime risk of developing CRC and a 2–3% risk of death from CRC. However, incidence and mortality from CRC have been steadily declining by about 2–3% per year for the last 15 years. These declines have been partially attributed to increasing rates of CRC screening leading to both prevention and early detection of CRC. Figure 16.1 demonstrates the increased uptake of CRC screening modalities over time compared to the incidence and mortality of CRC over time in the USA. CRC mortality among women began to decline in the 1950s, well before screening was available, suggesting that factors in addition to screening have been contributing to the decline in incidence and mortality, such as the use

S.G. Patel, M.S., M.D.
Fellow in Gastroenterology,
University of Colorado School of Medicine,
Aurora, CO, USA

D.J. Ahnen, M.D. (✉)
Denver Department of Veterans Affairs Medical Center,
University of Colorado School of Medicine,
Denver, CO, USA

S/M Gastroenterology, Gastroenterology Administration,
Campus Box A009/111E, VA Hospital Room 8C157, Denver, CO, USA
e-mail: Dennis.Ahnen@ucdenver.edu

A.B. Miller (ed.), *Epidemiologic Studies in Cancer Prevention and Screening*, Statistics for Biology and Health 79, DOI 10.1007/978-1-4614-5586-8_16,

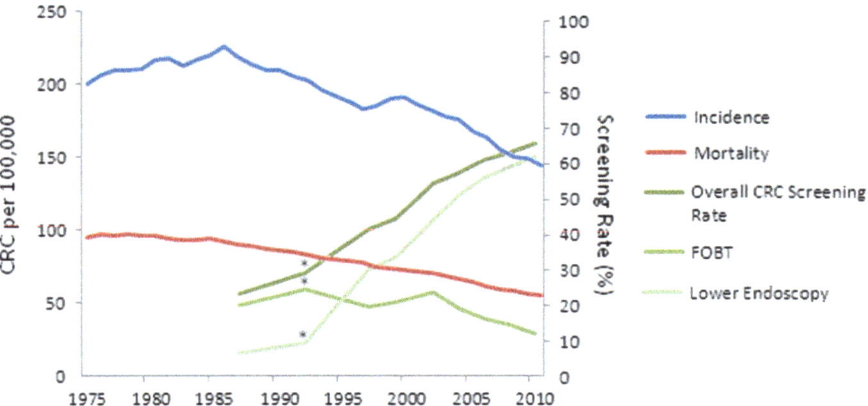

Fig. 16.1 Incidence/mortality of colorectal cancer and screening uptake rates over time. Incidence/mortality reported as rates among adults 50 or older Surveillance Epidemiology End Result (SEER), 2011 to reflect the screening population. CRC screening test uptake rates derived from National Health Information Survey (NHIS) prior to 1992 (*) from Center for Disease Control Morbidity and Mortality Weekly Reports. Behavioral Risk Factor Surveillance System (BRFSS) data used for 1997–2010, obtained from National Cancer Institute (Vital Signs 2002–2010). The surveys did not differentiate between FS and CS for "lower endoscopy"; however sharp rise is due almost entirely to an increased use of CS

of hormone replacement therapy among women and the widespread use of aspirin for cardiovascular health.

16.1.1 Rationale and History of CRC Screening

In the USA, screening for CRC had been promoted since the mid-1970s, but the tools that are currently used for screening have a much longer history. The digital rectal exam (Latin *palpatio per anum*) is a time-honored part of the physical examination. Although the *Corpus Hippocraticum,* dating back to the fourth and fifth centuries BC, recorded the first rudimentary attempt at endoscopy with a rectal speculum, most historians credit Philipp Bozzini (Fig. 16.2a) as the creator of the first modern endoscope in 1806—the *Lichtleiter* or light conductor (Fig. 16.2b). The device was constructed with double aluminum tubes (to be inserted in the body orifice being examined), angled mirrors to project internal structures to the human eye, and employed a single candle as a light source (Natalin and Landman 2009). Christian Friedrich Schonbein first recognized the chemical reaction causing rapid bluing of guaiac (a resin from the West Indian plant gouyacan) when exposed to ozonized air in the 1850s (Fruton 1999), and Van Deen discovered guaiac as a test for occult blood in 1863 (Massachusetts Medical Society 1907).

As early as 1977, the American Cancer Society (ACS) recommended CRC screening with digital rectal exam and rigid proctoscopy as part of a *cancer-related health checkup* (Eddy 1980). At that time, the rationale for screening was largely based on evidence that patients found to have earlier stage disease have a much

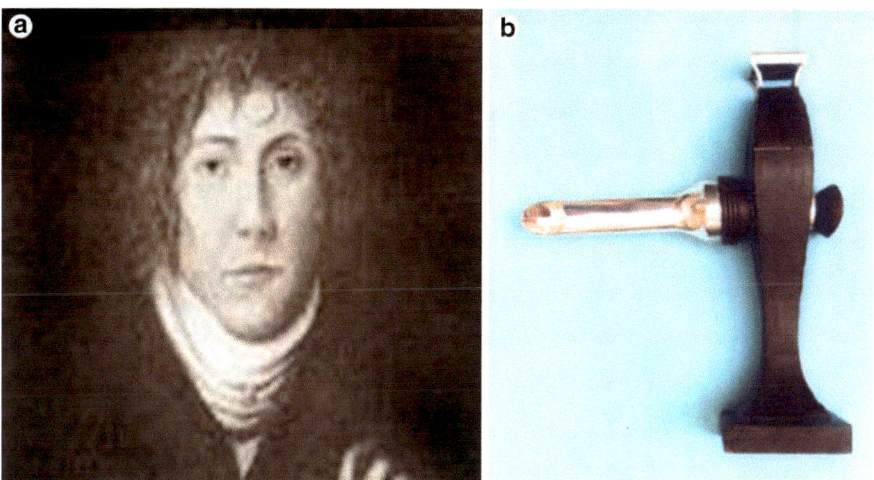

Fig. 16.2 (**a**) Philipp Bozzini (1773–1809). (**b**) The *Lichtleiter* or light conductor (Reprinted by permission from Macmillan Publishers Ltd.: Nature Reviews Urology reference (Natalin and Landman 2009), copyright 2009)

improved survival. Subsequent observations that patients with CRCs detected by screening had earlier stage disease as well as an improved survival compared to those who presented with symptoms seemed to support the value of screening. These types of observations are, of course, seriously biased; they are subject to both lead time and length bias, and compelling evidence of the effectiveness of screening awaited the completion of the randomized screening trials beginning in the 1990s. On the basis of these trials, the US Preventive Services Task Force (USPSTF) initially recommended CRC screening with annual fecal occult blood testing and/or sigmoidoscopy in 1995 with a grade B recommendation citing fair evidence of effectiveness (USPSTF 1995). In 2002, the USPSTF upgraded CRC screening to a grade A recommendation stating that the USPSTF "*strongly recommends that clinicians screen men and women aged 50 and older who are at average risk for colorectal cancer,*" and CRC screening became a Healthcare Effectiveness Data and Information Set (HEDIS) performance measure in 2004 essentially establishing that CRC screening is an accepted standard of care in the USA (HEDIS measures are said to be used by over 90% of US health plans to measure performance). CRC screening guidelines in the USA have evolved over time (Fig. 16.3), largely based on the results of the trials that will be described in this review.

16.2 Screening Options

Current CRC screening options can be categorized into stool-based testing and radiographic or endoscopic imaging. Stool-based tests detect the consequences of colonic neoplasia (bleeding or shedding of neoplastic cells into the stool) and are currently better at detecting cancers than precancerous colonic polyps, while imaging

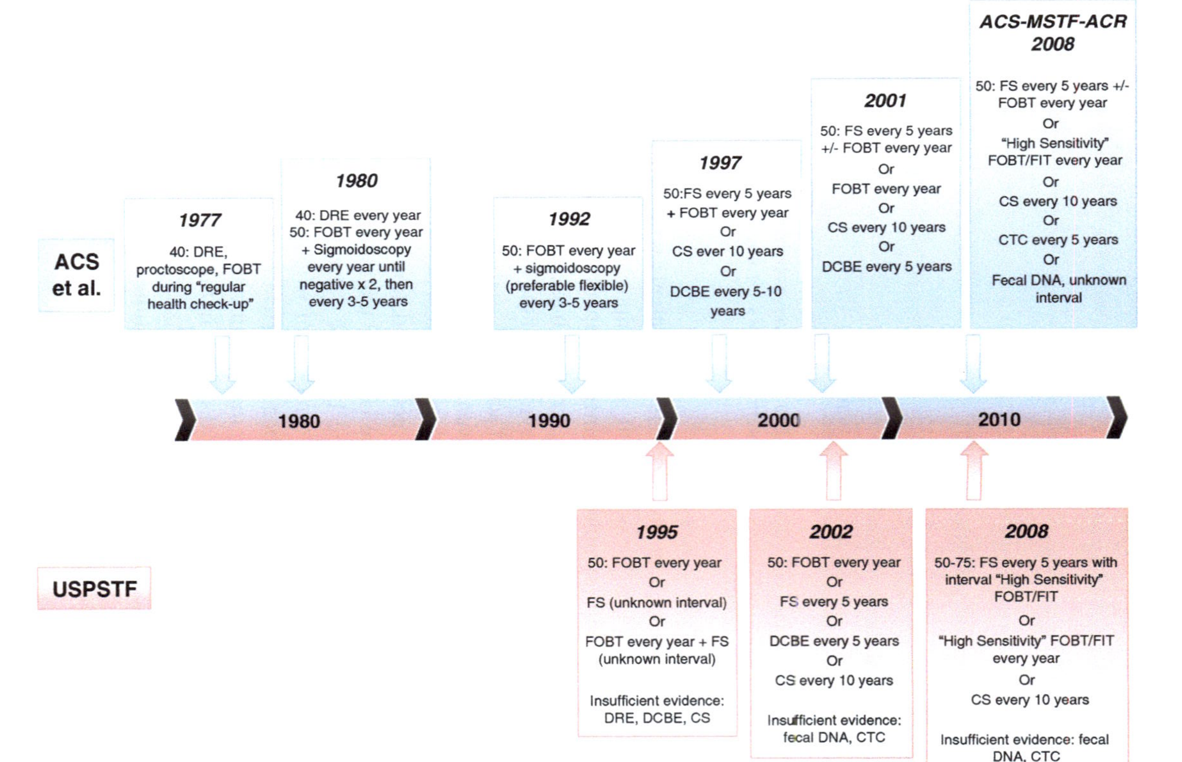

Fig. 16.3 Time line of colorectal cancer screening guidelines. ACS guidelines changed to ACS–MSTF–ACR guidelines in 2008. Prior to 2008, MSTF published independent guidelines. The 2008 USPSTF guidelines do not recommend routine screening for adults 75–85 years of age and recommend against screening adults older than 85 years of age (Levin and Murphy 1992; Byers et al. 1997; Smith et al. 2001; Levin et al. 2008; USPSTF 1995, 2002, 2008)

modalities (endoscopy, radiology) can directly visualize both colonic polyps and cancers. It is clinically more appealing to prevent CRC than to detect it early, so the imaging modalities have a decided conceptual advantage over the stool-based tests. The ability to identify and remove polyps of the colon, thus preventing the development of CRC, is a particular strength of endoscopic CRC screening; for this reason, it should perhaps be described as colon screening rather than CRC screening. A major disadvantage of imaging modalities is that polyps are very common (well over half the population will have polyps in their lifetime), while CRC is much less common (about 5% lifetime risk). Since the large majority of polyps do not progress to cancer, decisions need to be made about which polyps should be deemed important enough to remove.

The available colon screening tests will be described below with a brief summary of the evidence regarding their efficacy as a screening tool. Some of their performance characteristics are compared in Table 16.1. The discussion below is limited to screening of average-risk individuals. For more detailed reviews of each test and recommendations regarding high-risk groups (those with family history of CRC, familial cancer syndromes, or inflammatory bowel disease), see Levin et al. (2008) and USPSTF technical review (2008).

16.2.1 Stool-Based Tests

Stool-based CRC screening tests include guaiac-based and immunochemical fecal occult blood tests (FOBTs) and, more recently, stool DNA tests. The concept of stool testing is based on the observation that colonic neoplasms can both bleed and shed cells into the stool. Fecal occult blood testing is the most widely used CRC screening modality in the world (Von Karsa et al. 2008) and has been the most rigorously evaluated (Table 16.2a).

FOBT is an appealing screening option in that it is noninvasive, inexpensive, and generally simple to use and can be performed by the primary care provider. However, FOBTs have the distinct disadvantage that it is difficult to achieve adequate compliance, necessary for maximal effectiveness.

Stool DNA testing is conceptually appealing in that it measures genetic and epigenetic alterations of DNA that are thought to drive (or at least be directly related to) the process of carcinogenesis, and since these events occur in precancerous polyps as well as cancers, it might be able to detect precursor lesions (which typically do not bleed much) better than FOBT. Stool DNA testing also requires repeated testing and is currently more expensive than FOBTs. Any positive stool-based test requires an additional step (colonoscopy) as part of the screening program; thus, stool-based testing is by design a two-step program.

16.2.1.1 Guaiac Fecal Occult Blood Testing (gFOBT)

Guaiac-based tests detect heme in the stool by the presence of a peroxidase reaction, which turns the guaiac-impregnated paper blue. Appropriate testing requires

Table 16.1 Summary of colorectal cancer screening modalities

Test	Advantages	Disadvantages	Sensitivity	Specificity	Screening interval	Guideline support	Cost per test
Imaging tests							
FS	Minimal bowel preparation required Sedation not required Quick Performed every 5 years Does not require specialist or physician	Does not visualize entire colon Patient discomfort Risk of bleeding, perforation Two-step test Operator dependent, bowel preparation dependent	60–70% for "clinically significant neoplasia"[a]	Equivalent to CS for region visualized	5 years	Rex et al. (2009) Smith et al. (2001) Yee et al. (2010) USPSTF (2008) ASGE (2006) WGO (2007) ACN (2005)	$150–300[b]
CS	Can visualize entire colon Performed every 10 years Can remove/biopsy lesions Can diagnose other diseases Single-step diagnostic and treatment Minimal patient discomfort	Invasive Sedation required, patient must be accompanied Time consuming Expensive Full bowel preparation required Risk of bleeding, perforation Operator dependent, bowel preparation dependent	*Generally considered "gold standard"* 90% (when using CTC as standard) for adenoma >5 mm, 97% for advanced adenoma	*Generally considered "gold standard"*	10 years	Rex et al. (2009) Smith et al. (2001) Yee et al. (2010) USPSTF (2008) ASGE (2006) WGO (2007)	$>1,000[b]

DCBE	Small risk of perforation Performed every 5 years Does not require sedation Can visualize entire colon	Insensitive for lesions <1 cm Less training for technicians/radiologists administering and interpreting exam Full bowel preparation required Two-step test	50% for adenomas >1 cm 39% for all polyps	96% for adenomas >10 mm	5 years	Smith et al. (2001) Yee et al. (2010)	\$300–400[b]
CTC	Small risk of perforation Less time consuming than endoscopy No sedation required Performed every 5 years Can visualize entire colon	Can miss polyps <1 cm Full bowel preparation required Unclear how to follow extracolonic findings Two-step test Radiation exposure Operator dependent Expensive	6–9 mm: 23–86% >/= 10 mm: 52–92%	86–95%	5 years	0 Smith et al. (2001) Yee et al. (2010) USPSTF (2008) WGO (2007)	\$>1,000[b]
Stool based tests							
gFOBT	Low risk, noninvasive Widely available No bowel preparation Inexpensive Home testing	High false-positive rate Insensitive for adenomatous lesions Requires frequent testing Two-step test Pretest dietary limitations	For CRC: Single test: 30% Multiple non-rehydrated: 50–60% Multiple rehydrated: 80–90%	For CRC: 87–98%	1 year	Rex et al. (2009) Smith et al. (2001) Yee et al. (2010) USPSTF (2008) ASGE (2006) EU (2010) WGO (2007) ACN (2005)	\$13[d]

(continued)

Table 16.1 (continued)

Test	Advantages	Disadvantages	Sensitivity	Specificity	Screening interval	Guideline support	Cost per test
FIT/iFOBT	Low risk, noninvasive	High false-positive rate	81.9–94.1% for CRC	87.5% for CRC	1 year	Rex et al. (2009)	$20[d]
	Widely available	Insensitive for adenomatous lesions	25–27% for advanced adenoma	97–93% for advanced adenoma		Smith et al. (2001) Yee et al. (2010) USPSTF (2008)	
	No bowel preparation Inexpensive Home testing No pretest dietary restrictions More specific to lower GIT human globin	Requires frequent testing Two-step test	67% for "clinically significant neoplasia"	91.4% for "clinically significant neoplasia"		ASGE (2006) WGO (2007) ACN (2005)	

Stool DNA	Low risk, noninvasive	Cumbersome	25–51% for CRC	94–96% for CRC	Unknown	Rex et al. (2009)	$350[b]
	No bowel preparation	Expensive	20–41% for advanced adenomas + CRC		Rex et al. (2009) recommends 3 years	Smith et al. (2001)	
	Home testing	Unclear how to manage false-positive results				Yee et al. (2010)	
	No pretest dietary restrictions	Unknown surveillance interval				WGO (2007)	
		Two-step test					

FS flexible sigmoidoscopy, *CS* colonoscopy, *DCBE* double contrast barium enema, *CTC* computerized tomography colonography, *gFOBT* guaiac fecal occult blood testing, *FIT* fecal immunochemical testing, *iFOBT* immunochemical fecal occult blood testing, *ACG* American College of Gastroenterology, *ASGE* American Society for Gastrointestinal Endoscopy, *ACS–MSTF–ACR* American Cancer Society-Multi Society Task Force-American College of Radiology, *USPSTF* United States Preventative Services Task Force, *EU* European Guidelines for Quality Assurance in CRC screening and diagnosis, *WGO* World Gastroenterology Organization, *CCA/ACN* Cancer Council Australia/Australian Cancer Network

[a]Advanced adenoma or CRC

[b]American Cancer Society Colorectal Cancer Facts & Figures 2008–2010

[c]Advanced adenoma: significant villous features (>25%), size of 1.0 cm or more, high-grade dysplasia, or early invasive cancer

[d]Levi et al. 2007

Table 16.2a Summary of design of randomized screening trials of FOBT

<table>
<tr><th>Trial</th><th>Screening frequency</th><th>Follow-up (years)</th><th>Test</th><th>Participants</th><th>Attendance (first screen||at least 1||subsequent rounds)</th></tr>
<tr><td>Nottingham Scholefield et al. 2002</td><td>Biennial</td><td>11.7</td><td>Hemoccult not rehydrated</td><td>152,303</td><td>53.4% || 59.6% || ---</td></tr>
<tr><td>Funen Kronborg et al. 2004</td><td>Biennial</td><td>17</td><td>Hemoccult II not rehydrated</td><td>61,939</td><td>66.8% || --- || 91-94%</td></tr>
<tr><td>Goteborg Lindholm et al. 2008</td><td>Biennial</td><td>15.75</td><td>Hemoccult II rehydrated</td><td>23,916</td><td>63% || 70% || 60%</td></tr>
<tr><td>Minnesota Mandel et al. 1999, 2000</td><td>Annual (A) and biennial (B)</td><td>18</td><td>Hemoccult rehydrated</td><td>46,551</td><td>--- || 75% A, 78% B || ---</td></tr>
</table>

Table 16.2b Summary of results of randomized screening trials of FOBT

Trial	Sensitivity[a]	PPV[b] CRC	PPV adenoma	CRC incidence	CRC mortality[c]	All-cause mortality
Nottingham Scholefield et al. 2002	57.2%	9.9–17.1%	42.8–54.5%	1.51 vs. 1.53/1,000 person year	0.87 (0.78–0.97)	1.01 (0.96–1.05)
Funen Kronborg et al. 2004	55%	5.2–18.7%	14.6–38.3%	1.02 (0.93–1.12)	0.84 (0.73–0.96)	0.99 (0.97–1.02)
Goteborg Lindholm et al. 2008	82%	4.8%	14%	0.96 (0.86–1.06)	0.84 (0.71–0.99)	1.02 (0.99–1.06)
Minnesota Mandel et al. 1999, 2000	92.2%	0.9–6.1%	6–11%	A: 0.8 (0.73–0.94) B: 0.83 (0.73–0.94)	A: 0.67 (0.51–0.83) B: 0.79, (0.62–0.97)	342 (334–350)[d] A: 340 (333–348) B: 343 (336–351)

[a]Proportion of all CRC that were detected by screening, where "all CRC" was the sum of screen-detected cancers (TP) and interval cancers within 1 or 2 years of screening (FN)

[b]Positive predictive value

[c]Reported as odd ratio with 95% confidence interval

[d]Mortality per 1,000

collecting stool samples from three consecutive bowel movements at home to improve sensitivity. Patients are typically instructed to avoid aspirin and other nonsteroidal anti-inflammatory drugs (NSAIDs) for 7 days and vitamin C, raw vegetables, red meat, poultry, and fish for 3 days prior to testing to theoretically improve specificity. However, a systematic review indicated that a recommended restricted diet did not decrease FOBT false-positivity rates, but did decrease compliance to testing (Pignone et al. 2001). There are a variety of commercial FOBTs available; the initial tests such as Hemoccult and Hemoccult II have been shown to be effective in screening trials (Table 16.2b) and are the standard by which subsequent FOBTs have been compared, but they have substantially lower sensitivity for CRC than Hemoccult SENSA (see below). The current US CRC screening guidelines (USPSTF and ACS–MSTF–ACR) recommend the use of only high-sensitivity FOBTs.

Performance Characteristics

The performance characteristics of gFOBTs can be assessed as a one-time test for the detection of CRC or adenomas of the colon, but since gFOBTs are recommended to be repeated every 1–2 years, the performance of a program of gFOBT testing is also important (this distinction highlights the critical importance of ongoing compliance as an issue for stool testing). As would be expected, the performance characteristics of any gFOBT will vary with the age and prevalence of CRC in the population screened, but there is even greater performance variability among the types of gFOBTs (Winawer et al. 1993; Allison et al. 1996, 2007; Hewitson et al. 2008; Kronborg et al. 2004; Lansdorp-Vogelaar et al. 2009; Mandel et al. 1999). Of all the commercial kits available, Hemoccult SENSA is the most sensitive (64–80%) but the least specific (87–90%) of the gFOBT (Whitlock et al. 2008). Despite the lower specificity, Hemoccult SENSA has recently become the most widely recommended gFOBT kit in the United States. In 2008, both the USPSTF (2008) and the ACS–MSTF–ACR (Levin et al. 2008) published consensus guidelines endorsing fecal tests with 50% or greater one-time sensitivity, and HemeSensa is the only gFOBT that was mentioned as meeting this threshold. Since both of these guidelines also endorse colonoscopy as an acceptable screening test for the average-risk population in the USA, the lower specificity of HemeSensa becomes less important since the result of a positive test is a recommendation for colonoscopy. In this context, stool testing can be viewed as a way of identifying a subset of the average-risk population that is more likely to benefit from colonoscopic evaluation.

Efficacy

Despite the current recommendations for the use of a highly sensitive FOBT, the clinical efficacy of FOBT has only been established by prospective trials using the lower sensitivity Hemoccult or Hemoccult II tests. The first trial, reported by Mandel et al. (2000) from the University of Minnesota, randomized 46,551 patients to annual FOBT, biennial FOBT, or a control arm. Mortality due to colorectal cancer was decreased by 33% at 13 years in the annual screening group and 21% at 18 years in the biennial screening group when compared to the control arm. Subsequently, three European trials also demonstrated a CRC mortality benefit ranging from 13% to 16% using biennial screening (Scholefield et al. 2002; Kronborg et al. 2004; Lindholm et al. 2008). Longer-term follow-up of the Minnesota study showed that gFOBT screening led to a 17–20% lower incidence of CRC (Mandel et al. 2000), (Table 16.2a). Since FOBT screening is not therapeutic, this observation remains among the strongest evidence that the colonoscopic identification and removal of polyps can prevent the future development of CRC. Overall, there is a solid evidence base for gFOBT screening for CRC; the 33% reduction in mortality with annual gFOBTs is similar to that seen for regular mammography screening, and the decrease in incidence established the role of screening for the prevention as well as the early detection of CRC. It is only fair to note that there is no evidence that screening with FOBT decreases all-cause mortality (Table 16.2b); in fact a meta-analysis of the three major controlled trials (Moayyedi and Achkar 2006) found that screening was associated with a significant decrease in CRC mortality, a significant increase in non-CRC mortality, and no impact on overall mortality.

16.2.1.2 Fecal Immunochemical Tests (iFOBT or FIT)

Immunochemical tests for blood in the stool have several theoretical and practical advantages over gFOBTs. FITs specifically detect human globin, so they do not require dietary restriction of meat or peroxidase-rich food, and FITs typically require one to two stool samples rather than the three recommended for gFOBTs, making the test easier for patients to complete. Not surprisingly, participation rates have been reported to be significantly higher for FIT than gFOBT, 61.5% versus 49.5% (Hol et al. 2010a). In addition, globin protein is digested in the stomach and proximal small bowel, so FIT should be more specific for bleeding from the colon than gFOBTs. There are multiple FDA-approved FIT kits commercially available; the major technical differences among the tests are whether they can report quantitative as well as qualitative results and whether they can be performed in an individual laboratory or require central processing. Analysis of reported data with FITs is complicated by the fact that the level of sensitivity can be adjusted and the number of tests recommended is not uniform—the performance characteristics of the test vary substantially by adjusting either or both of these parameters. FIT is typically more expensive than gFOBT.

Performance Characteristics

FIT is thought to have a similar sensitivity for CRCs and advanced adenomas as Hemoccult SENSA, and both have improved sensitivity over other gFOBTs like

Hemoccult II. Allison et al. (2007) reported that FIT sensitivity was higher than Hemoccult SENSA for distal CRCs (81.9% vs. 64.3%) but lower for advanced adenomas (29.4% vs. 41.3%). Similarly, Levi et al. (2007) analyzed 1,000 consecutive average-risk patients undergoing colonoscopy, 17 of whom were found to have cancer. Using three immunochemical FOBTs and a hemoglobin threshold of 75 ng/mL, they calculated a sensitivity of 94.1% and specificity of 87.5% for cancer. Using the same testing parameters, they calculated a sensitivity and specificity of 67% and 91.4%, respectively, for clinically significant neoplasia (advanced adenoma and cancer). Hundt et al. (2009) examined the testing characteristics of six different FIT kits and found great variability in performance. For the two best performing tests (immoCARE-C [CARE diagnostica, Voerde, Germany] and FOB advanced [ulti med, Ahrensburg, Germany]), the sensitivity for detection of advanced adenomas was 25% and 27% with a specificity of 97% and 93%, respectively.

Efficacy

There are no long-term data of the impact of screening with FIT on CRC mortality or incidence.

Guidelines

Annual FOBT screening with a high (>50%)-sensitivity guaiac-based or immunochemical test is included among the recommended options in both the USPSTF (2008) and ACS–MSTF–ACR (Levin et al. 2008) guidelines and is a covered benefit by the Center for Medicare & Medicaid Services (CMS) and most US insurance plans. FOBTs are the most commonly used colon screening tests worldwide with national population-based screening programs in most developed nations.

16.2.1.3 Fecal DNA Testing

Fecal DNA testing is a new and evolving stool-based screening test based on the observations that colonic neoplasms have altered DNA compared to normal cells, that colonic neoplasms shed cells into the stool, and that their altered DNA can be detected in the stool. Fecal DNA testing has the theoretical advantage of identifying a marker thought to be in the causal pathway to CRC (mutations or mutation-like events) rather than the less-specific finding of blood in the stool. There is currently one commercially available stool DNA test in the USA (PreGen-Plus™) that tests for a panel of 21 specific mutations as well as a marker of microsatellite instability and DNA integrity. For this test, patients receive a kit to collect an entire bowel movement into a container which is shipped to a central laboratory for processing.

Performance Characteristics

Stool DNA testing is a very active area of ongoing research, and there are numerous studies reporting high sensitivity and specificity of various stool DNA tests in selected patient populations. In the screening setting, there are two controlled trials of PreGen-Plus™ which reported a sensitivity for CRC of 25–51% and for clinically significant neoplasia (CRC plus advanced adenomas) of 20–41% with specificities of 94–96%* (Imperiale et al. 2004; Ahlquist et al. 2008).

Efficacy

There are no long-term data available upon which to draw conclusions regarding the efficacy of fecal DNA testing on CRC mortality or incidence.

Guidelines

Fecal DNA testing was included as a recommended option in the current ACS–MSTF–ACR guidelines (Levin et al. 2008); however, it was concluded that there was insufficient evidence to recommend a surveillance interval. The USPSTF (2008), on the other hand, concluded that there was insufficient evidence to recommend the test and CMS ruled in 2007 that the only fecal DNA test commercially available at the time (PreGen Plus) required premarket approval by the FDA prior to consideration of Medicare/Medicaid coverage. There would appear to be a large potential upside for stool DNA testing as more informative molecular markers (mutations, epigenetic markers such as gene hypermethylation, microRNAs) of the adenoma–carcinoma sequence are identified.

16.2.2 Imaging Tests

Colonic imaging tests used for screening include radiologic (barium enema and CT colonography) as well as endoscopic (flexible sigmoidoscopy and colonoscopy) tests.

16.2.2.1 Double Contrast Barium Enema (DCBE)

Clinically, DCBE is not a very appealing option for colon screening; it has never been tested for this purpose and it is not often used. DCBE has the advantage of being a time-honored imaging modality of the entire colon, but it requires fluoroscopy which in the United States is being supplanted by cross-sectional imaging techniques such as CT colonography. Routine bowel preparation is required; the examination is un-sedated and can be painful. Abnormal results should be followed by direct endoscopic visualization via colonoscopy.

Performance Characteristics

There have been no large prospective controlled trials of DCBE in screening populations. In retrospective analyses, DCBE has been reported to have a sensitivity for cancer of 85–97% (Levin et al. 2008). In two small studies, the sensitivity for adenomas greater than 7–10 mm in size was 48–73% (Winawer et al. 2000; Williams et al. 1982), and one study reported that DCBE has a specificity of 96% for large adenomas (Yee et al. 2010).

Efficacy

There are no studies evaluating the effectiveness of DCBE on CRC mortality or incidence.

Guidelines

DCBE is included as a recommended option in the current ACS–MSTF–ACR guidelines (Levin et al. 2008) but was dropped without comment from the most recent USPSTF guidelines (2008).

16.2.2.2 Computerized Tomography Colonography (CTC)

CT colonography first emerged as a possible tool for colorectal cancer screening in the mid-1990s, and the technology has rapidly evolved since. CTC is an attractive screening approach in that, like colonoscopy, it visualizes polyps as well as cancer throughout the colon, but it does not require sedation; it takes less time and is associated with a lower complication rate than colonoscopy. Current protocols require patients to undergo a standard bowel preparation, and the colon is inflated using a rectal catheter prior to imaging, which can cause discomfort.

Performance Characteristics

Estimating sensitivity and specificity for CTC is more complicated than for any of the other screening modalities since the current radiologic practice is not to report polyps less than 5 mm in size. The rationale for this policy appears to be that these diminutive polyps are thought to be of little clinical importance and the sensitivity and specificity of CTC is low for diminutive polyps. Thus, the true sensitivity for small but histologically advanced adenomas cannot be calculated. In addition, the reported sensitivities for CTC studies are quite varied. Sensitivity for polyps sized 6–9 mm has ranged from 23% to 86% and from 52% to 92% for polyps ≥10 mm (Pickhardt et al. 2003; Cotton et al. 2004; Rockey et al. 2005; Johnson et al. 2008). This wide variability is likely due to differences in technology and operator dependence.

There is a concern that operator dependence could be even a bigger issue in the general community than that reported in the controlled trials. Pickhardt et al. (2003) utilized "very highly skilled readers," and Johnson et al. (2008) required their study radiologists to have experience with greater than 500 cases and to pass a qualifying examination (90% detection rate); 25% of invited readers failed the exam and were not allowed to participate in the study. Thus, the data in the studies reflects highly skilled readers and may not be generalizable to the community. At present, although professional society guidelines exist, there are no clear minimal standards and no requirements to document or regulate competence in the performance of CTC, and even non-radiologists are being offered training in CTC. Despite these concerns, the best CTC studies (Pickhardt et al. 2003 and Johnson et al. 2008) reported a sensitivity of CTC for cancer and for polyps larger than 1 cm that was high (93.8% and 90%, respectively) equivalent to that of colonoscopy, and the images can be strikingly similar (Fig. 16.4).

Specificity is important with regard to CTC because a certain polyp size threshold is generally used to trigger referral for endoscopic evaluation. Early studies (Pickhardt et al. 2003; Cotton et al. 2004; Rockey et al. 2005) reported specificities above 95% for polyps greater than 1 cm. More recent studies have reported lower specificities, likely in attempts to capture a higher sensitivity. For instance, Johnson et al. (2008), in the American College of Radiology Imaging Network (ACRIN) study, reported a specificity of 86% for polyps larger than 10 mm.

There are several important caveats to consider when interpreting the CTC data. First, the CTC studies either did not report or had very low sensitivity and specificity for detection of polyps less than 5 mm. Even though only a small percentage of polyps less than 5 mm have advanced histology (only 1 of 966 diminutive polyps found in Pickhardt's trial had villous features), it is unclear if leaving these polyps undetected and unremoved is an acceptable practice. Secondly, there are little data about the performance of CTC for the detection of flat lesions in the colon which are increasingly reported as having a substantial cancer risk (Soetikno and Kaltenbach 2010). To be fair, small and flat lesions are also missed frequently by endoscopy.

Among the colon screening tests, CTC is second only to colonoscopy in cost. There are conflicting data regarding the cost-effectiveness of CTC compared with colonoscopy (Ladabaum et al. 2004; Hassan et al. 2007; Hur et al. 2007; Vijan et al. 2007; Pickhardt et al. 2008). Most of these modeling studies assumed use of the recommendation to only routinely refer patients for colonoscopy if polyps greater than 1 cm are found. In practice, Shah et al. (2009) found that both patients and physicians preferred to follow even small polyps with colonoscopic examination. If all detected polyps led to colonoscopy, the cost of primary CTC screening would go up substantially.

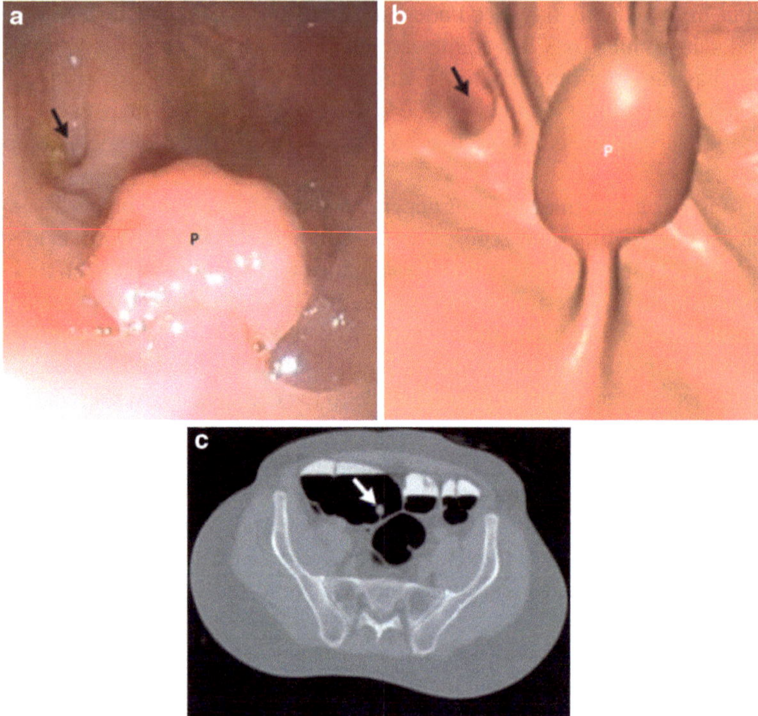

Fig. 16.4 Fifty-five-year-old male with 16-mm pedunculated cecal polyp. *Panel A* shows endoscopic view of insufflated cecum with polyp. *Panel B* is three-dimensional endoluminal "fly-through" view of CTC showing same polyp. *Panel C* is axial, two-dimensional CT image with patient in prone position showing air-filled colon and polyp. In panel A and B, appendiceal orifice marked with *arrow*, polyp labeled "P." In panel C, *arrow points* out polyp (Adapted from Pickhardt et al. 2003 with permission from the Massachusetts Medical Society)

Efficacy

There are no long-term data available to assess CTC screening on CRC mortality.

Guidelines

CTC is included among the recommended options in the ACS–MSTF–ACR (Levin et al. 2008), but the USPSTF (2008) concluded there was insufficient evidence to recommend CTC screening and CMS ruled in 2009 that CTC screening would not be covered by Medicare or Medicaid. Both the USPSTF and CMS raised concerns about the variability in the literature on CTC performance characteristics, radiation exposure, and the high frequency of non-colonic findings on CTC in their recommendations. Although none of these concerns are unique to CTC (Garg and Ahnen 2010), the combination was deemed a significant limitation of CTC screening.

CTC is sporadically reimbursed by insurance programs, and the CMS ruling precludes offering CTC to Medicare/Medicaid recipients. It seems likely that these limitations can be overcome with ongoing standardization of techniques, performance, and training and as more efficacy and safety data emerges. There would seem to be a lot of upside potential for technology to improve CTC characterization of colonic lesions and to decrease the need for a bowel preparation by stool tagging.

16.2.2.3 Flexible Sigmoidoscopy (FS)

FS is generally performed with a 60 cm sigmoidoscope which typically allows visualization to the descending colon or splenic flexure (less than half of the colonic length). The bowel preparation for FS is usually enemas alone, so the preparation may not be as good as with the more extensive preparations used for CTC or colonoscopy. FS typically does not require sedation which is a major advantage for patient convenience and capacity in that it allows FS to be performed by nonphysicians (nurses, mid-levels), but it also leads to substantially more patient discomfort than with sedated procedures. Polyps can be removed during FS to determine their histology, and in the United States, the finding of an adenoma prompts referral for colonoscopy (guidelines in the United Kingdom allow for no surveillance for patients with 1–2 small [<1 cm] adenomas).

Performance Characteristics

Within the whole colon, sensitivity of FS for advanced adenomas and CRC is approximately 60–70% (when compared to colonoscopy as gold standard) (Imperiale et al. 2000). Provided good bowel preparation, the sensitivity and specificity for detecting lesions in the distal bowel is assumed to be equivalent to colonoscopy.

Efficacy

The initial evidence supporting CRC screening with FS came from case–control studies that demonstrated a CRC-related mortality benefit in people who had undergone FS within the previous 6–10 years compared to those who had not (Newcomb et al. 1992; Selby et al. 1992; Müller and Sonnenberg 1995). There have been three randomized screening trials that have examined the effect of FS on CRC incidence and mortality (Table 16.3), with several more trials underway (Prostate, Lung, Colon, and Ovarian [PLCO] trial in US and Italian National Trial).

The first trial of FS screening, the Norwegian Telemark Polyp Study I (Thiis-Evensen et al. 1999), was a small (799 participants) single-center randomized comparison of FS to no screening. The authors reported a remarkably high screening rate in this study (81%), and all patients with any polyp were referred for colonoscopy at 2 and 6 years, with an 86% and 75% attendance rate, respectively. After 13 years of follow-up, the authors reported a stunning 80% reduction in CRC incidence.

Table 16.3 Summary of randomized controlled trials for flexible sigmoidoscopy: CRC incidence, mortality, and all-cause mortality

Trial	Participants	Follow-up (years)	CRC incidence	CRC mortality[a]	All-cause mortality
Telemark Thiis-Evensen et al. 1999	799	13	0.2 (0.03–0.95, $p=0.02$)*	No patients died of CRC in either arm	1.57 (1.03–2.4, $p=0.02$)*
NorCCaP[b] Hoff et al. 2009	55,736	7	134.5 vs. 131.9/100,000 person-year	0.73 (0.47–1.13, $p=0.16$) ITT[c] 0.41 (0.21–0.82, $p=0.011$) per protocol*	1.02 (0.98–1.07, $p=0.28$)
UK FS trial	113,195	11.2	0.77 (0.7–0.84, $p<0.0001$) ITT*	0.69 (0.59–0.82, $p<0.0001$) ITT*	0.97 (0.94–1, $p=0.0519$)
Atkin et al. 2010			0.67 (0.6–0.76, $p<0.0001$) per protocol*	0.57 (0.45–0.72, $P<0.0001$) per protocol*	

*Statistically significant
[a]Reported as odds ratio with 95% confidence interval
[b]Norwegian Colorectal Cancer Prevention
[c]Intention to treat

A decade later, Hoff et al. (2009) reported much less promising results from their larger (55,736 participants) Norwegian Colorectal Cancer Prevention (NorCCaP) trial. At 7-year follow-up, there was no difference in the cumulative CRC incidence (134.5 vs. 131.9 cases per 100,000 person-years for screening group and control group, respectively) or mortality (HR 0.73, CI 0.47–1.13) in the intention to treat analysis. Most recently, Atkin et al. (2010) reported results from the very large (113,195 participants) multicenter randomized UK sigmoidoscopy trial of FS versus no screening. Within the intervention group, 71% underwent FS, 5% of which were referred for colonoscopy because of multiple adenomas or large adenomas. After a mean follow-up of 11.2 years, they found that FS reduced CRC incidence by 23% (HR 0.77, 95% CI 0.70–0.84) and CRC mortality was reduced by 31% (HR 0.69, 95% CI 0.59–0.82) in the intention to treat analysis.

Guidelines

FS is included as a CRC screening option in both the USPSTF (2008) and the ACS–MSTF–ACR (Levin et al. 2008) guidelines. FS is covered by CMS and most US insurance plans. The UK has announced a nationwide FS screening program through their National Health Service.

16.2.2.4 Colonoscopy

Colonoscopy is thought by many to be the most effective and appealing CRC screening test available given its ability to visualize and simultaneously remove/sample lesions throughout the entire colon. There are not, however, any controlled trials to establish the effect of colonoscopy on CRC incidence and mortality. Although colonoscopy has been accepted as the gold standard for evaluation of other screening tests, it is important to acknowledge that this assumption is seriously flawed given evidence that colonoscopy quality is highly operator dependent; it varies greatly among endoscopists (Rex et al. 1997) in large part due to differences in the training, experience, and skill of the endoscopist. Although various benchmarks have been set to assess the quality of colonoscopy such as cecal intubation rates, adequate withdrawal times and more recently adenoma detection rates, none of these measures directly assess an endoscopist's ability to ultimately detect and completely remove potentially neoplastic lesions.

Colonoscopy is certainly the most expensive screening test that has ever been recommended for average-risk individuals. Colonoscopy also carries more risk in comparison to other modalities with an overall perforation rate of 0.6 per 1,000 (up to four times higher in patients undergoing polypectomy) and a bleeding risk as high as 8.7 per 1,000 procedures in which a polypectomy is performed (Warren et al. 2009). The examination is performed after a full bowel preparation requiring patients to remain on clear liquids the day prior to the procedure and ingest a large volume saline laxative to cleanse the colon. It is generally performed with conscious sedation or anesthesia, which provides an amnesic benefit so that most patients report that the preparation is the most difficult and unpleasant part of the procedure.

Performance Characteristics

Because colonoscopy has been viewed as the gold standard in CRC screening, there are no robust estimates as to test characteristics in terms of sensitivity and specificity. Initially, tandem colonoscopy studies (two complete colonoscopies by different endoscopists during the same session) (Hixson et al. 1990, 1991; Van Rijn et al. 2006) estimated miss rates of 2% for adenomas 10 mm or greater, 13% for adenomas 5–10 mm, and 25% for adenomas less than 5 mm, with a 22% overall miss rate for all polyps. Studies performing both CTC and colonoscopy estimate that the miss rate for colonoscopy is substantially higher (11.8% miss rate for polyps greater than or equal to 10 mm) than those found in the tandem colonoscopy trials (Pickhardt et al. 2003).

Efficacy

There have been no randomized screening trials demonstrating that colonoscopy confers a decreased CRC incidence or mortality. Nonetheless, there is substantial indirect evidence to support the use of colonoscopy as a screening tool. The efficacy of colonoscopic polypectomy was initially highlighted by the National Polyp Study (NPS) which estimated a 76–90% reduction in incidence of colorectal cancer after polyp removal compared to historic controls (Winawer et al. 1993). Similarly, a case–control study by Müller and Sonnenberg (1995) reported that having had a lower endoscopy within the previous 6 years was associated with a 60% reduced CRC mortality (OR 0.41, 95% CI 0.33–0.50). Efficacy can also be extrapolated from randomized controlled trials performed for other screening modalities that eventually referred patients for colonoscopy. The reduction in CRC mortality and incidence in the FOBT and FS trials has been largely attributed to the colonoscopy and polypectomy performed for positive screening results. Thus, although no direct evidence is available to date regarding the efficacy of colonoscopy, there is still a compelling body of indirect evidence to support its use as a screening modality.

However, recent studies have called into question the ability of colonoscopy to prevent CRC throughout the entire colon. Baxter et al. (2009) performed a case–control study in Canada demonstrating that colonoscopy resulted in a significant decrease in mortality from distal colon cancers (OR 0.33, CI 0.28–0.39), but had no effect on death from proximal colon cancers (0.99, 0.86–1.14). Similarly, Brenner et al. (2010) reported that previous colonoscopy was associated with a 67% reduction in advanced neoplasia in the left colon but no risk reduction for right-sided lesions. Interestingly, the same group (Brenner et al. 2011) reported a population-based case–control study from a different region of Germany showing colonoscopy in the preceding 10 years was associated with an overall 77% lower risk of CRC. A varied reduction in CRC was seen when stratified by location with adjusted odds ratios for any CRC, right-sided CRC, and left-sided CRC were 0.23 (95% CI, 0.19–0.27), 0.44 (CI, 0.35–0.55), and 0.16 (CI, 0.12–0.20). Regardless of the magnitude of the effect, in all these studies colonoscopy was less effective in reducing risk of right- than left-sided CRC. Possible reasons for these marked regional differences include differences in biology of right-sided tumors (shortened adenoma–carcinoma sequence), higher proportion of flat lesions, and higher likelihood of poor bowel preparation, among others. It will be of interest when US data on this issue is reported as colonoscopy is much more widely used in the USA than in Canada or Germany.

Three randomized trials are currently underway to directly examine the efficacy of colonoscopy in reducing CRC incidence and mortality. Both the US Department of Veterans Affairs CONFIRM (Colonoscopy vs. Fecal Immunochemical Test in Reducing Mortality from Colorectal Cancer) trial and a Spanish trial will be comparing colonoscopy to FIT, while the Nordic-European Initiative on Colorectal Cancer will compare colonoscopy to no screening. These trials are expected to take another decade to complete.

Guidelines

Colonoscopy is included as an acceptable screening option in both the USPSTF (2008) and ACS–MSTF–ACR (Levin et al. 2008) guidelines with a 10- year interval if no adenomas are found. In the USA, colonoscopic surveillance is recommended (usually at 3–5 year intervals) if adenomas are found on a screening exam. Colonoscopic screening is a covered benefit by CMS and most US insurance plans. Poland is the only country that offers colonoscopy as the only CRC screening option, but it is done on an opportunistic rather than population screening basis (Hol et al. 2010a). In 2002, Germany became the first country to offer colonoscopy screening to the general population, but the uptake rates have been low (<10%) (Hol et al. 2010b) and well below the reported rates in the US.

16.3 Current Screening Practices

Currently, the two most widely quoted sets of guidelines in the USA, the United States Preventive Services Task Force (USPSTF) and the joint guideline of the American Cancer Society (ACS), the US Multi-Society Task Force on CRC (USMSTF) and the American College of Radiology (ACR), both endorse a panel of colon screening options (Table 16.1) including high-sensitivity FOBT, flexible sigmoidoscopy, barium enema, or colonoscopy. The latter group also recommended CT colonography and stool DNA tests as acceptable options, but the USPSTF concluded that there was insufficient evidence to recommend these tests.

CRC screening rates in the USA have been tracked through self-report surveys by the National Health Interview Service (NHIS) of the National Center for Health Statistics, Centers for Disease Control and Prevention since 1987 and by the Behavioral Risk Factor Survey System (BRFSS) since 1997 (Breen et al. 2001). Overall screening rates have been steadily rising (Fig. 16.1), and the most recent BRFSS reports that about 65% of Americans are current with screening recommendations. It seems very likely that the Healthy People 2020 goal (healthypeople.gov2011) of a 75% CRC screening adherence rate will be met. CRC screening rates vary greatly around the world with generally higher compliance with FOBT than endoscopic programs (Hol et al. 2010a).

Colonoscopy is by far the most popular colon screening approach in the USA despite its high cost, invasiveness, and inconvenience; despite the lack of convincing trials showing that colonoscopy is superior to other screening modalities; and despite modeling studies that suggest that an annual high-sensitivity FOBT program would be as or more effective (Zauber et al. 2008). Nevertheless, colonoscopic screening rates have been steadily increasing in the USA, while FOBT use has been slowly declining, and FS has been rapidly declining (Fig. 16.1). The reasons for colonoscopy's dominance are not totally clear but are likely due to a combination of numerous incentives and essentially no disincentives to colonoscopic screening in the USA.

The incentives for colonoscopic screening include the fact that colonoscopy is the final common pathway of all CRC screening programs and it is the only screening test that examines the entire colon and allows polypectomy during the same procedure. Thus, colonoscopy is considered, by many, to be the definitive "gold standard" for CRC screening, and it is conceptually appealing to do the definitive test initially rather than to use a two-step approach. The incentives for the primary care provider (PCP) to choose colonoscopy include that it can be simply ordered by a referral and is then taken off the PCP plate and performance becomes the endoscopists' responsibility. If the colonoscopy is negative, no further testing needs to be done for 10 years as opposed to annual testing with FOBT, thus relieving the PCP as well as the patient from an annual responsibility. There are strong financial incentives for the endoscopist to offer colonoscopic screening since screening colonoscopies are covered by almost all insurance plans in the USA, they are well reimbursed, and, not surprisingly, colonoscopy accounts for a large proportion of the average US gastroenterologist's revenue stream.

There are also substantial disincentives to all of the non-colonoscopic screening tests in the USA. The difficulty of ensuring annual compliance is a major disincentive for FOBT. The USPSTF (2008) and ACS–MSTF–ACR (Levin et al. 2008) recommendations that favor imaging tests that have the potential for prevention over tests that they view as primarily early detection tests for CRC are a disincentive for stool-based tests. The lack of a USPSTF endorsement for stool DNA, CTC, or DCBE is a major disincentive. These roadblocks leave the endoscopic tests; endoscopists would much rather do colonoscopy than FS due to a variety of reasons including the prominently displayed sentiment by the GI community that "flexible sigmoidoscopy is the intellectual equivalent of mammography of one breast"

(Podolsky 2000). In addition, the greater discomfort, inferior bowel preparation, and the low reimbursement rate for FS are major disincentives.

In contrast, there are few disincentives to colonoscopy screening in the USA. One would think that cost would be a major issue; however, cost-effectiveness models have argued that the increased cost of colonoscopy is justified by its estimated increased effectiveness. There are, however, a number of trends in the use of colonoscopy that are impacting its cost-effectiveness in a negative manner including increasing adenoma detection rates which will identify a larger portion of the screened population that will require more frequent surveillance and increase in the pathology costs associated with colonoscopy, the tendency of endoscopists to schedule follow-up colonoscopies at intervals substantially shorter than the guidelines recommend, and the increasing use of anesthesia-directed propofol for routine colonoscopies. Interestingly, all screening and preventive approaches look more attractive (Luo et al. 2009) and even cost-effective (Lansdorp-Vogelaar et al. 2009) as the cost of CRC treatment with the addition of biologics has skyrocketed.

16.4 Conclusions

Colon screening is arguably one of the greatest cancer prevention success stories of the last 25 years contributing substantially to over a 40% reduction in CRC mortality in the USA since 1975. Screening rates are currently over 60% in the USA and are steadily increasing. The field is continuing to move from early detection of CRC to identification and removal of precancerous colonic polyps. High-sensitivity FOBTs (Hemoccult SENSA and FITs) have a higher sensitivity for CRC and advanced adenomas than traditional gFOBTs and are now the only recommended FOBT for screening in the USA. Colonoscopy is the dominant screening test used in the USA, despite limitations including its high cost and lack of data demonstrating that it is more effective than other screening approaches. Colonoscopy is appealing because it can simultaneously identify, diagnose, and treat (remove) colonic neoplasia throughout the entire colon, thus preventing CRC as well as detecting it early. There are few disincentives to its use in the United States. CTC and stool DNA testing may have the highest upside potential for technological advancement in the short term and will likely emerge as contending colon screening modalities.

References

Ahlquist DA, Sargen DJ, Loprinzi CL, Levin TR, Douglas K. Rex DK, Ahnen DJ et al. Stool DNA and occult blood testing for screen detection of colorectal neoplasia. *Ann Intern Med* 2008;149:441–450.

Allison JE, Sakoda LC, Levin TR, Tucker JP, Tekawa IS, Cuff T et al. Screening for colorectal neoplasms with new fecal occult blood tests: update on performance characteristics. *J Natl Cancer Inst* 2007; 99:1462–1470.

Allison JE, Tekawa IS, Ransom LJ, Adrain AL. A comparison of fecal occult-blood tests for colorectal-cancer screening. *N Engl J Med* 1996; 334:155–160.

ASGE. Colorectal Cancer Screening and Surveillance. *Gastrointestinal Endoscopy* 2006; 4:546–557.

Atkin WS, Edwards R, Kralj-Hans I, Wooldrage K, Hart AR, Northover JMA, et al. Once-only flexible sigmoidoscopy screening in prevention of colorectal cancer: a multicentre randomised controlled trial. *Lancet* 2010; 375:1624–1634.

ACN (Australian Cancer Network Colorectal Cancer Guidelines Revision Committee). *Guidelines for the Prevention, Early Detection and Management of Colorectal Cancer*. The Cancer Council Australia and Australian Cancer Network, Sydney 2005.

Baxter NN, Goldwasser MA, Paszat LF, Saskin R, Urbach DR, Rabeneck L. Association of colonoscopy and death from colon cancer. *Ann Intern Med* 2009; 150:1–8.

Breen N, Wagener DK, Brown ML, Davis WW, Ballard-Barbash R. Progress in Cancer Screening Over a Decade: Results of Cancer Screening From the 1987, 1992, and 1998 National Health Interview Surveys. *J Natl Cancer Inst* 2001; 93:1704–1713.

Brenner H, Chang-Claude J, Seiler CM, Rickert A, Hoffmeister M. Protection from colorectal cancer after colonoscopy: a population-based, case-control study. *Ann Intern Med.* 2011;154(1):22–30.

Brenner H, Hoffmeister M, Arndt V, Stegmaier C, Altenhofen L, Haug U. Protection from right- and left-sided colorectal neoplasms after colonoscopy: population-based study. *J Natl Cancer Inst.* 2010; 102:89–95.

Byers T, Levin B, Rothenberger D, Dodd GD, Smith RA. American Cancer Society Guidelines for Screening and Surveillance for Early Detection of Colorectal Polyps and Cancer: Update 1997. *CA Cancer J Clin* 1997; 47:154–160.

Center MM, Jemal A, Smith RA, Ward E. Worldwide variations in colorectal cancer. *CA Cancer J Clin.* 2009; 59:366–378.

Colorectal Cancer Facts and Figures 2008–2010. American Cancer Society. Retrieved 12/29/2011 from http://www.cancer.org/acs/groups/content/@nho/documents/document/f861708finalforwebpdf.pdf.

Cotton PB, Durkalski VL, Pineau BC, Palesch YY, Mauldin PD, Hoffman B et al. Computed tomographic colonography (virtual colonoscopy): a multicenter comparison with standard colonoscopy for detection of colorectal neoplasia. *JAMA* 2004; 291:1713–1719.

Eddy D. ACS report on the cancer-related health checkup. *CA Cancer J Clin.* 1980;30:193–240.

EU (European Guidelines for quality assurance in colorectal cancer screening and diagnosis, first edition). European Union Health Programme 2010.

Fruton JS. Proteins, Enzymes, Genes: the Interplay of Chemistry and Biology. New Haven, Connecticut: Yale University 1999.

Garg S, Ahnen DJ. Is computed tomographic colonography being held to a higher standard? *Ann Intern Med.* 2010; 152:178–181

Hassan C, Zullo A, Laghi A, Reitano I, Taggi F, Cerro P et al. Colon cancer prevention in Italy: cost-effectiveness analysis with CT colonography and endoscopy. *Dig Liver Dis* 2007; 39:242–250.

Hewitson P, Glasziou P, Watson E, Towler B, Irvig L. Cochran systematic review of colorectal cancer screening using the fecal occult blood test (Hemoccult): an update. *Am J Gastroenterol* 2008; 103:1541–1549.

Hixson LJ, Fennerty MB, Sampliner RE, Garewal HS. Prospective blinded trial of the colonoscopic missrate of large colorectal polyps. *Gastrointestinal Endoscopy* 1991; 37:125–127.

Hixson LJ, Fennerty MB, Sampliner RE, McGee D, Garewal H. Prospective study of the frequency and size distribution of polyps missed by colonoscopy. *J Natl Cancer Inst.* 1990; 82:69–1772.

Hoff G, Grotmol T, Skovlund E, Bretthauer M. Risk of colorectal cancer seven years after flexible sigmoidoscopy screening: randomized controlled trial. *BMJ* 2009; 338:b1846.

Hol L, van Leerdam ME, van Ballegooijen M, van Vuuren AJ, van Dekken H, Reijerink JCIY et al. Screening for colorectal cancer: randomised trial comparing guaiac-based and immunochemical faecal occult blood testing and flexible sigmoidoscopy. *Gut* 2010a; 59:62–68.

Hol L, de Jonge V, van Leerdam ME, van Ballegooijen M, Looman CWM, van Vuuren AJ et al. Screening for colorectal cancer: Comparison of perceived test burden of guaiac-based faecal occult blood test, faecal immunochemical test and flexible sigmoidoscopy. *Eur J Cancer* 2010b; 46:2059–2066.

Hundt S, Haug U, Brenner H. Comparative evaluation of immunochemical fecal occult blood tests for colorectal adenoma detection. *Ann Intern Med* 2009;150:162–169.

Hur C, Chung DC, Schoen RE, Gazelle GS. The management of small polyps found by virtual colonoscopy: results of a decision analysis. *Clin Gastroenterol Hepatol* 2007; 5:237–244.

Imperiale TF, Wagner DR, Lin CY, Larkin GN, Rogge JD, Ransohoff DF. Risk of advanced proximal neoplasms in asymptomatic adults according to the distal colorectal findings. *N Engl J Med* 2000; 343:169–174.

Imperiale TF, Ransohoff DF, Itzkowitz SH, Turnball BA, Ross ME. Fecal DNA versus Fecal Occult Blood for Colorectal Cancer Screening in an Average Risk Population. *N Engl J Med* 2004; 351:2704–2714.

Johnson CD, Chen MH, Toledano AY, Heiken JP, Dachman A, Kuo MD et al. Accuracy of CT colonography for detection of large adenomas and cancers. *N Engl J Med* 2008; 359:1207–1217.

Kronborg O, Jorgensen OD, Fenger C, Rasmussen M. Randomized study of biennial screening with a faecal occult blood test: results after nine screening rounds. *Scand J Gastroenterol* 2004; 39:846–851.

Ladabaum U, Song K, Fendrick AM. Colorectal neoplasia screening with virtual colonoscopy: when, at what cost, and with what national impact? *Clin Gastroenterol Hepatol* 2004; 2:554–563.

Lansdorp-Vogelaar I, van Ballegooijen M, Zauber AG, Boer R, Wilschut J, Habbema JD. At what costs will screening with CT colonography be competitive? A cost-effectiveness approach. *Int J Cancer.* 2009;124:1161–1168.

Levi Z, Rozen P, Hazazi R, Vilkin A, Waked A, Maoz E et al. A quantitative immunochemical fecal occult blood test for colorectal neoplasia. *Ann Intern Med* 2007; 146:244–255.

Levin B, Lieberman DA, McFarland B, Smith RA, Brooks D, Andrews KS et al. Screening and surveillance for the early detection of colorectal cancer and adenomatous polyps, 2008: a joint guideline from the American Cancer Society, the US Multi-Society Task Force on Colorectal Cancer, and the American College of Radiology. *CA Cancer J Clin* 2008; 58:130–160.

Levin B, Murphy GP. Revision in American Society Recommendations for the Early Detection of Colorectal Cancer. *CA Cancer J Clin* 1992; 42:296–99.

Lindholm E, Brevinge H, Haglind E. Survival benefit in a randomized clinical trial of faecal occult blood screening for colorectal cancer. *Br J Surg* 2008; 95:1029–1036.

Luo Z, Bradley CJ, Dahman BA, Gardiner JC. Colon cancer treatment costs for Medicare and dually eligible beneficiaries. *Health Care Financing Review* 2009; 31:35–50.

Mandel JS, Church TR, Bond JH, Ederer F, Geisser MS, Mongin SJ et al. The effect of fecal occult-blood screening on the incidence of colorectal cancer. *N Engl J Med* 2000; 343:1603–1607.

Mandel JS, Church TR, Ederer F, Bond JH. Colorectal cancer mortality: effectiveness of biennial screening for fecal occult blood. J Natl Cancer Inst. 1999; 91:434–7.

Massachusetts Medical Society. New England Surgical Society (digitized 2007). *Boston medical and surgical journal.* 1907; 157:170–74. Boston, Mass. Harvard University.

Moayyedi P, Achkar E. Does fecal occult blood testing really reduce mortality? A reanalysis of systematic review data. *Am J Gastroenterol.* 2006; 101:380–384.

Müller AD, Sonnenberg A. Protection by endoscopy against death from colorectal cancer. A case-control study among veterans. *Arch Intern Med* 1995; 155:1741–1748.

National Cancer Institute. Colon and Rectal Cancer. Retrieved 12/29/2011 from http://www.cancer.gov/cancertopics/types/colon-and-rectal.

Natalin RA, Landman J. Where next for the endoscope? *Nature Reviews Urology* 2009; 6:622–628.

Newcomb PA, Norfleet RG, Storer BE, Surawicz TS, Marcus PM. Screening sigmoidoscopy and colorectal cancer mortality. *J Natl Cancer Inst* 1992; 84:1572–1575.

Pickhardt PJ, Choi JR, Hwang I, Butler JA, Puckett ML, Hildebrandt HA et al. Computed tomographic virtual colonoscopy to screen for colorectal neoplasia in asymptomatic adults. *N Engl J Med* 2003; 349:2191–2200.

Pickhardt PJ, Hassan C, Laghi A, Zullo A, Kim DH, Iafrate F et al. Small and diminutive polyps detected at screening CT colonography: a decision analysis for referral to colonoscopy. *Am J Roentgenol* 2008; 190:136–144.

Pignone M, Campbell MK, Carr C, Phillips C. Meta-analysis of dietary restriction during fecal occult blood testing. *Eff Clin Pract* 2001; 4:150–156.

Podolsky DK. Going the distance - the case for true colorectal cancer screening. *N Engl J Med.* 2000; 343:207–208.

Rex DK, Cutler CS, Lemmel GT, Rahmani EY, Clark DW, Helper DJ et al. Colonoscopic miss rates of adenomas determined by back-to-back colonoscopies. *Gastroenterology* 1997; 112: 24–28.

Rex DK, Johnson DA, Anderson JC, Schoenfeld PS, Burke CA, Inadomi JM. American College of Gastroenterology Guidelines for Colorectal Cancer Screening 2008. *American Journal of Gastroenterology* 2009; 104:739–750.

Rockey DC, Paulson E, Niedzwiecki D, Davis W, Bosworth HB, Sanders L et al. Analysis of air contrast barium enema, computed tomographic colonography, and colonoscopy: prospective comparison. *Lancet* 2005; 365:305–311.

Rockey DC. Computed Tomographic Colonography: Current Perspectives and Future Directions. *Gastroenterology* 2009; 137:7–17.

Scholefield JH, Moss S, Sufi F, Mangham CM, Hardcastle JD. Effect of faecal occult blood screening on mortality from colorectal cancer: results from a randomized controlled trial. *Gut* 2002; 50:840–844.

Selby JV, Friedman GD, Quesenberry CP Jr, Weiss NS. A case-control study of screening sigmoidoscopy and mortality from colorectal cancer. *N Engl J Med* 1992; 326:653–657.

Shah JP, Hynan LS, Rockey DC. Management of small polyps detected by screening CT colonography: patient and physician preferences. *Am J Med* 2009; 122:687. E1-9.

Smith RA, von Eschenbach AC, Wender R, Levin B, Byers T, Rothenberger D et al. American Cancer Society Guidelines for the Early Detection of Cancer: Update for early detection guidelines for Prostate, Colorectal and endometrial cancers. *CA Cancer J Clin* 2001; 51:38–75.

Soetikno R, Kaltenbach T. High-quality CT Colonography can detect nonpolypoid colorectal neoplasm (NP-CRN)-science or rhetoric? *Academic Radiology*. 2010;17:1317–1318.

Surveillance Epidemiology End Result (SEER). National Cancer Institute. Retrieved 12/29/2011 from http://seer.cancer.gov/faststats/selections.php?series=cancer.

Thiis-Evensen E, Hoff GS, Sauar J, Langmark F, Majak BM, Vatn MH. Population-based surveillance by colonoscopy: effect on the incidence of colorectal cancer. Telemark Polyp Study I. *Scand J Gastroenterol* 1999;34:414–420.

USPSTF. *Guide to clinical preventive services (2nd edition), Report of the U.S. Preventive Services Task Force.* Department of Health and Human Services, Washington, DC 1995. Retrieved 12/29/2011 from http://odphp.osophs.dhhs.gov/pubs/guidecps/.

USPSTF. Screening for colorectal cancer: Recommendation and Rationale. *Ann Intern Med* 2002; 137:129–131.

USPSTF. Screening for Colorectal Cancer: U.S. Preventive Services Task Force Recommendation Statement. *Ann Intern Med* 2008; 149:627–38.

Van Rijn JC, Reitsma, JB, Stoker, J, Bossuyt PM,van Deventer SJ,Dekker E. Polyp miss rate determined by tandem colonoscopy: a systematic review. *Am J Gastroenterol* 2006; 101:343–350.

Vijan S, Hwang I, Inadomi J, Wong RKH, Choi JR, Napierkowski J et al. The cost-effectiveness of CT colonography in screening for colorectal neoplasia. *Am J Gastroenterology* 2007; 102:380–390.

Vital Signs: Colorectal Cancer Screening, Incidence, and Mortality --- United States, 2002–2010. Morbidity and Mortality Weekly Report (MMWR) Center for Disease Control and Prevention (CDCP). Retrieved 12/29/2011 from http://www.cdc.gov/mmwr/preview/mmwrhtml/mm6026a4.htm.

Von Karsa L, Anttila A, Ronco G, Ponti A, Malila N, Arbyn M, et al. *Cancer screening in the European Union. Report on the implementation of the Council recommendation on cancer screening – First Report.* Luxembourg: European Commission; 2008.

Warren, JL, Klabunde, CN, Mariotto, AB, Meekins A, Topor M, Brown ML et al. Adverse events after outpatient colonoscopy in the Medicare population. *Ann Intern Med* 2009; 150:849–857.

Whitlock EP, Lin JS, Liles E, Beil TL, Fu R. Screening for colorectal cancer: a targeted, updated systematic review for the U.S. Preventive Services Task Force. *Ann Intern Med* 2008; 149:638–658.

Williams CB, Macrae FA, Bartram CI. A Prospective Study of diagnostic methods in adenoma follow-up. *Endoscopy* 1982; 14:74–78.

Winawer SJ, Stewart ET, Zauber AG, Bond JH, Ansel H, Waye JD et al. A comparison of colonoscopy and double-contrast barium enema for surveillance after polypectomy. National Polyp Study Work Group. *N Engl J Med* 2000; 342:1766–1772.

Winawer SJ, Flehinger BJ, Schottenfeld D, Miller DG. Screening for colorectal cancer with fecal occult blood testing and sigmoidoscopy. *J Natl Cancer Inst* 1993; 85:1311–1318.

WGO (World Gastroenterology Organization/International Digestive Cancer Alliance). *Practice Guidelines: Colorectal cancer screening.* 2007.

Yee J, Rosen MP, Blake MA, Baker ME, Cash BD, Fidler JL et al. ACR Appropriateness Criteria® *Colorectal cancer screening.* [online publication]. Reston (VA): American College of Radiology (ACR); 2010.

Zauber AG, Lansdorp-Vogelaar I, Knudsen AB, Wilschut J, van Ballegooijen M, Kuntz KM. Evaluating test strategies for colorectal cancer screening: a decision analysis for the U.S. Preventive Services Task Force. *Ann Intern Med.* 2008; 149:659–669.

Chapter 17
Breast Cancer Screening

Anthony B. Miller

17.1 Introduction

There have been more randomized trials evaluating breast screening than for any other cancer, yet controversy over its efficacy and effectiveness persists.

In part, the controversy results from confusing case detection with efficacy. Detecting a case of breast cancer "early" before it becomes metastatic is a prerequisite for effective screening, but is not sufficient (Miller 2010). Demonstrating improved stage distribution and survival of screen-detected cancers compared to that in the absence of screening is also not sufficient. Such "improvements" are inevitable with screening largely because of the four established biases associated with screen detection: lead time bias, length bias, selection bias, and overdiagnosis (Miller 1996). A marker of probable efficacy is reduction in the cumulative prevalence of advanced disease (Prorok et al. 1984), but demonstrating that following screening takes time, and in populations, such data may not be available or, if available, recorded with sufficient consistency for validity.

The other central difficulty is that screening alone does not reduce breast cancer mortality. To obtain mortality reduction requires effective treatment for the detected cancers. Treatment for breast cancer is itself evolving, and much of this evolution has postdated the majority of the screening trials generally cited in support of breast screening. When all breast cancers can be cured, whatever their stage at diagnosis, there will be no role for screening at all. Until this happens, we have to consider screening, but in planning programs take cognizance of the fact that as treatment

A.B. Miller (✉)
Dalla Lana School of Public Health, University of Toronto,
155 College Street, Toronto, ON M5T 3M7, Canada
e-mail: ab.miller@sympatico.ca

A.B. Miller (ed.), *Epidemiologic Studies in Cancer Prevention and Screening*, Statistics for Biology and Health 79, DOI 10.1007/978-1-4614-5586-8_17,

improves, the absolute effect of screening will be less and less (Glasziou and Houssami 2011).

I have discussed elsewhere many of the issues I shall consider in this chapter (Miller 2012), and they also considered in a special issue on breast screening in preventive medicine I edited (Miller 2011a, b).

17.2 The Screening Trials

The first randomized screening trial was conducted within the Health Insurance Plan of Greater New York (HIP) (Shapiro et al. 1988). This trial included women ages 40–64 and was individually randomized: 30,239 to the screening and 30,256 to the control groups. Sixty-five percent of those allocated to screening had at least one combined mammography and clinical breast examination screen. There were four annual screening rounds. The mammography was primitive by today's standards, and it was estimated that over 70 % of the screen-detected cancers were identified by the clinical breast examinations, which were conducted by surgeons and of a high standard (Miller 1989). Initially, a reduction in breast cancer mortality in women 50–64 years was seen; only later was there a reduction for women ages 40–49, although it was not significant. The hypothesis that there was a difference in screening efficacy for younger compared with older women was raised by this trial. Such a hypothesis has a strong biological foundation; as on average, the breasts of younger women are denser than those of postmenopausal women, and the sensitivity of mammography screening is lower in women with dense breasts (IARC 2002).

Following the HIP trial, the American Cancer Society and the US National Cancer Institute initiated the Breast Cancer Detection Demonstration Project. Eventually, more than 280,000 women ages 35–74 were screened by mammography and clinical breast examination in 29 centers (Baker 1982). The project demonstrated that it was possible to recruit women for screening, though in centers specifically sited to recruit African-Americans, their recruitment proved difficult. A higher proportion of breast cancers was detected by mammography than with breast examination compared with the HIP trial, but this might have been due to lower quality breast examinations rather than superior mammography. Morrison et al. (1988) attempted an indirect evaluation of effectiveness, using a method described by Moss et al. (1987). This depends on estimating the expected incidence of breast cancer, the survival of incident cases, and computing the cumulative numbers of expected deaths from breast cancer over the duration of the projects. Using this approach, Morrison et al. (1988) concluded that the projects appeared to be achieving their desired objectives in reducing breast cancer mortality. However, the main contribution of these projects was to raise the specter of mammography causing more harm than good because of the carcinogenic effects of the radiation that are inseparable from mammography itself (Bailar 1976). A working group established to evaluate the projects recommended the cessation of mammography screening in women ages 40–49 and "a trial to evaluate the net benefit of mammography screening should be conducted" (Beahrs et al. 1979).

A quasi-experimental study of mammography, clinical breast examination, and breast self-examination was established in the UK (UK Trial of Early Detection of Breast Cancer Group 1999) with a randomized component in Edinburgh (Roberts et al. 1984). These studies suggested similar efficacy of mammography plus clinical breast examination as seen in the HIP trial, though none for breast self-examination alone. The randomized component tends to be discounted, as it was based upon cluster randomization of family practices, and it became apparent that there was a major baseline discrepancy in cardiovascular disease events suggesting that the groups were not similar in factors that could be related to breast cancer mortality (Alexander et al. 1989).

Several trials of mammography alone were established in Sweden (Andersson et al. 1988; Bjurstam et al. 2003; Frisell et al. 1986; Tabár et al. 1992). Although the population registers in Sweden enabled the investigators to identify and invite for screening the women included in the trials, and subsequently determine the occurrence of breast cancer and deaths by record linkage with the national cancer register and vital statistics system, women in the control groups were not contacted until a decision was taken to offer them screening at the end of the intervention period which was usually 5 years or less, except for Malmö where screening of controls was delayed for 10 years (Andersson et al. 1988). Randomization was at the individual level in Malmö and for women under the age of 50 in Gothenberg (Bjurstam et al. 2003), but cluster randomization was used in the two-county trial (Tabár et al. 1992), Stockholm, where only two screens were offered (Frisell et al. 1986) and older women in Gothenberg (Bjurstam et al. 2003). The age range, frequency of rescreening, duration of screening, and other specific features also varied. These differences have complicated meta-analysis or overview analyses of these trials. The two-county trial has tended to be the most influential, though it has been severely criticized on methodological grounds (Olsen and Gotzsche 2001). However, the question as to whether earlier analyses of the two-county trial, which did not specifically take account of the cluster randomization, overestimated the benefit was answered by a special analysis which took account of the method of randomization and found results similar to those previously reported (Nixon et al. 2000). There have been two attempts to perform an overview analysis of all the Swedish trials combined (Nyström et al. 1993, 2002). For the second, the principal investigator refused to provide updated data for the component (Kopparberg) of the two-county trial he supervised, thus preventing Nyström et al. (2002) from addressing most of the methodological issues for this component, most importantly, to confirm that the randomized groups were evenly balanced.

Trials in Canada were designed to respond to the review of the US BCDDP in women ages 50–59 and to address screening efficacy in women aged 40–49 (Miller et al. 1992a, b, 2000, 2002). A total of 50,430 women aged 40–49 and 39,405 aged 50–59 were enrolled in 15 centers from 1980 to 1985. Each woman provided data on risk factors for breast cancer on a self-administered questionnaire, checked by the coordinator in the screening center before she received her initial breast examination, and then was randomized irrespective of the findings on examination. The intervention included both two-view mammography and clinical breast examination. The control group for women ages 40–49 received a clinical breast examination only at the time of randomization and then no screening, whereas the control group for women ages 50–59 received annual clinical breast examinations alone. In both components of the trial, screening was offered on five occasions for all except those recruited in the final year, for whom only four screens were offered. Compliance with screening was high. All women were taught breast self-examination as part of the clinical breast examination, which followed a special protocol (Bassett 1985).

The UK age trial was designed to assess the efficacy of mammography screening for women in their 40s. Women aged 39–41 were identified from lists stratified by general practitioner, two-thirds (106,956 women) were randomized to the unscreened group and 53,884 women to the screened group, with mammography offered annually for 7 years. Women allocated to be screened were invited to attend the regional screening center of the UK National Health Service (NHS) Breast Screening Program, and 70 % accepted the invitation. The women in the unscreened group were not contacted. Both groups were followed through the NHS register and were invited to enter the UK screening program at the age of 50 (Moss et al. 2006).

No other trials of breast screening with mammography have been initiated. Increasingly, evaluation has focused on measuring the impact of population-based screening programs.

17.3 Efficacy of Breast Screening

17.3.1 The Evidence on Mammography Screening

Most evidence on the efficacy of mammography alone comes from the last overview analysis of the trials in Sweden (Nyström et al. 2002). In the "follow-up" model, events were defined as all breast cancer diagnoses after the date of randomization, with breast cancer as the underlying cause of death before the closing date of follow-up. The "evaluation model" ignored breast cancer deaths among women whose breast cancer diagnosis was made after the first completed screening round of the control group. The results were similar, with a slightly greater estimated benefit for the evaluation than the follow-up model. From the evaluation model, the age-adjusted results for all ages (40–74) were a significant reduction in breast cancer mortality in the screened group compared to the control – RR 0.80 (95 % CI 0.71–0.90). Within 5-year age groups, there was no benefit for women ages 50–54 or 70–74. For women ages 40–49, the RR was 0.80 (95 % CI 0.63–1.01). These results are similar to those from a meta-analysis computed by an IARC working group (2002) which also included data from the Kopparberg component of the two-county trial. For women ages 40–49, the RR was 0.81 (95 % CI 0.65–1.01), but for those aged 50–69, there was a significant reduction in risk (0.75, 95 % CI 0.67–0.85).

The IARC working group (2002) also produced a meta-analytic result for all valid trials using mammography for women ages 40–49, thus including the HIP trial and the relevant Canadian trial, both evaluating combined screening with mammography and breast examinations. This reduced the estimated benefit to an RR of 0.88 (95 % CI 0.74–1.04), probably because the Canadian data showed no benefit from screening.

The UK age trial also found a statistically nonsignificant reduction for mammography alone screening initiated at ages 39–41 (RR 0.83, 95 % CI 0.66–1.04) (Moss et al. 2006). The UK investigators also performed a meta-analysis combining their data with all other valid screening trials in women ages 40–49, resulting in a RR of 0.84 (95 % CI 0.74–0.95). Thus, the combined analyses performed to date agree on less benefit of mammography screening among women ages 40–49 than among those ages 50–69.

In a review for the US Preventive Services Task Force (2009), a similar effect among women ages 40–49 was estimated (RR 0.85, 95 % CI 0.75–0.96) (Nelson et al. 2009). The lower incidence of breast cancer among women at these ages and the frequency of unnecessary surgery consequent on screening led to a recommendation against routine mammography screening among women ages 40–49 (US Preventive Services Task Force 2009). Although the Task Force's meta-analysis indicated a similar degree of efficacy for women ages 50–59 as for 40–49 (RR 0.85, 95 % CI 0.75–0.99), lower than that for women ages 60–69 (RR 0.68, 95 % CI 0.54–0.87), and no effect for women ages 70–74 (RR 1.12, 95 % CI 0.73–1.72) (Nelson et al. 2009), their recommendation included biennial screening mammography for women between the ages of 50 and 74 years (US Preventive Services Task Force 2009). These US recommendations are therefore now in line with most organizations in other countries, though many countries only offer screening for women older than 69 if they request it. They were also mirrored by the Canadian Task Force on Preventive Health Care (2011).

The recommendations have largely ignored the finding from the second Canadian trial. By 1980, when the CNBSS was initiated, the HIP trial had demonstrated the efficacy of screening by mammography and breast physical examinations in women ages 50–69 in an era when adjuvant therapy for stage II breast cancer was unavailable (Shapiro et al. 1988), so an unscreened control group in the Canadian trial was considered unethical. Therefore, the trial was designed to evaluate the additional benefit of mammography in women ages 50–59 who also received annual clinical breast examinations, in line with the recommendation of the working group that reviewed the BCDDP (Beahrs et al. 1979). Mammography in the CNBSS resulted in many additional false positives and detection of small tumors, but no reduction in breast cancer mortality (Miller et al. 1992a, b, 2000, 2002). The trial thus casts doubt upon the common assumption that the benefit from mammography resides in detecting impalpable breast cancers (including ductal carcinomas in situ), and it was initially challenged (Boyd et al. 1993; Kopans and Feig 1993). However, the cancer detection rates were at least as good as those achieved by modern mammography, and the trial met other quality evaluation criteria (Fletcher et al. 1993). Importantly, the trial was conducted when adjuvant chemotherapy and tamoxifen were standard for stage II breast cancer in Canada, though that was not so in the Swedish two-county trial (Holmberg et al. 1986; Tabár et al. 1999).

In an update of the follow-up to 29 years of the Swedish two-county trial, Tabár et al. (2011) reported that the difference between the intervention and control arms in breast cancer mortality continued to widen throughout the period of follow-up and that "most prevented breast cancer deaths would have occurred (in the absence of screening) after the first 10 years of follow-up." This is an unusual finding and suggests, far from showing a benefit of screening, that the compared groups were unbalanced at the time of the cluster randomization.

The randomized screening trials can only provide limited data to support recommendations on policy. To fill the gap, modeling is now being increasingly used. Please see Chap. 21 by Stout et al. (this volume) on how modeling was used to inform the development of policy in the United States and particularly, to guide the deliberations of the US Preventive Services Task Force (2009).

17.3.2 Evidence on Screening by Clinical Breast Examination

No trial has yet reported benefit from clinical breast examination (CBE) alone. Nevertheless, there is indirect or observational evidence on the effectiveness of CBE, as well as some emerging evidence from trials in developing countries.

As previously indicted, it seems probable that most of the benefit from screening in the HIP trial came from the good CBEs performed (Miller 1989). Further, a model-based evaluation of the likely efficacy of breast examinations in the Canadian trial suggested a 20 % reduction in breast cancer mortality compared with no screening (Rijnsburger et al. 2004). However, the model used data from the Swedish two-county trial to estimate breast cancer mortality in the absence of screening, so it did not adequately consider the contribution of better treatment in Canada than in Sweden.

A population-based breast screening trial in Cairo, Egypt, has shown that women will attend primary health centers for screening breast examinations (Boulos et al. 2005), while there is preliminary indication that a stage shift in diagnosis has been achieved (Miller 2008).

In Mumbai, India, a large cluster-randomized controlled trial evaluating screening for breast and cervix cancer was started in 1978 using trained primary health workers to provide health education, visual inspection of the cervix (with 4 % acetic acid) and clinical breast examination in the screening arm, and only health education in the control arm (Mittra et al. 2010). After three rounds of screening, an excess of early stage breast cancers had been diagnosed in the screened compared with the control group (78 vs. 38) but similar numbers of advanced breast cancers (47 and 49, respectively). At the time of completion of the report, 22 deaths out of the total 125 (18 %) breast cancer cases were recorded in the screening arm, and 10 deaths out of the 87 (12 %) reported breast cancer cases in the control arm. It is not yet clear whether this difference was due to a delay in receiving reports on deaths from the control arm, though an excess of early deaths from breast cancer has been noted in some of the randomized trials of breast screening, which later disappeared (Fletcher et al. 1993). A major issue in a breast screening trial conducted in the Philippines was that women detected with an abnormality largely failed to attend a center for diagnosis, such that the trial was abandoned after the first round (Pisani et al. 2006). In the Mumbai trial, considerable effort was made to avoid this problem, but as the main mechanism used to identify new cancers in the control group was through the cancer registry, it may not be surprising that there could be delay in identifying cases in the control group.

At least two countries in the Middle East (Morocco and Oman) are initiating breast screening based upon clinical breast examination. It will be some time before the results of these programs can be evaluated.

In Ontario, Canada, a provincial breast screening program for women ages 50–69 was initiated in 2000 based upon biennial mammography and clinical breast examination, though later, some centers were incorporated that utilized mammography alone. Women attending a regional cancer center or affiliated centers providing nurse-administered clinical breast examinations had higher breast cancer detection rates (Chiarelli et al. 2009) and were significantly more likely to make a timely return within the recommended biennial screening interval (Chiarelli et al. 2010) than women attending affiliated centers without nurses providing clinical breast examination. This experience suggests that clinical breast examination could increase the effectiveness of mammography screening.

17.3.3 Evidence on Breast Self-examination

Two large trials were initiated on BSE, one in China (Thomas et al. 1997) and one in Russia (Semiglazov et al. 1993). No breast cancer mortality reduction was found in the Chinese trial (Thomas et al. 2002). To date, an adequate analysis taking note of the cluster randomization performed in the Russia/WHO trial has not been reported, and the findings of the Moscow component have only been reported in Russian, though no benefit was noted.

Nevertheless, there is indirect or observational evidence on the effectiveness of BSE. Evidence that BSE, when practiced well, contributes to reduction in breast cancer mortality has been derived from a case-control study within the Canadian trial which showed that BSE compliers have lower predictors of mortality from breast cancer than non-compliers (Harvey et al. 1997). Concerns over recall bias and selection bias that tend to affect case-control studies were overcome as the measure of BSE performance was recorded by nurses when women attended their screening clinical breast examination, while information on risk factors for breast cancer, collected at baseline, enabled the analysis to be adjusted for any differences between good and poor BSE compliers. The magnitude of benefit seems similar to that derived from a cohort study of nearly 30,000 women in Finland (Gastrin et al. 1994), where information on BSE was obtained by calendars sent to the investigator and breast cancer incidence and mortality was compared to the general population. In both studies, BSE seemed equally effective in women under and over the age of 50.

17.4 Harms from Breast Cancer Screening

One reason to seek screening is to be reassured that one does not have cancer. Although a screening appointment requires time and some expense, in general, women are prepared to accept this for the comfort reassurance brings. However, they do not expect to be inconvenienced by unnecessary diagnostic tests and even more so by unnecessary surgery (Nelson et al. 2009; US Preventive Services Task Forcc 2009).

In addition to the harms associated with false-positive screening tests, there is another category, not often recognized by women nor advocates of screening – unnecessary early detection of cancers that would be cured even after clinical detection and unnecessary detection of cancers not destined to present in a woman's lifetime. This overdiagnosis has been estimated to be about 11–15 % of cancers in the screening arms compared to the control arm in the Canadian trial (Moss 2005). Ductal carcinoma in situ (DCIS) detection falls under this category but deserves special consideration. The frequency of DCIS reporting has increased in the USA since the introduction of mammography screening, and the probability that a woman will die within 10 years of such detection has fallen (Ernster et al. 2000). However, there has been no evidence published from any of the screening trials that the detection of DCIS by mammography and subsequent treatment has resulted in a reduction in breast cancer incidence in screened women. This suggests that DCIS is not a classic cancer precursor on the lines of carcinoma in situ of the cervix or advanced adenomas of the colon.

17.5 Impact of Breast Screening in Populations

Trends in breast cancer mortality have been used to measure the effectiveness of a breast screening program in the relevant population. Inferences are complicated when therapy for breast cancer improves at the same time. This began to occur about the mid-1980s when trials of the treatment of stage II breast cancer found benefit from adjuvant chemotherapy in premenopausal women and tamoxifen in postmenopausal women. Therefore, analyses must assess the impact of both screening and treatment. Subsequent to 1990, breast cancer mortality has fallen in many countries; the falls seem more related to improved therapy than screening (Jatoi 2011).

Blanks et al. (2000) used data for 1971–1989 from the UK to predict breast cancer mortality for 1990–1998, assuming no major effect from screening or improvements in treatment until after 1989. The total reduction in mortality from breast cancer to 1998 in women aged 55–69 was estimated as 21.3 %. The direct effect of screening was estimated as 6.4 % (range of estimates from 5.4 % to 11.8 %). The effect of all other factors (improved treatment with tamoxifen and chemotherapy and earlier presentation outside the screening program) was estimated as 14.9 % (range 12.2–14.9 %). Nyström (2000) concluded this result matched expectation, but the expectation of an eventual 30 % reduction in breast cancer mortality probably overestimated benefit (Miller 2000).

Berry et al. (2005) reported the findings from a major evaluation of the impact of screening and treatment on breast cancer mortality in the USA for the Cancer Intervention and Surveillance Modeling Network (CISNET) Collaborators. Seven different statistical models were applied to the same mortality, mammography use, and treatment data. The models varied in the efficiency with which they predicted the observed trends in breast cancer mortality. The percent reduction attributable to screening varied in the seven models from 7.5 % to 22.7 %. This translates into the proportion of the total reduction in breast cancer mortality attributable to screening varying from 28 % to 65 %, with adjuvant treatment contributing the rest. A major difficulty with this analysis was the assumption that breast cancer mortality rates would have risen in the absence of screening and improved treatment as breast cancer incidence was rising. In fact, some of the previous increase was due to the use of mammography (Miller et al. 1991). Further, within a short period it became apparent that breast cancer incidence fell in the USA (Ravdin et al. 2007) with cessation of hormone replacement therapy by many women after the Women's Health Initiative investigators reported that such therapy increased breast cancer risk (Rossouw et al. 2002). As most of the breast cancers induced by hormone replacement therapy are estrogen receptor positive, which respond well to tamoxifen, it seems likely that the assumption of Berry et al. (2005) that breast cancer mortality would have risen absent screening and improved treatment was invalid. As this assumption was necessary to make the models fit the data, the effect of screening may have been substantially overestimated by Berry et al. (2005). Unfortunately, there appears to have been no attempt so far to address this in other analyses.

An attempt has been made to evaluate the impact of breast screening in Norway, capitalizing on the delay in introducing screening (Kalager et al. 2010). The authors used a historical comparison of breast cancer incidence and mortality in the non-screened counties to evaluate the effect of improvements in management and treatment of breast cancer, and compared these trends to a similar historical comparison in the screened areas. They found that the rate of death was reduced by 7.2 deaths per 100,000 person-years in the screening group as compared with the historical screening group (rate ratio, 0.72; 95 % CI 0.63–0.81) and by 4.8 deaths per 100,000 person-years in the non-screening group as compared with the historical non-screening group (rate ratio, 0.82; 95 % CI 0.71–0.93; $P<0.001$ for both comparisons), for a nonsignificant relative reduction in mortality of 10 % in the screening group ($P=0.13$). There are often problems in historical comparisons, and the assumption that the effect of improvements in management and treatment in breast cancer would be identical in screened and non-screened counties can be challenged, as counties not introducing screening may have made less effort to improve breast cancer management. Therefore, it is possible that even a 10 % reduction in breast cancer mortality attributable to screening is an overestimate.

Harris et al. (2011) systematically reviewed the observational evidence concerning the effect of screening in various populations on breast cancer mortality among women ages 50–69 years. They concluded that breast cancer mortality has been reduced, but the magnitude of the effect is probably smaller than predicted in the randomized screening trials, and assumed by the US Preventive Services Task Force (2009). There was insufficient evidence to determine whether the effectiveness of screening is decreasing over time (see Chap. 20 by Autier, this volume, for a further discussion of this issue).

17.6 Discussion

Cancer screening in general, and breast cancer screening in particular, has been an emotionally charged topic. A woman whose breast cancer has been detected by mammography, and apparently cured, will be convinced that her life was saved by the screening. Raffle and Gray (2007) have coined the term "the popularity paradox" for this situation: "The greater the harm from overdiagnosis and overtreatment from screening, the more people there are who believe they owe their health, or even their life, to the programme." Yet the marginal benefit from earlier detection by screening for women ages 40–49 has lessened as treatment for breast cancer has improved considerably (US Preventive Services Task Force 2009). Even for older women, the harm from overdiagnosis, false positives, and unnecessary surgery may also, on average, outweigh possible benefit from screening (Gøtzsche 2011).

In the controversy over at what age mammography screening should start, there has been an implicit suggestion by the critics of the US Preventive Services Task Force recommendation (2009) that a life "saved" from screening women in their 40s will result in more life-years saved per death prevented than from screening women in their fifties or sixties. I have pointed out that if the findings from the trials on which Nelson et al. (2009) based their meta-analysis still apply in the present therapeutic era, then there seems little justification in terms of life-years saved not to screen women ages 40–49 if the decision is made to screen women ages 50–59 rather than focusing on women ages 60–69 where the major benefit can be anticipated (Miller 2012). However, this does not address the major issue not fully considered by the US Preventive Services Task Force (2009) and the Canadian Task Force on Preventive Health Care (2011); should we really base screening policy on the trials conducted before the present therapeutic era?

Lack of data has precluded full evaluation of many of the trials of breast screening, especially those conducted in Sweden based upon cluster randomization of areas. In addition to the possible lack of balance in possible confounders in the compared groups discussed earlier, Black et al. (2002) suggested the possibility of bias in attribution of cause of death, which could be avoided if the endpoint of the trials was all-cause, rather than breast cancer mortality. In two of the Swedish trials that reported a breast cancer mortality reduction, the two-county and the Gothenburg trials, the reduction was offset by greater mortality from all causes other than breast cancer in the intervention group offered screening than in the usual care control groups. As breast cancer is only one of the many causes of death in screened women, and therefore differences in all-cause mortality are rarely significant, it is now recognized that a full exploration of the potential reasons for apparent compensating increases of mortality from other causes is necessary, and trials which have such increases may be far less valid than those which do not. This issue remains unresolved but adds to the uncertainty of making decisions based on the affected trials.

Given the requirement that screening can only be effective if treatment is curative for the discovered lesions but that treatment as it improves will reduce the impact of screening, it is difficult to justify the use of data from the trials that were conducted before adjuvant therapy for breast cancer was available to make policy decisions in the present era. Only one other trial was conducted after the Canadian trials that benefited from the availability of adjuvant therapy for breast cancer, the UK age trial, and although it suggested a screening benefit in younger women, it was not conclusive and could possibly have been confounded by differences in management between the two arms.

Breast cancer screening, like screening for prostate cancer, suffers from the lack of a detectable, precancerous phase whose elimination results in reduction in disease incidence, unlike screening for cervical and colorectal cancer. We may have reached the point of negligible benefit in screening for invasive breast cancer. If so, we should be turning our efforts to primary prevention, early diagnosis through public and professional education for breast awareness, and the provision of adequate diagnosis and management.

References

Alexander F, Roberts MM, Lutz W, Hepburn W. Randomisation by cluster and the problem of social class bias. *J Epidemiol Commun Hlth* 1989; 43:29-36.

Andersson I, Aspegren K, Janzon L, Landberg T, Lindholm K, Linell F et al. Mammographic screening and mortality from breast cancer: The Malmö mammographic screening trial. *Br Med J* 1988; 297:943-948.

Bailar JC. Mammography: a contrary view. *Ann Intern Med* 1976; 84: 77-84.

Baker, L. Breast Cancer Detection Demonstration Project: five-year summary report. *CA* 1982; 32:194-225.

Bassett AA. Physical examination of the breast and breast self-examination. In Miller AB (ed), *Screening for Cancer*. Orlando Fla, Academic Press Inc, 1985, pp 271-291.

Beahrs O, Shapiro S, Smart C. Report of the working group to review the National Cancer Institute American Cancer Society Breast Cancer Detection Demonstration Projects. *J Natl Cancer Inst*, 1979; 62:640-709.

Berry DA, Cronin KA, Plevritis SK, Fryback DG, Clarke L, Zelen M et al. Effect of Screening and Adjuvant Therapy on Mortality from Breast Cancer. *N Engl J Med* 2005;353:1784-1792.

Bjurstam N, Björneld L, Warwick J, Sala E, Duffy SW, Nyström L, et al. The Gothenburg Breast Screening Trial. *Cancer*. 2003; 97:2387-2396.

Black WC, Haggstrom DA, Welch HG. All-cause mortality in randomized trials of cancer screening. *J Natl Cancer Inst*. 2002;94:167-173.

Blanks RG, Moss SM, McGahan CE, Quinn MJ, Babb PJ. Effect of NHS breast screening programme on mortality from breast cancer in England and Wales, 1990-8: comparison of observed with predicted mortality. *BMJ* 2000; 321:665-669.

Boulos S, Gadallah M, Neguib S, Essam Ea, Youssef A, Costa A et al. Breast screening in the emerging world: High prevalence of breast cancer in Cairo. *The Breast* 2005; 14:340-346.

Boyd NF, Jong RA, Yaffe MJ, Tritchler D, Lockwood G, Zylak CJ. A critical appraisal of the National Breast Cancer Screening Study. *Radiology* 1993;189:661-663.

Canadian Task Force on Preventive Health Care. Recommendations on screening for breast cancer in average-risk women aged 40–74 years. *CMAJ* 2011. DOI:10.1503/cmaj.110334

Chiarelli AM, Majpruz V, Brown P, Thériault M, Shumak R, Mai V. The Contribution of Clinical Breast Examination to the Accuracy of Breast Screening. *J Natl Cancer Inst* 2009;101:1236–1243.

Chiarelli AM, Majpruz V, Brown P, Theriault M, Edwards S, Shumak R et al. Influence of Nurses on Compliance with Breast Screening Recommendations in an Organized Breast Screening Program. *Cancer Epidemiol Biomarkers Prev* 2010; 19: 697–706.

Ernster VL, Barclay J, Kerlikowske K, Wilkie H, Ballard-Barbash R. Mortality among women with ductal carcinoma in situ of the breast in the population-based surveillance, epidemiology and end results program. *Arch Intern Med* 2000;160:953-958.

Fletcher SW, Black W, Harris R, Rimer BK, Shapiro S. Report on the International Workshop on Screening for Breast Cancer. *J Natl Cancer Inst* 1993;85:1644–1656.

Frisell J, Glas U, Hellstrom L, Somell A. Randomized mammograohic screening for breast cancer in Stockholm. Design, first round results and comparisons. *Breast Cancer Res Treat* 1986; 8: 45-54.

Gastrin G, Miller AB, To T, Aronson KJ, Wall C, Hakama M et al. Incidence and mortality from breast cancer in the Mama program for breast screening in Finland, 1973-1986. *Cancer* 1994; 73:2168-2174.

Glasziou P, Houssami N. The evidence base for breast cancer screening. *Preventive Medicine* 2011; 53: 100-102.

Gøtzsche PC. Time to stop mammography screening? *CMAJ* 2011. DOI:10.1503/cmaj.111721

Harris R, Yeatts J, Kinsinger L. Breast cancer screening for women ages 50 to 69 years a systematic review of observational evidence. *Preventive Medicine* 2011; 53:108-114.

Harvey BJ, Miller AB, Baines CJ, Corey PN. Effect of breast self-examination techniques on the risk of death from breast cancer. *Can Med Assoc J* 1997;157:1205-1212.

Holmberg LH, Tabar L, Adami HO, Bergstrom R. Survival in breast cancer diagnosed between mammographic screening examinations. *Lancet* 1986; (ii): 27-30.

IARC Handbooks on Cancer Prevention, Vol 7, *Breast cancer screening*. Lyon, IARC Press, 2002.

Jatoi I. The impact of advances in treatment on the efficacy of mammography screening. *Preventive Medicine* 2011; 53:103-104.

Kalager M, Zelen M, Langmark F, Adami H-O. Effect of Screening Mammography on Breast-Cancer Mortality in Norway. *N Engl J Med* 2010;363:1203-1210.

Kopans DB, Feig SA. The Canadian National Breast Screening Study: a critical review. *Am J Radiol* 1993; 161:755-760.

Miller AB. Mammography: a critical evaluation of its role in breast cancer screening, especially in developing countries. *J Publ Hlth Policy* 1989; 10: 486-98.

Miller AB. Fundamental issues in screening for cancer. In Schottenfeld D & Fraumeni JF, Jr. Eds *Cancer Epidemiology and Prevention*, Second Edition. New York, Oxford, Oxford University Press, 1996, pp 1433-52.

Miller AB. Benefit of 30% may be substantial overestimate. *BMJ* 2000; 321:1527.

Miller A. Practical applications for clinical breast examination (CBE) and breast self-examination (BSE) in screening and early detection of breast cancer. *Breast Care* 2008; 3:17-20.

Miller AB. Conundrums in screening for cancer. Mini Review. *Int J Cancer* 2010; 126: 1039-46.

Miller AB. Breast cancer screening: Introduction. *Preventive Medicine* 2011a; 53: 99.

Miller AB. Breast cancer screening: Commentary and Conclusions. *Preventive Medicine* 2011b; 53: 147-148.

Miller AB. Breast cancer screening. In Goldman MB, Troisi R, Rexrode KM, Eds. *Women and Health*, Second Edition Elsevier 2012, In press.

Miller AB, Baines CJ, To T, Wall C. Canadian national breast screening study: 1. Breast cancer detection and death rates among women age 40-49 years. Can Med Assoc J 1992a; 147: 1459-1476 (published erratum in Can Med Assoc J 1993; 148:718).

Miller AB, Baines CJ, To T, Wall C. Canadian National Breast Screening Study 2. Breast cancer detection and death rates among women aged 50 to 59 years. Can Med Assoc J 1992b; 147: 1477-88 (published erratum in Can Med Assoc J 1993; 148:718).

Miller AB, To T, Baines CJ, Wall C. Canadian National Breast Screening Study - 2.: 13-year results of a randomized trial in women aged 50-59 years. *J Natl Cancer Inst* 2000; 92:1490-1499.

Miller AB, To T, Baines CJ, Wall C. The Canadian National Breast Screening Study-1: Breast cancer mortality after 11 to 16 years of follow-up. A randomized screening trial of mammography in women age 40 to 49 years. *Ann Intern Med* 2002; 137: 305-312.

Miller BA, Feuer EJ, Hankey BF. The increasing incidence of breast cancer since 1982: relevance of early detection. *Cancer Causes Control* 1991; 2:67-74.

Mittra I, Mishra GA, Singh S, Aranke S, Notani P, Badwe R et al. A cluster randomized, controlled trial of breast and cervix cancer screening in Mumbai, India: methodology and interim results after three rounds of screening. *Int J Cancer* 2010; 126: 976–984.

Morrison AS, Brisson J, Khalid N. Breast cancer incidence and mortality in the breast cancer detection demonstration project. *J Natl Cancer Inst*, 1988; 80:1540-7.

Moss S. Overdiagnosis in randomised controlled trials of breast cancer screening. *Breast Cancer Research* 2005; 7: 230-234.

Moss SM, Cuckle H, Evans A, Johns L, Waller M, Bobrow L, for the Trial Management Group. Effect of mammographic screening from age 40 years on breast cancer mortality at 10 years' follow-up: a randomised controlled trial. *Lancet* 2006; 368: 2053–2060.

Moss S, Draper GJ, Hardcastle JD, Chamberlain J. Calculation of sample size in trials of screening for early diagnosis of disease. *Int J Epidemiol* 1987; 16:104-10.

Nelson HD, Tyne K, Naik A, Bougatsos C, Chan BK, Humphrey L. Screening for Breast Cancer: An Update for the U.S. Preventive Services Task Force. *Ann Intern Med* 2009;151:727-737.

Nixon RM, Prevost TC, Duffy SW, Tabar L, Vitak B, Chen HH. Some random-effects models for the analysis of matched-cluster randomised trials: application to the Swedish two-county trial of breast-cancer screening. *J Epidemiol Biostat* 2000; 5:349-358.

Nyström L. How effective is screening for breast cancer? Reductions in mortality should not be the only marker of success. *BMJ* 2000;321:647–648.

Nyström L, Andersson I, Bjurstam N, Frisell J, Nordenskjold B, Rutqvist, L-E. Long-term effects of mammography screening: updated overview of the Swedish randomized trials. *Lancet* 2002; 359:909-919.

Nyström L, Rutqvist LE, Wall S, Lindgren A, Lindqvist M, Ryden S et al. Breast cancer screening with mammography: overview of Swedish randomized trials. *Lancet* 1993; 341:973-978.

Olsen O, Gotzsche PC. Screening for breast cancer with mammography (Cochrane Review). In: *The Cochrane Library*, Issue 4, 2001. Oxford: Update software.

Pisani P, Parkin DM, Ngelangel C, Esteban D, Gibson L, Munson M et al. Outcome of screening by clinical examination of the breast in a trial in the Philippines. *Int J Cancer* 2006;118:149–154.

Prorok PC, Chamberlain J, Day NE, Hakama M, Miller AB. UICC Workshop on the evaluation of screening programmes for cancer. *Int J Cancer* 1984; 34: 1-4.

Raffle AE, Gray JAM. Screening: Evidence and Practice. Oxford, *Oxford University Press*, 2007, pp 366.

Ravdin PM, Cronin KA, Howlader N, Berg CD, Chlebowski RT, Feuer EJ et al. The Decrease in Breast-Cancer Incidence in 2003 in the United States. *N Engl J Med* 2007; 356:1670-1674.

Rijnsburger AI, van Oortmarssen GJ, Boer R, Draisma G, To T, Miller AB et al. Mammography benefit in the Canadian National Breast Screening Study-2: a model evaluation. *Int J Cancer* 2004; 110: 756-762.

Roberts MM, Alexander FE, Anderson TJ, Forrest AP, Hepburn W, Huggins A et al. The Edinburgh randomised trial of screening for breast cancer: description of method. *Br J Cancer* 1984; 50: 1-6.

Rossouw JE, Anderson GL, Prentice RL, LaCroix AZ, Kooperberg C, PhD, Stefanick ML et al. Risks and benefits of estrogen plus progestin in healthy postmenopausal women: principal results from the Women's Health Initiative randomized controlled trial. *JAMA* 2002;288:321-333.

Semiglazov VF, Sagaidack VN, Moiseyenko VM, Mikhailov EA. Study of the role of breast self-examination in the reduction of mortality from breast cancer. *Eur J Cancer* 1993; 29A: 2039-2046.

Shapiro, S, Strax P, Venet L, Venet W. Periodic screening for breast cancer. The Health Insurance Plan Project and its Sequelae, 1963-1986. Baltimore: *The Johns Hopkins University Press*; 1988.

Tabár L, Chen H-H T, Duffy SW, Kruesmo UB. Primary and adjuvant therapy, prognostic factors and survival in 1053 breast cancers diagnosed in a trial of mammography screening. *Jpn J Clin Oncol* 1999; 2129:608-616.

Tabár L, Fagerberg G, Duffy SW, Day NE, Gad A, Grontoft O. Update of the Swedish two county program of mammographic screening for breast cancer. *Radiol Clin N Am* 1992; 30:187-210.

Tabár L, Vitak B, Chen TH-H, Yen AM-Y, Cohen A, Tot T et al. Swedish Two-County Trial: Impact of Mammographic Screening on Breast Cancer Mortality during 3 Decades. *Radiology* 2011 doi: 10.1148/radiol.11110469

Thomas DB, Gao Dl, Ray, RM, Wang WW, Allison CJ, Chen FL et al. Randomized trial of breast self-examination in Shanghai: Final results. *J Natl Cancer Inst* 2002; 94:1445-1457.

Thomas DB, Gao Dl, Self EG, Allison CJ, Tao Y, Mahloch J et al. Randomized trial of breast self-examination in Shanghai: Methodology and preliminary results. *J Natl Cancer Inst* 1997; 89:355-365.

UK Trial of Early Detection of Breast Cancer Group. 16-year mortality from breast cancer in the UK trial of early detection of breast cancer. *Lancet* 1999; 353:1909-14.

US Preventive Services Task Force. Screening for Breast Cancer: U.S. Preventive Services Task Force Recommendation Statement. *Ann Intern Med* 2009;151:716-726.

Chapter 18
Prostate Cancer Screening

Anthony B. Miller

18.1 Introduction

Two tests have been advocated for screening for prostate cancer, the digital rectal examination (DRE) and the determination of the amount of prostate-specific antigen (PSA) in the blood. Although there has been a tendency to use both tests together, experience has shown the DRE is unreliable and fails to detect many early prostate cancers detected by PSA. Further, the evidence available on the efficacy of prostate screening relates largely to PSA. Therefore, in this chapter, I shall concentrate on the evidence relating to the effectiveness of screening with PSA.

Since the introduction of the PSA test, with wide adoption for screening in the United States, a number of jurisdictions in other countries with publicly funded or insurance-based health systems have agreed that PSA testing would be funded, though in many parts of Canada, the funding is for tests ordered for diagnosis and not screening by a physician. However, such types of funding are difficult to monitor, and it seems probable that the majority of the tests now performed in Canada and other countries are for screening. This is because the public and many of their physicians believe that the early detection and proper treatment of prostate cancer must be beneficial. A significant proportion of the male population, as well as many advocacy groups, have agreed testing for elevated PSA levels is good. For example, over 25 % of men over the age of 40 reported they had had a PSA screening test in a 2003 Canadian survey (Canadian Cancer Society 2006).

However, the release of mortality results on prostate cancer from two large screening trials, the prostate component of the Prostate, Lung, Colon and Ovary (PLCO) trial in the United States (Andriole et al. 2009) and the European Randomized Study of Screening for Prostate Cancer (ERSPC) (Schröder et al. 2009), and their

A.B. Miller, M.D., FRCP (✉)
Dalla Lana School of Public Health, University of Toronto,
155 College Street, Toronto, ON M5T 3M7, Canada
e-mail: ab.miller@sympatico.ca

A.B. Miller (ed.), *Epidemiologic Studies in Cancer Prevention and Screening*,
Statistics for Biology and Health 79, DOI 10.1007/978-1-4614-5586-8_18,

recent update (Andriole et al. 2012; Schröder et al. 2012) has served to fuel the debate. In this chapter, I shall try and clarify the present situation and address the issue as to whether, and if so at what ages, PSA testing should be offered.

18.2 The Potential Benefits of PSA as a Screening Test

Prostate cancer is the most common cause of death from cancer in men in most technically advanced countries. It is by far the most prevalent cancer with 30–40 % of men over 60 found to have prostate cancer at autopsy (Miller 2007). The lifetime risk of a man developing microscopic prostate cancer has been estimated to be 42 % (Frankel et al. 2003). The sensitivity of the PSA tests depends on the cutoff level selected. If the cutoff for an abnormal PSA test is 4 ng/ml, then the sensitivity of a PSA test is about 75 %, rising to over 80 % if the cutoff is lowered to 3 ng/ml. However, there is a reciprocal relationship between sensitivity and specificity. The specificity if the cutoff is 3 ng/ml is approximately 80 %, i.e., 20 % of those screened would have a false-positive result, resulting in substantial numbers of men placed under supervision and many unnecessary biopsies. At the cutoff level of 4 ng/ml, the specificity rises to about 90 %, making it a more reasonable test as a false-positive PSA test leads only to temporary anxiety while awaiting a negative biopsy, and the unnecessary biopsies can be accepted if there is benefit from the test. Physicians console themselves that patients are always grateful for early detection of disease especially with a good outcome which they believe is more likely than not with early detection of cancer. These arguments have made the PSA test attractive to many patients and their physicians.

18.3 The Risks of PSA as a Screening Test

Although the PSA screening test can detect most men with prostate cancer with some accuracy, over 80 % of them will die with the disease but from another cause, and only a small proportion of men with prostate cancer will die from the disease. The treatment of prostate cancer has modestly lowered the mortality rate, but as screening rates have risen, prostate cancer detection has increased quite dramatically, but with little improvement in mortality. Recent declines in prostate cancer mortality in many countries are probably attributable to prolongation of life from hormone therapy of more advanced cases, with most of them dying from other causes. Frankel et al. (2003) estimated if 1 million men over 50 were screened with a PSA test cutoff at 4 ng/ml, 110,000 would have elevated PSA on the first test, 90,000 would have a biopsy, and 20,000 will be found to have cancer. Of this group, 10,000 will have a prostatectomy, of whom 300 will be left with chronic incontinence, 4,000 will be impotent, and 10 will die from the surgery. In Finland, component of the ESPC trial 12.5 % of the screened men had at least one false-positive PSA test during the three rounds of 4-yearly screening (Kilpeläinen et al. 2010). Thus, evidence of benefit is necessary to justify all this morbidity and mortality.

18.4 The ERSPC and PLCO Randomized Screening Trials

Both trials commenced in the early 1990s. The ERSPC trial enrolled more than 260,000 men from 8 countries (Belgium, Finland, France, Italy, the Netherlands, Spain, Sweden, Switzerland) (Schröder 2008). In all countries, men ages 55–69 were included; in Sweden, men ages 50–54 were also included, and in four countries, men up to age 74. The PLCO trial enrolled nearly 77,000 men ages 55–74 from 10 centers across the United States. In both trials, many have been followed for more than 13 or more years. There have been reports on screening from both trials (Crawford et al. 2006; Grubb et al. 2008; Schröder 2008; Schröder and Roobol 2009). The mortality results in PLCO were related to all subjects randomized (Andriole et al. 2009, 2012), in ERSPC to a subgroup of 182,160 men (Schröder et al. 2009, 2012). The difference between this number and the total randomized as previously reported (Schröder 2008) is unexplained, apart from the absence of those recruited in France, where randomization did not begin until 2001.

The PLCO trial was conducted on a background of persistent, long-term advocacy of PSA screening for prostate cancer in the United States (American Urological Association 2000; American Cancer Society 2008), though not all organizations shared the view that screening should be offered (US Preventive Task Force 2008). In contrast, in the ERSPC trial, PSA screening in the population was infrequent in most countries when the trial was initiated, though that situation probably changed during the course of the trial. The two trials differ in some other important respects. In PLCO, annual PSA screening to a total of 6 screens and 4 annual DRE were offered to the intervention group; in the ERSPC trial, in most countries, two or more PSA screens at 4-year intervals were offered, though the interval was two yearly in Sweden. The cutoff for a positive PSA was 4 ng/ml in PLCO, and in general 3 ng/ml in ERSPC, though the use of ancillary tests such as DRE and transrectal ultrasound (TRUS) varied between countries, sometimes being applied to those with a PSA <3 ng/ml. PLCO was an individually randomized trial following informed consent, as was the case in Belgium, the Netherlands, Spain, and Switzerland in ERSPC, but in the other four countries (France, Finland, Italy, Sweden), randomization on the basis of population registers was performed prior to consent, which was only obtained in those who accepted the offer of screening. In PLCO, the results of screening were reported to the participant and their physicians, and they decided on subsequent management. This resulted in many being placed on regular PSA surveillance, rather than immediate biopsy, though by 4 years, over 80 % of those with positive tests had achieved resolution (biopsy or PSA falling to lower levels) (Grubb et al. 2008). In ERSPC, immediate biopsy of those with an abnormal test result was encouraged, treatment of those found to have cancer often being conducted under the supervision of the trial investigators. In the control groups, care of prostate cancers that were diagnosed occurred in the community.

In both trials, there was no reduction in prostate cancer mortality in the first 7 years after randomization in the screened groups compared to the control (Andriole et al. 2009; Schröder et al. 2009). After that, there was a difference between the trials. In PLCO, with 92 % of those enrolled followed to 10 years and 57 % to 13 years, there was if anything higher mortality from prostate cancer in the intervention arm (the screened group) than in the usual care control group, though the difference was nonsignificant (rate ratio 1.09, 95 % confidence intervals 0.87–1.36) (Andriole et al. 2012). Mortality from all causes other than prostate, lung, and colorectal cancer was identical in both arms. In ERSPC with a median follow-up of 11 years, the reverse occurred, with lower prostate cancer mortality observed in the screened group than the control group (RR 0.79, 95 % CI 0.69–0.91) (Schröder et al. 2012). As the confidence intervals surrounding the point estimates of the reported mortality rate ratios in the two trials overlap, chance cannot be excluded as an explanation for the differences between them.

However, there are other major differences between the US and European trials that need to be considered. The first relates to the degree of background screening that occurred in the control groups. In PLCO, 45 % of those randomized had had at least one PSA test in the 3 years preceding randomization, and screening in the usual care group (opportunistic screening in the community) reached an estimated 52 % by the time screening came to an end in the intervention group. Nevertheless, the level of screening in the intervention arm was substantially higher than that in the usual care arm in the early study years, and throughout, screening levels remained distinctly higher. In ERSPC, the degree of contamination was certainly less, though details are not provided in the reports. The second is the different PSA cutoff level applied in the trials. This seems to have resulted in a higher detection rate of prostate cancer following screening in ERSPC than PLCO and substantially more overdiagnosis. It seems unlikely that this resulted in a mortality differential in ERSPC being missed in PLCO, however, as the lethality of prostate cancer increases with increasing PSA levels (as well as the converse), while it has been shown in ERSPC that cancers detected by screening with a PSA of <4 ng/ml have a favorable prognosis (Schröder 2008). The third possible reason for the difference in the results is differences in the application of treatment for prostate cancer. Given the way the ERSPC trial was conducted, with treatment of screen-detected cancers directly controlled by trial investigators, but carried out in the community for those diagnosed in the control group, the potential for treatment differences existed (Barry 2009), and in a publication by some of the ERSPC investigators, it was reported that men diagnosed with prostate cancer were more likely to be treated at an academic center in the screening arm than men diagnosed in the control arm (Wolters et al. 2010). To the extent that outcomes after major surgery may be better in major referral centers than in community hospitals, this difference in place of treatment may have favored the screening arm. Further, trial arm was associated with treatment choice, especially in men with high-risk prostate cancer. Thus, a control subject with high-risk prostate cancer was more likely than a screen subject to receive radiotherapy (OR 1.43, 95 % CI 1.01–2.05), expectant management (OR 2.92, 95 % CI 1.33–6.42), or hormonal treatment (OR 1.77, 95 % CI 1.07–2.94) instead of radical prostatectomy. In contrast, the policy in the PLCO trial not to mandate specific therapies after screen detection resulted in substantial similarity in treatment by stage between the two arms (Andriole et al. 2009, 2012).

A report of follow-up through to 14 years of the Goteborg component of ERSPC has been published, combined with findings from some subjects who were not part of the ERSPC analysis (Hugosson et al. 2010). Comparing the earlier ERSPC report (Schröder et al. 2009) with this manuscript, it seems reasonable to conclude that 60 % of the Goteborg cohort was included in the core age group (55–69) of ERSPC. Of the 122 deaths from prostate cancer reported in the Goteborg trial, 109 (89 %) occurred in those 55–64 at entry. Schröder et al. (2012) only reported deaths by country in an appendix figure, while Hugosson et al. (2010) did not report how many of the Goteborg deaths were included in the core age-group analysis of ERSPC, so the extent of the overlap in deaths between the two analyses is unclear; it seems reasonable, though, to assume that most or all of these 109 were included in the core group analyses of Schröder et al. (2009, 2012). Thus, the Goteborg study's finding concerning a prostate cancer mortality reduction seems largely derived from previously reported ERSPC data and cannot be regarded as independent validation of the findings of Schröder et al. (2009, 2012). Further, as the control group in the Goteborg trial were followed passively through national registers, probably did not know they were part of a trial and were treated in community centers, it seems likely that differences in treatment had a major impact upon the reported results.

Crawford et al. (2011) utilizing PLCO prostate mortality data through to 10 years reported a statistically significant interaction of trial arm by comorbidity status. However, a similar analysis using a modified Charlson score of comorbidity through to 13 years did not confirm this (Andriole et al. 2012), casting substantial doubt on the claim by Crawford et al. (2011) that those with no comorbidity at baseline derive a benefit from PSA screening.

In the USA, men are often advised to have annual PSA tests, yet if the ERSPC result is accepted, annual testing is unnecessarily frequent. But before accepting these results to guide policy, we need further clarification on what actually happened in the trial, especially with regard to treatment, and confirmation that the compared arms were balanced (Miller 2012a).

Reconciling the ERSPC results with the results of PLCO is difficult. What PLCO seems to show is that adding organized screening to opportunistic screening will result in no benefit and many adverse effects. Those effects include false-positive screening tests, unnecessary biopsies, overdiagnosis, and impaired quality of life. The latter will be the subject of a later report from ERPSC as it will from PLCO. In ERSPC, 13 % of the screening tests were false positives compared to 7 % in PLCO, 76 % of biopsies did not result in the diagnosis of prostate cancer in ERSPC compared with 62 % in PLCO, and overdiagnosis approximated to 50 % and 17–30 %, respectively (Miller 2012a).

Although the natural history of prostate cancer is believed to be long, leading many to suggest that the follow-up in PLCO has been too short to show a benefit, the likelihood of a change in its negative findings if follow-up was extended has been reduced by the negative finding from a 20-year follow-up of a community based trial from Sweden (Sandblom et al. 2011). The participants were all men aged 50–69 in the city of Norrköping, identified in 1987 in the National Population Register ($n = 9026$). From the study population, 1494 men were randomly allocated to be screened by including every sixth man from a list of birth dates who were invited to be screened every third year from 1987 to 1996; the remainder served as controls. DRE was used for the first two tests, and PSA was added for the next two. There were 85 cases (5.7 %) of prostate cancer diagnosed in the screened group and 292 (3.9 %) in the control group. The risk ratio for death from prostate cancer in the screened group was 1.16 (95 % confidence interval 0.78–1.73).

18.5 Discussion

In PLCO, the screening that occurred in the usual care arm was not enough to eliminate the expected impacts of the annual screening in the intervention arm such as earlier diagnosis and a persistent excess of cases. Therefore, what the trial was evaluating was the effect of adding an organized component of annual screening to the opportunistic screening already in place, and even with the extension of the follow-up to 13 years, there is no evidence of a benefit; indeed there are major harms, in part, associated with the false-positive screening tests but also with the overdiagnosis inseparable from PSA screening, especially in older men. What the trial does seem to confirm, however, would be the futility of making any attempt to set up organized screening programs in addition to what is currently ongoing in any country. This seems to be a generally accepted conclusion. Even when authors conclude that PSA screening reduces prostate cancer mortality, they also conclude that screening cannot be justified yet in the context of public health policy (van Leeuwen et al. 2010; Chou and LeFevre 2011).

Nevertheless, the question that has to be addressed is whether the European trial results support the continuation of the opportunistic screening that is ongoing in North America and some other countries. The uncertainty that surrounds the validity of the results of ERSPC makes that difficult to answer with certainty. The delay in seeing a possible benefit is certainly compatible with what is known about the long natural history of prostate cancer. Although the separation of the mortality curves in ERSPC beyond 10 years has been confirmed with more data (Schröder et al. 2012), it is still necessary to be certain that other factors, especially treatment differences between the randomized groups, are not responsible for the benefit seen. However, it is important to note that both trials support the recommendation of the US Preventive Services Task Force (2008) against screening men older than 69.

The harms from prostate screening are considerable. In addition to the complications associated with false-positive diagnoses, and the risk of postoperative mortality in elderly men subjected to prostatectomy, there is evidence of substantial overdiagnosis, estimated in ERSPC to be 27 % from a single screening test at age 55 to 56 % for a single screening test at age 75 (Draisma et al. 2003). These harms have to be set against a low probability of benefit. Even if the ERSPC findings of benefit represent the truth, the investigators estimated that to prevent one death from prostate cancer at 11 years of follow-up, 1055 men would need to be invited for screening and 37 cancers would need to be detected (Schröder et al. 2012). Thus, the large majority of men who believe that their lives have been saved by PSA testing have been deceived. Raffle and Gray (2007) have coined the term "the popularity paradox" for this situation: "The greater the harm from overdiagnosis and overtreatment from screening, the more people there are who believe they owe their health, or even their life, to the programme."

I conclude that from our present knowledge of risks and benefits attributable to prostate cancer screening and treatment, we cannot justify advocating screening programs for prostate cancer. Each physician has an ethical responsibility to inform their patients of potential risks and benefits of any procedure. There is a great need for alignment of all organizations with currently available evidence. Mass PSA screening cannot be justified, and most PSA screening should be stopped to prevent more unjustified death and morbidity. So the answer to the question men often ask their physician as to whether they should have a PSA test is "Do not Screen for Prostate cancer with PSA" (Rosser W, personal communication 2010).

Acknowledgements The initial version of the manuscript that formed the basis for this chapter was jointly written by the present author together with emeritus professor of family medicine of Queen's University, Ontario, Canada, Walter Rosser, subsequently published as Miller (2012b). Since then, the publications of Andriole et al. (2012) and Schröder et al. (2012) have appeared, and the manuscript was extensively revised for the present chapter.

I should like to express my indebtedness to my colleagues in the PLCO trial, especially Barry Kramer, Paul Pinsky, and Philip Prorok, for many useful discussions on the issues considered in this chapter.

Potential Conflicts of Interest The author declares that he has no financial relationship with any commercial organization concerned with prostate cancer screening. However, he has been a consultant to the Division of Cancer Prevention of the US National Cancer Institute since 1996, was chair of the Death Review Committee of the PLCO trial 1998–2004, has been chair of the Analysis Cost-effectiveness and Modeling Committee of the PLCO trial since 2004, and is coauthor of a number of publications on the PLCO trial (including Grubb et al. 2008; Andriole et al. 2009, 2012).

References

American Cancer Society, Cancer Screening Guidelines 2008. at: http://www.cancer.org/docroot/ped/content/ped_2_3x_acs_cancer_detection_guidelines_36.asp

American Urological Association (AUA). Prostate-specific antigen (PSA) best practice policy. *Oncology* 2000;14:267–272, 277–278, 280 passim.

Andriole GL, Grubb RL, Buys SS, Chia D, Church TR, Fouad MN et al. Mortality results from a randomized prostate-cancer screening trial. *New Eng J Med* 2009; 360: 1310–1319.
Andriole GL, Crawford ED, Grubb RL, Buys SS, Chia D, Church TR, et al. Prostate Cancer Screening in the Randomized Prostate, Lung, Colorectal, and Ovarian Cancer Screening Trial: Mortality Results after 13 Years of Follow-up. *J Natl Cancer Inst* 2012;104:1–8.
Barry M. Screening for prostate cancer – the controversy that refuses to die. *New Eng J Med* 2009; 360: 1351–1354.
Canadian Cancer Society/National Cancer Institute of Canada: Canadian Cancer Statistics 2006, Toronto, Canada, 2006.
Chou R, LeFevre ML. Prostate Cancer Screening-The Evidence, the Recommendations, and the Clinical Implications. *JAMA* 2011; 306: 2721–2722.
Crawford ED, Pinsky PF, Chia D, Kramer BS, Fagerstrom RM, Andriole G, et al. Prostate specific antigen changes as related to the initial prostate specific antigen: data from the prostate, lung, colorectal and ovarian cancer screening trial. *J Urol.* 2006; 175:1286–1290.
Crawford ED, Grubb RL, Black A, Andriole GL, Chen M-H, Izmirlian G et al. Comorbidity and Mortality Results from a Randomized Prostate Cancer Screening Trial. *J Cin Oncol.* 2011; 29:355–361.
Draisma G, Boer R, Otto SJ, van der Cruijsen IW, Damhuis RAM, Schröder FH et al. Lead Times and Overdetection Due to Prostate-Specific Antigen Screening: Estimates From the European Randomized Study of Screening for Prostate Cancer. *J Natl Cancer Inst* 2003; 95:868–878.
Frankel S, Smith GD, Donovan J, Neal D. Screening for prostate cancer. *Lancet* 2003; 361:1122–1128.
Grubb RL, Pinsky PF, Greenlee RT, Izmirlian G, Miller AB, Hickey TP et al. Prostate cancer screening in the Prostate, Lung, Colorectal and Ovarian cancer screening trial: update on findings from the initial four rounds of screening in a randomized trial. *BJU International* 2008; 102: 1524–1530.
Hugosson J, Carlsson S, Aus G, Bergdahl S, Khatami A, Lodding P, et al. Mortality results from the Göteborg randomized population-based prostate-cancer screening trial. *Lancet Oncol.* 2010; 11:725–732.
Kilpeläinen TP, Tammela TLJ, Määttänen L, Kujala P, Stenman U-H, Ala-Opas M et al. False-positive screening results in the Finnish prostate cancer screening trial. *Br J Cancer* 2010; 102: 469–474.
Miller AB. Commentary: Implications of the frequent occurrence of occult carcinoma of the prostate. *Int J Epidemiol* 2007; 36: 282–284.
Miller AB. New data on prostate cancer mortality after PSA screening *N Engl J Med* 2012a;366:1047–1048.
Miller AB. Chapter 12. Prostate Cancer Screening. In *Cancer and Aging: Research and Practice.* Bellizzi K, Gosney M, Eds. New York: Wiley-Blackwell. In press, 2012 b.
Raffle AE, Gray JAM. Screening: Evidence and Practice. Oxford, Oxford University Press, 2007, pp 366.
Sandblom G, Varenhorst E, Rosell J, Lo¨fman O, Carlsson P. Randomised prostate cancer screening trial: 20year follow-up. *BMJ* 2011; 342:d1539 doi:10.1136/bmj.d1539
Schröder FH. Screening for prostate cancer (PC) – an update on recent findings of the European Randomized Study of Screening for Prostate Cancer (ERSPC). *Eur Oncol* 2008; 26:533–541.
Schröder FH, Hugosson J, Roobol MJ, Tammela TLJ, Ciatto S, Nelen V et al. Screening and prostate-cancer mortality in a randomized European study. *New Engl J Med* 2009; 360: 1320–1328.
Schröder FH, Hugosson J, Roobol MJ, Tammela TLJ, Ciatto S, Nelen V et al. Prostate Cancer Mortality at 11 years of Follow-up in the ERSPC. *N Engl J Med* 2012; 366:981–990.
Schröder FH, Roobol MJ. A comment on prostate cancer screening in the Prostate, Lung, Colorectal and Ovarian cancer screening trial: update on findings from the initial four rounds of screening in a randomized trial. *BJU Int* 2009; 103: 143–144.

van Leeuwen PJ, van Vugt HA, Bangma CH. The implementation of screening for prostate cancer. *Prostate Cancer and Prostatic Diseases* 2010; **13**: 218–227.

Wolters T, Roobol MJ, Steyerberg EW, van den Bergh RCN, Bangma CH, Hugosson J, et al. The effect of study arm on prostate cancer treatment in a large screening trial (ERSPC). *Int J Cancer* 2010; 126: 2387–2393.

US Preventive Task Force. Screening for prostate cancer: U.S. Preventive Services Task Force recommendation statement. *Annals of Int Med* 2008;149:185–191.

Chapter 19
Applying Cancer Screening in the Context of a National Health Service

Julietta Patnick

19.1 The Decision to Screen

National Health Services provide to their eligible populations a range of health care either through directly funded care or by reimbursing the population for defined care. The UK has a health-care system which is totally free at the point of delivery and which traditionally has owned all the health-care providers. This system has rationed care by making people wait, sometimes for months or years in the past. Other countries, such as Canada, operate their free at the point of care service through private providers who bill and are reimbursed directly from the health-care system. There are various models, and in many of these national health services, cancer screening is paid for by the state.

This does not mean, however, that individuals can simply decide to have a test and the state will automatically pay. There is always a process to determine which screening activities will be covered and which not. The UK has the National Screening Committee which makes these decisions (NSC 2012); the Netherlands has the Health Council (Health Council of the Netherlands 2012). There is a major difference between these decisions and decisions made, for example, by the Preventive Services Task Force in the United States of America, since the USPSTF offers advice which it is then up to individual clinicians and patients to take or not (USPSTF 2009). In those countries where there is a national health service, these decisions have a very practical effect.

J. Patnick (✉)
NHS Cancer Screening Programmes,
Fulwood House, Old Fulwood Road, Sheffield, S10 3 TH, UK
e-mail: julietta.patnick@cancerscreening.nhs.uk

A.B. Miller (ed.), *Epidemiologic Studies in Cancer Prevention and Screening*, Statistics for Biology and Health 79, DOI 10.1007/978-1-4614-5586-8_19,

In order to make decisions and recommendations, the process begins in the same place, with the evidence. Thus, most countries will screen for breast, cervix and bowel cancer, and where there is a national health system, this will be covered. There will be variation in the age-group targeted and frequency of screening, and it cannot be ignored that when the public purse is involved, the cost of screening is a factor in what may be provided. Where resources are limited and there are competing demands, as is generally the case in a publicly funded service, there is consequently the question of getting the best value for available money and manpower and of achieving the greatest gain in public health for the funding and resources available.

Evidence is not always clear. There is a particular debate about prostate cancer screening. Evidence came in 2009 from the European Randomised Study of Screening for Prostate Cancer (ERSPC) that screening with PSA reduced mortality by 20 % at 12 years follow-up (and see Miller, this volume). However, the number needed to treat to save a life as computed from the ERSPC results was 48 (Schröder et al. 2009). There has been debate about PSA testing for many years, and sometimes PSA testing is provided on request, while there are no organised programmes as there are for breast, cervix and bowel cancer. This may change in the next few years as longer follow-up provides more information about the effects of prostate screening.

While evidence leads and resources, both financial and clinical, permit, political support is vital in a publicly funded setting. Screening is always controversial as it is health care intervening in the lives of people who have not asked for assistance and promising them benefits. When it is the state supporting that intervention or even providing it itself, then the controversy is magnified. Political support is thus vital before a new screening programme can be introduced. At the same time, screening is very popular with the general public, and screening can attract a great deal of attention from politicians. This can have benefits when the introduction of a new screening programme which is supported by strong evidence is being advocated. For example, in England, the prime minister made plain his support for a new flexible sigmoidoscopy colorectal cancer screening programme within 6 months of the research being published (BBC1 2010). But it can also focus attention on the shortcomings of screening programmes when there is a failing or when there is some change being made to a previously provided service (see below). Finally, sometimes politicians can push for screening to take place when the evidence is not in place to justify it. In these circumstances, public servants have to be very firm and very skilled.

19.2 Running the Programme

The ethics of screening have been discussed at great length, and in 1968, the seminal work of Wilson and Jungner (1968) laid down ten principles to help support policymakers in deciding whether to screen for a disease or not. Chief amongst these is that the chance of benefit should be greater than the chance of harm. Further ethical issues are overlaid once the state becomes involved since there is the extra dimension of state interference in the lives of its citizens. This is tolerated to a greater or lesser extent in different societies, and generally where there is a national health service, there is a greater tolerance. But there are also greater expectations. The state should ensure not only that the service is offered but that it is a service of the requisite quality. In order, then, to avoid things going wrong and to protect both the public to whom screening is offered and the political paymasters, quality assurance is generally a major component of a publicly funded service.

The ethical underpinning of a screening programme comes to the fore particularly prominently in the area of invitations for screening and the information given to those invited by the public service. An individual doctor will make recommendations to an individual patient and can temper the strength of the recommendation with knowledge of the patient's particular circumstances. When it is a national programme that is inviting people to be screened, the information given can become a highly charged issue.

Operating cancer screening in the context of a national health service allows a population-based approach to be taken. Having an organised programme requires having an infrastructure to build on, and this is more readily available where there is a national health service. The first requirement is a register of those eligible. In some countries, such as the Republic of Ireland, this may be the electoral roll, but legislation might be needed in order to access this for the purpose of inviting people for cancer screening. In other countries, this might be a register of people enrolled in an insurance plan. In the UK, it is the list of those registered with the National Health Service which is available to all those ordinarily resident there. Taking a population-based approach brings advantages in terms of quality assurance and audit, equity across society and cost-effectiveness.

19.3 Quality Assurance and Audit

Minimum quality control standards are often laid down for cancer screening services, sometimes in legislation if the country concerned requires this. However, in the context of a national health service, quality assurance can often go into great depths. The Council of Europe (2003) recommends that member states "offer evidence-based cancer screening through a systematic population-based approach with quality assurance at all appropriate levels .....(and) implement screening programs in accordance with European guidelines on best practice". These have now been published for breast, cervical and colorectal cancer screening and cover quality assurance of all aspects of a screening programme (Perry et al. 2006; Arbyn et al. 2008; Segnan et al. 2010). In the context of breast screening, for example, it is not only the number of mammograms read but also the expected pickup rate of cancers, the dose of radiation given, timescales for results, the accuracy of localisation procedures and of pathology reporting and so on for many other aspects of the process. In cervical screening and colorectal screening, similar detail is gone into and standards suggested for all aspects of the programme from testing through to diagnosis and including the epidemiology and evaluation of screening when delivered on a population basis. It is up to each member state whether to follow these guidelines or not, but they have been well adopted by those countries within the European Union which have national health services and can offer screening on a population basis.

A screening programme operating within a national health service can be required to operate using a single information technology (IT) system with single definitions to be applied. All units in a service can be required to operate to a single set of protocols agreed between the service and the professionals to be appropriate. Taken together, all this supports detailed quality control on a population basis and allows great facility for auditing and developing the evidence underpinning the programmes. There can be local and national comparison of performance across a large number of parameters, and when quality control is organised at a national level, there can be a degree of externality applied. This, of course, can happen without a national health service, but where this exists, there is usually greater confidence that like is being compared with like, detail in what is audited beyond the individual unit and a degree of compulsion for local units about compliance with both quality assurance activities and any subsequent recommendations. There may also be less emphasis on the process and facilities and greater emphasis on clinical outcomes since linking data and following patients up is easier within one unified system than where there are completely separate providers of care. The numbers involved in a service which is organised on a whole population basis can be very large. Thus, differences which are small and can appear to be immaterial at a local level can be seen to have an effect when observed across many thousands and even millions of people. This generates a scientific basis for developments in programme delivery which can improve quality. These developments can be recommended wherever in the world a screening technology is applied, but in a national health service, not only can recommendations then be made, but action can be guaranteed. An early example of this is the move to an optimal optical density in the UK breast cancer screening programme (Young et al. 1994). When the programme started, the density of the image was left to individual radiologist's discretion, with some preferring darker and others lighter films. Pulling together data on a number of parameters, including this one, across all the screening units demonstrated that those with lighter films found fewer cancers and, after a certain point, the darker film gave a greater dose of radiation, but with no increase in sensitivity. An optimal density range was then set, and all units in the country were required to operate within the specified range. Adherence to the policy was then monitored through the quality assurance infrastructure.

19.4 Cost-Effectiveness

There is now a body of evidence that organised screening is more cost-effective than opportunistic screening. Indeed, the European Council notes "the public health benefits and cost efficiency of a screening programme are achieved if the programme is implemented systematically, covering the whole target population and following best-practice guidelines". A direct comparison was made in France in the 1990s looking at opportunistic versus organised cervical screening and concluded that opportunistic screening costs three times as much as an organised system (Schaffer et al. 1995).

From lists of those eligible, it is possible to send invitations for screening or notifications that screening is due, to calculate the denominator population necessary to calculate programme reach and to look at the population which will shortly meet the entry criteria for a population screening programme based on age and thus plan services accordingly. Planning is much easier when the likely participation rate is known and particularly if there is central provision of services with timed appointments. This allows a very efficient service to be delivered where people and equipment are available at the appropriate level to meet demand. A highly efficient service is less demanding on the public purse.

19.5 Access to Screening and Informed Choice

One advantage that accrues with organised population-based screening services provided in the context of a national health service is that they can be more easily accessed by the less affluent parts of the population who might not access screening in an opportunistic setting where they would have to pay. Countries which have organised screening programmes have fewer inequalities in their participation patterns (Palència et al. 2010). Nevertheless, even in the UK where screening is provided totally free of charge, the less affluent, less well-educated groups within society are less likely to attend. This is further influenced by other factors such as ethnicity (Moser et al. 2009; Szczepura et al. 2008; von Wagner et al. 2011). Clearly where there is some alienation felt from mainstream society, this is not totally ameliorated by the fact that screening is provided free of charge.

High uptake indicates that the service is largely acceptable to those to whom it is offered and also uptake can be an indicator of accessibility of the service to all parts of society. Uptake can be monitored by area, by household or by individual depending on information available and legally accessible within a society; it can be analysed by socio-economic status or educational attainment, by ethnicity or religious affiliation and by language group or place of birth in societies which are interested in those factors. Participation rates are generally lower for minority groups within any society. Organised population-based screening has been shown to reduce inequalities, but not to eliminate them altogether. Screening services operating within national health service systems are well placed to address these inequalities, but more may be asked of them in this respect than in those health systems which are entirely opportunistic or at the discretion of the individual clinician or patient.

A disadvantage of a highly centralised, highly organised service is that it is difficult to take account of individual preferences. The screening test may require attendance at a time and place which is not convenient but which is allocated perhaps according to address of residence. Women may prefer to have their screening mammograms reported immediately, but this is probably not possible in a population service. When services are planned on a population not an individual basis, and the individual is not the financial client, then it is not always possible to tailor a screening episode to individual requirements within the constraints of the nationally prescribed service.

Where there is a national health service which offers screening, there will generally be nationally approved, or nationally produced, information which supports that offer. Often, in order to ensure equity and cost-effectiveness, those controlling the funding are concerned to see that participation or uptake/acceptance rates for the service offered are high. So there is an in-built tension between achieving the high acceptance rates generally required by, or of, those offering the service and offering informed choice to those invited for screening, while respecting the decision not to participate. The information given to accompany breast screening appointments in England has been the subject of a much-heated debate with allegations that information is deliberately withheld in order to drive up participation (Gøtzsche and Jørgensen 2011). This has led to a major review not only of the information given but of the evidence on which the programme is based (CRUK 2011). It is difficult to produce information for everyone in a society which is accessible to all and almost impossible to do that without it seeming patronising to the better educated.

19.6 When Things Go Wrong

When a screening programme is provided with public funding, and certainly when it is directly provided by a national health service, politicians are generally held to be accountable by the public and the media. Thus, when things go wrong as well as the issues of looking after the patients affected, learning from the error, handling the publicity and scrutiny from health authorities, it may also be necessary to deal with political questions. Questions have been asked in the House of Commons about failures in breast screening in England, for example, and the Public Accounts Committee (PAC) has demanded explanations for limitations in cervical screening (Hansard 1997; PAC 1997). This can be helpful since changes can be made with political momentum that could not otherwise happen. An example would be the introduction of national coordination into the cervical screening programme in England on the breast screening model. The cervical screening programme was older and more established, but those organising it were reluctant in the mid-1990s to change its modus operandi and structure. Problems in Scotland in cervical screening together with an earlier PAC report critical of the programme created the situation where change could be made which was not possible, or perhaps the need not perceived, beforehand. Once it was desired that the systems should change however, the fact that the programme operated within a national health service allowed those changes to be put in place.

19.7 Withdrawal of Screening

Recently, there has been reconsideration about the harms of screening in many countries. This particularly applies to breast and cervical screening which have been operating for decades. In several settings, this has led to a recommendation that there should be a reduced amount of screening, usually at the edges of the eligibility age range. The USPSTF in 2009 issued revised guidelines which recommended against routine mammography screening for women younger than 50 years old and suggested that screening end at age 74 years (USPSTF 2009). It also recommended screening every two years rather than annually as previously. The new recommendations contrasted with guidelines from many other organisations such as the American Cancer Society (ACS). The ACS has not changed its recommendation for annual mammograms from 40 (ACS 2010), and in the US health-care system, it is up to each clinician and each woman to decide on an individual basis whether to follow the USPSTF recommendation or not.

In contrast when the Advisory Committee on Cervical Screening in England recommended raising the age of first invitation for cervical screening to 25, this had a very real effect. This recommendation was based on growing evidence of the harms of treating the cervix for subsequent pregnancies and growing recognition of a lack of effectiveness of cervical screening in the younger woman. Since the screening programme is delivered by the NHS, the recommendation had to be agreed by health ministers, and the decision was then announced in October 2003. The Committee's scientific recommendation had a practical effect.

The withdrawal of screening from women under 25 gradually filtered through as women either reached the age of 20 and were not invited for screening or, if they had been screened below the age of 25, they were not rescreened until reaching that age. As growing numbers of women were not screened, a major campaign began to reinstate screening from 20, despite the fact that participation at that age had been no more than 50 % and falling and despite the evidence supporting the decision growing firmer. In these circumstances, ministers asked the Committee to think again. The original decision still stood, however, and a ministerial statement was then made to announce this (Keen 2012). The practical implementation by the NHS of the Committee's decision had repercussions which involved ministers. The Committee's view was not simply a recommendation to doctors but had practical consequences. Vocal opposition to the decision by a campaigning group did not affect the scientific decision but did affect how that decision was handled politically.

19.8 A National Office

In order for advantage to be taken of having a national approach to cancer screening, some sort of national coordination will be necessary. If it is a large country, either in population or geographic terms, there may also be regional offices. The relationship between the national office, any regional teams and local screening units and the balance of power between them will be set by the local health system. The national function could be relatively weak if there is some sort of federated arrangement for health care or stronger in a more centralised state. The functions that a national or large regional office will have could include overseeing the development of professional protocols and definitions, of the IT system to support them, and collating and analysing the information that is eventually produced by that system. National information can be produced or commissioned by this office, and there could be large-scale purchasing of equipment to increase the cost-effectiveness of the service. There could be support for decision-making bodies about introducing, amending or withdrawing screening and coordination of responses to problems in the service based in a national office. Over time, the national or regional office can also become the repository of the programme's memory with files and expertise going back over many years. The cost of this office and any bureaucracy has to be included in calculations about the cost-effectiveness of the programme and balanced against clinicians' needs for local autonomy when dealing with patients on a day to day basis.

19.9 Conclusion

The context of a national health service affects not only the science underpinning screening but also how that science is applied. Decisions taken about the introduction of screening need to be tempered by the availability of resources, and the withdrawal of screening can have political ramifications. It can be difficult to tailor screening to an individual's preferences or to pitch the information given to accompany screening at the optimal level. However, applying screening in this context allows a population approach to be taken which can have many advantages in terms of the ability to quality assure a programme, to use the programme to develop knowledge about screening and the disease screened for, to have an equitable approach to screening across all groups in society and to operate a highly efficient and cost-effective service.

References

American Cancer Society Guidelines for the Early Detection of Cancer. last medical review 25 February 2010 http://www.cancer.org/Healthy/FindCancerEarly/CancerScreeningGuidelines/american-cancer-society-guidelines-for-the-early-detection-of-cancer last accessed 3 February 2012

Arbyn M, Anttila A, Jordan J, Ronco G, Schenck U, Segnan N et al. *European guidelines for quality assurance in cervical cancer screening.* Second Edition Luxembourg: Office for Official Publications of the European Communities, 2008

BBC1 Andrew Marr Show October 3 2010 interview with Prime Minister Rt Hon David Cameron MP http://www.bbc.co.uk/programmes/b00v4pmt last accessed 22 January 2012

CRUK. Cancer Research UK. *Breast Screening Review.* December 15 2011 http://info.cancerresearchuk.org/publicpolicy/ourpolicypositions/symptom_Awareness/cancer_screening/breast-screening-review/ last accessed 22 January 2012

Council of Europe. *Recommendation of 2 December 2003 on Cancer Screening* (2003/878/EC) http://eur-lex.europa.eu/LexUriServ/LexUriServ.do?uri=OJ:L:2003:327:0034:0038:EN:PDF last accessed 22 January 2012

Gøtzsche PC, Jørgensen KJ. The breast screening programme and misinforming the public. *J R Soc Med.* 2011;104:361-369.

Hansard 9 June 1997, vol 295 col 793 *Breast Screening.* http://www.publications.parliament.uk/pa/cm199798/cmhansrd/vo970609/debtext/70609-05.htm#70609-05_head0 last accessed 22 January 2012

Health Council of the Netherlands http://www.gezondheidsraad.nl/en/publications/prevention last accessed 22 January 2012

Keen A. Written Ministerial Statement. *Cervical screening for women aged under 25 years.* http://www.cancerscreening.nhs.uk/cervical/news/012.html last accessed 3 February 2012

Moser K, Patnick J, Beral V. Inequalities in reported use of breast and cervical screening in Great Britain: analysis of cross sectional survey data. *BMJ.* 2009;338:b2025. doi: 10.1136/bmj.b2025

NSC. National Screening Committee http://www.screening.nhs.uk/about last accessed 22 January 2012

Palència L, Espelt A, Rodríguez-Sanz M, Puigpinós R, Pons-Vigués M, Pasarín MI et al. Socio-economic inequalities in breast and cervical cancer screening practices in Europe: influence of the type of screening program. *Int J Epidemiol.* 2010; 39:757-765.

Perry N, Broeders M. de Wolf C. Törnberg S. Holland R. von Karsa L Eds. *European guidelines for quality assurance in breast cancer screening and diagnosis* 4th Edition Luxembourg: Office for Official Publications of the European Communities, 2006

Public Accounts Committee. PAC 69th report. HC757 *The Performance of the NHS Cervical Screening Programme in England.* Her Majesty's Stationery Office London 1997

Schaffer, P., Anthony, S. & Allemand, H. Would a higher frequency of tests leadto the prevention of cervical cancer? In: Monsonego, J., ed., *Papillomavirus in HumanPathology,* Rome, Ares Serona Symposia, 1995; pp.193–204

Segnan N, Patnick J, von Karsa Eds. *European guidelines for quality assurance in colorectal cancer screening and diagnosis.* First Edition Luxembourg: Publications Office of the European Union, 2010

Schröder FH, Hugosson J, Roobol MJ, Tammela TL, Ciatto S, Nelen V et al. Screening and prostate-cancer mortality in a randomized European study. *N Engl J Med.* 2009; 360:1320-8.

Szczepura A, Price C, Gumber A. Breast and bowel cancer screening uptake patterns over 15 years for UK south Asian ethnic minority populations, corrected for differences in socio-demographic characteristics. *BMC Public Health* 2008; 8: 346.

United States Preventive Services Task Force http://www.uspreventiveservicestaskforce.org/ last accessed 22 January 2012

USPSTF Screening for Breast Cancer: U.S. Preventive Services Task Force. Recommendation Statement *Ann Intern Med.* 2009;151:716-726.

von Wagner C, Baio G, Raine R, Snowball J, Morris, S, Atkin, W et al. Inequalities in participation in an organised national colorectal cancer screening programme: results from the first 2.6 million invitations in England. *Int J. Epidemiol.* 2011; 40: 712-718.

Wilson JM, Jungner YG. *Principles and practice of mass screening for disease.* Public Health Paper 34 1968. Geneva,World Health Organization Geneva.

Young KC, Wallis MG, Ramsdale ML. Mammographic film density and detection of small breast cancers. *Clin Radiol.* 1994; 49:461-465.

Part III
Impact of Prevention and Screening in Populations

Chapter 20
Do International Trends in Cancer Incidence and Mortality Reflect Expectations from Cancer Screening?

Philippe Autier

20.1 Introduction

A wealth of clinical data demonstrates that the prognosis of cancerous diseases is directly associated with two types of characteristics: the extent of the disease at diagnosis and the histological characteristics of the cancer. In the absence of efficient treatment, the prognosis is poor when a cancer has extended beyond the organ of origin or, when at histology, the cells and tissues constituting the cancerous lesions no longer display the features of the organ of origin (i.e., the degree of dedifferentiation of cancerous tissues).

Cancer extent is summarized by the TNM stage (T for tumor size, N for node status, and M for evidence of metastases in distant organ(s)), and the histological characteristics are specific to the various cancers that develop in each organ (UICC 2002; AJCC 2002). Staging provides an estimate of the cancer extent (e.g., still local, regional nodes invaded, or already evidence of distant metastases), and the histological characteristics provide an estimate of the cancer aggressiveness. Local extension of a cancer is a strong predictor of metastases in the lymph nodes or in distant organs. For instance, the probability of positive axillary lymph nodes (i.e., presence of metastases in the lymph nodes) steadily increases with the size of invasive breast cancer. In addition, the extent of the cancer and the histological characteristics are correlated because in patients diagnosed with tumors of similar size, tumors with bad prognosis are more likely to have metastases in regional lymph nodes or in distant organs.

P. Autier, M.D., MPH, Ph.D. (✉)
International Prevention Research Institute (iPRI),
95 Cours Lafayette, 69006 Lyon, France

Chemin du Saquin, Espace Européen, batiment G,
69130 Ecully (Lyon), France
e-mail: philippe.autier@i-pri.org

A.B. Miller (ed.), *Epidemiologic Studies in Cancer Prevention and Screening*,
Statistics for Biology and Health 79, DOI 10.1007/978-1-4614-5586-8_20,

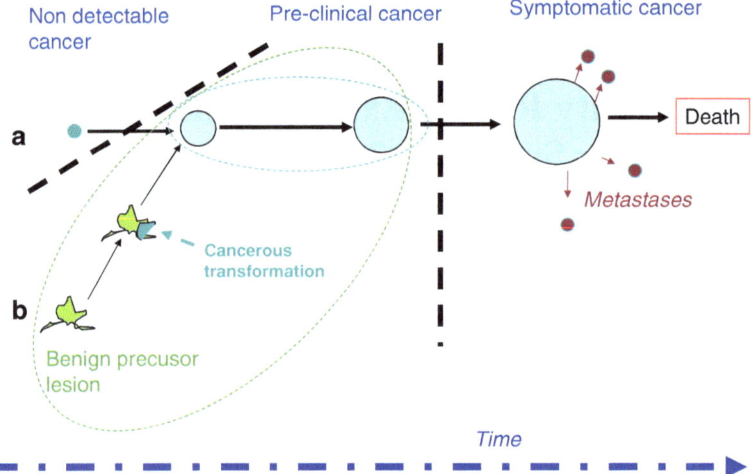

Fig. 20.1 Evolution of cancer, developing from a clonal expansion of an initiated cell or from a benign precursor lesion that undergoes cancerous transformation. The *dotted ellipses* indicate the window of opportunity for detecting precursor lesions of preclinical cancers

The correlation between cancer extent and histological features typical of cancer is in line with the classic paradigm of chronological development of cancer according to which if nothing opposes a cancerous process, the cancer growth will occur in successive steps during which molecular abnormalities accumulate and interact, which leads to increasingly aggressive malignant lesions, with ultimately metastases released in the lymphatic fluid or in the blood stream. The chronological development paradigm assumes that a time window exists between the start of the clonal expansion of a single transformed cell into a tumor and the time the tumor could be spotted by an early detection method, followed by another time window between the time the tumor can be detected by an early detection method and the time the tumor becomes symptomatic or clinically apparent (Fig. 20.1). The latter time window is called the preclinical detectable period (PCDP) or the sojourn time. The PCDP represents the window of opportunity during which an early detection method can identify subjects possibly having the cancer.

Following the chronological development paradigm, the goal of cancer screening is to reduce the risk of cancer death by detecting cancers when they are not yet clinically apparent, at a stage they are less life threatening and more curable. An immediate consequence of this goal is that the ability of a cancer-screening test to reduce the risk of cancer death is tightly bound to its capacity to prevent the occurrence of advanced (or late-stage) cancer. So, if screening for a specific cancer works, then reductions in mortality rates from that cancer should be preceded by reductions in the incidence rates of patients diagnosed with advanced stage.

20.2 Two Type of Cancers

From a screening point of view, cancer can be classified in two broad categories. The first category includes cancers that develop from a known benign precursor lesion. Treatment (most usually by removal) of the precursor lesion prevents both cancer occurrence and mortality. In this group of cancers, the most efficient screening consists in detecting the precursor lesions. Three common cancers fall in this category: cervical cancer, whose precursor lesion is cervical intraepithelial neoplasia (CIN); colorectal cancer, whose precursor lesion is an adenomatous polyp (having a size of at least 1 cm); and oral cancer, whose precursor lesion is leukoplakia. The majority of precursor lesions do not progress into invasive cancer, but it is their systematic detection and removal that ultimately impacts on cancer incidence and mortality.

The second category includes cancers for which no real precursor lesion is known. Screening aims at preventing late-stage cancer and thus tries to detect invasive cancers when still at an early stage. Breast, thyroid, and prostate cancers; cutaneous melanoma; and neuroblastoma belong to this second category.

Cancers of the first category can also be screened with methods detecting them when they are already invasive, but at an early stage of its development, for instance, the fecal-occult-blood test that detects blood leaks caused by the penetration of colorectal cancer into the surrounding tissues.

20.3 Published Data on Advanced Cancer Incidence

The data related to cervical, colorectal, breast, and prostate cancer are summarized, as relevant data from randomized trials, population-based cancer registries, and mortality were available for these cancers.

20.3.1 Cervical Cancer

Cytology screening of the uterine cervix allows the early detection of invasive cervical cancer as well as the detection of cervical intraepithelial neoplasia (CIN). The treatment of early invasive cervical cancer may reduce the incidence of advanced cancer, and removal of CIN lesions may reduce the incidence of both early and advanced cancer. Other screening methods exist, like visual inspection, cervicography, and HPV testing.

Cervical cancer screening has been implemented in many countries without prior evidence from randomized trials that it was actually able to reduce cervical cancer mortality. Two randomized trials have been conducted in the last decade in India that evaluated the influence of visual inspection, cytology screening, and HPV testing on the risk of cervical cancer death (Sankaranarayanan et al. 2007; 2009). A good correlation exists between the reduction in the risk of being diagnosed with an advanced cervical cancer and the reduction in the risk of cervical cancer death (Fig. 20.2).

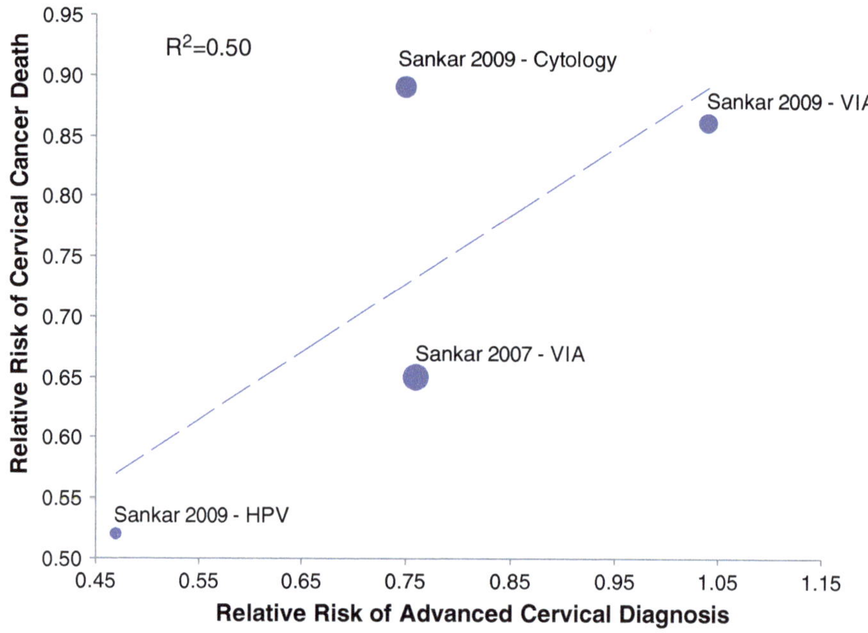

Fig. 20.2 Changes in risks of being diagnosed with an advanced cervical cancer and risks of cervical cancer death in two randomized trials in India (Sankaranarayanan et al. 2007, 2009; VIA: visual inspection; HPV: test for detection of HPV)

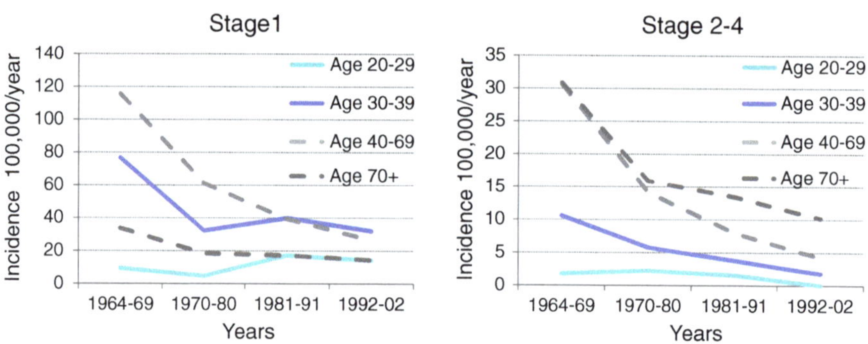

Fig. 20.3 Cervical cancer incidence in Iceland (Adapted from Sigurdsson and Sigvaldason, 2006)

In Iceland, a population-based program of cytology screening was introduced in 1969 that rapidly covered 100 % of the female adult population (Läärä et al. 1987). The Icelandic cancer registry has collected data on cervical cancer by stage from 1964 onward. The incidence of stage 2–4 cancer dropped dramatically in years following screening introduction (Fig. 20.3). Of note, the fall in stage 1 cancer incidence illustrates that the incidence of that cancer has considerably declined in Iceland.

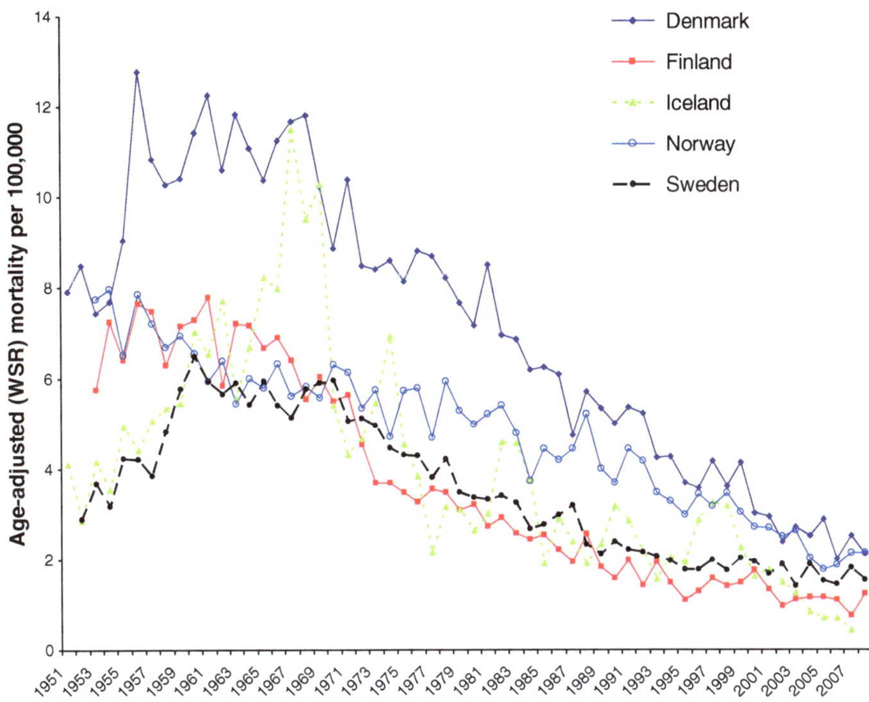

Fig. 20.4 Trends in mortality from cervical cancer in Nordic countries (Engholm et al. 2010). Full population coverage with cytology screening was achieved in 1969–1973 in Iceland, Sweden, and Finland; 7–10 years later in Denmark; and 10–15 years later in Norway (Läärä et al. 1987)

Mortality statistics show that cervical cancer mortality reductions in Nordic countries from 1965 to 1980 were related to nationwide screening programs from the 1960s (Fig. 20.4). In countries where screening programs were delayed (Norway and Denmark), the mortality reductions were also delayed and never reached those observed in other Nordic countries. Access to surgery and radiotherapy was comparable between the Nordic countries, and the clear differences in mortality trends could be attributed to time differences in the implementation of cervical cancer screening. For years, these data have remained the most compelling evidence that cytology screening reduces mortality from this cancer (IARC 2005).

20.3.2 *Colorectal Cancer*

Three randomized trials on fecal-occult-blood test (Hardcastle et al. 1996; Kronborg et al. 1996; Mandel et al. 1999) and one of the randomized trials on sigmoidoscopy (Segnan et al. 2011) have shown reduced risk of colorectal cancer death associated with being allocated to the screening group. These trials also showed a correlation

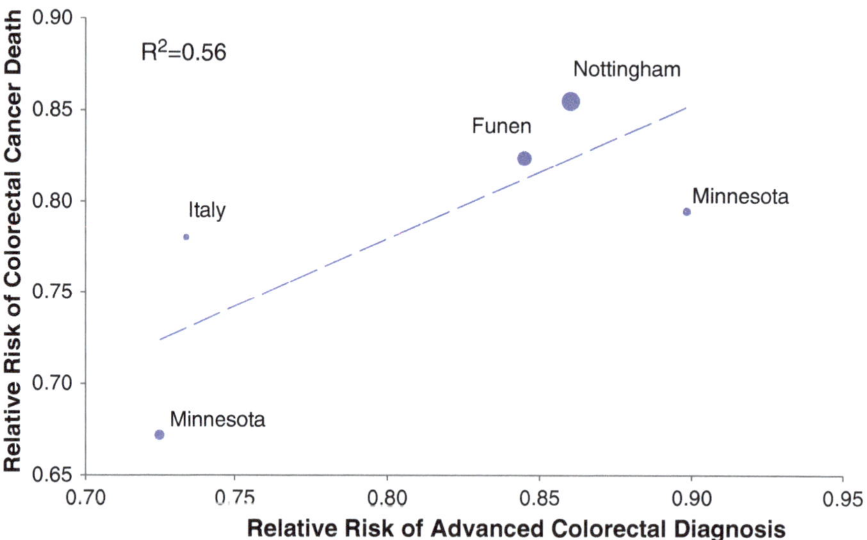

Fig. 20.5 Changes in risks of being diagnosed with an advanced colorectal cancer and risks of colorectal cancer death in the three randomized trials on fecal-occult-blood test in Nottingham (United Kingdom) (Hardcastle et al. 1996), Funen (Denmark) (Kronborg et al. 1996), and Minnesota (USA) (Mandel et al. 1999) and one trial on sigmoidoscopy in Italy (Segnan et al. 2011)

between reductions in the risk of being diagnosed with an advanced colorectal cancer and reductions in the risk of colorectal cancer death (Fig. 20.5).

The US Surveillance, Epidemiology, and End Results Program (SEER) data show sharp declines in advanced as well as in early stage colorectal cancer (Fig. 20.6), indicating that incidence is also declining. In fact, major contrasts in colorectal cancer and in screening for that cancer exist between high-income countries. A plot of changes in colorectal cancer mortality in European and US men ≥50 (Fig. 20.7) shows marked reductions in mortality that are well correlated with past exposure to endoscopic examination of the large bowel. Similar reductions and correlations are observed among women ≥50 (data not shown). Mortality reductions are also correlated with past exposure to fecal-occult-blood test, but the strength of the association is not as high (data not shown).

20.3.3 Breast Cancer

A systematic review of breast screening randomized trials using mammography has shown a one-to-one correlation between the risk of advanced breast cancer and of breast cancer death (Autier et al. 2009).

Another systematic review found that in areas in Europe, North America, and Australia where screening was widespread for a long time, no or small decreases in the incidence of advanced and of very advanced breast cancer were observed

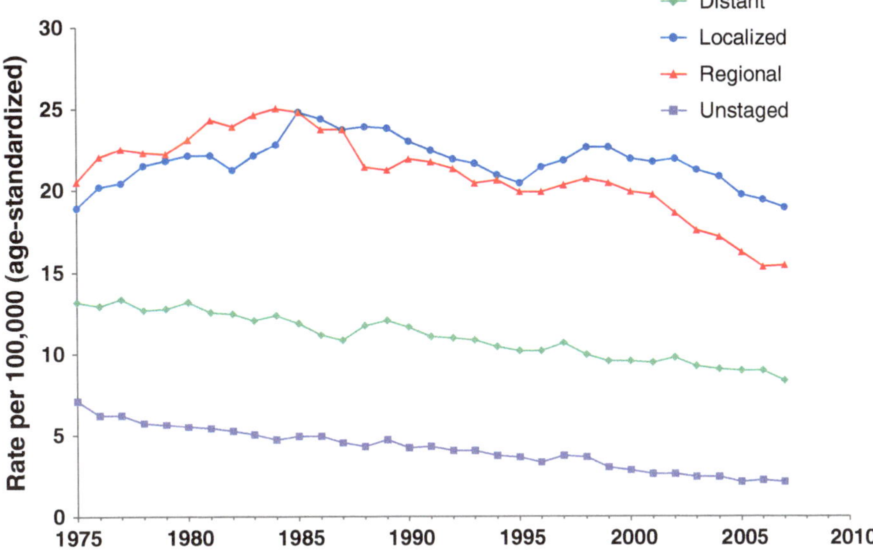

Fig. 20.6 Incidence trends of local, regional, or distant CRC in the US SEER 9 older cancer registries (Edwards et al. 2010)

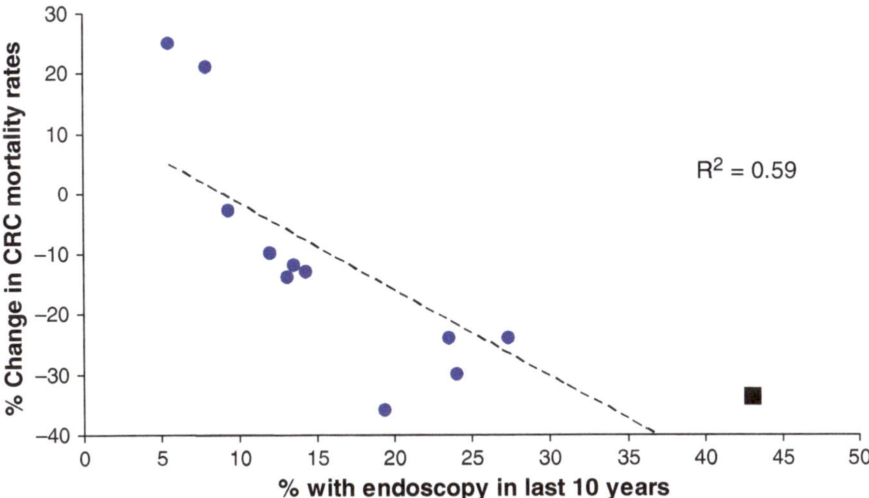

Fig. 20.7 Percent changes in colorectal cancer mortality and percent of European and US men ≥50 who had an endoscopic examination (sigmoidoscopy or colonoscopy) of the large bowel in the last 10 years. European countries (plain circles) are Austria, Belgium, Denmark, France, Germany, Greece, Italy, Spain, Sweden, Switzerland, and the Netherlands. The plain square represents the US data. Data for Europe were collected in 2004–2005 (Stock and Brenner, 2010), and US data are those from the BRFSS (Behavioral Risk Factor Surveillance System) survey of 2002 (Stock et al. 2010). For European countries, mortality changes from 1988–1990 to 2005–2007 were derived from the WHO mortality database; for the USA, changes in mortality were those reported in Jemal et al. (2010)

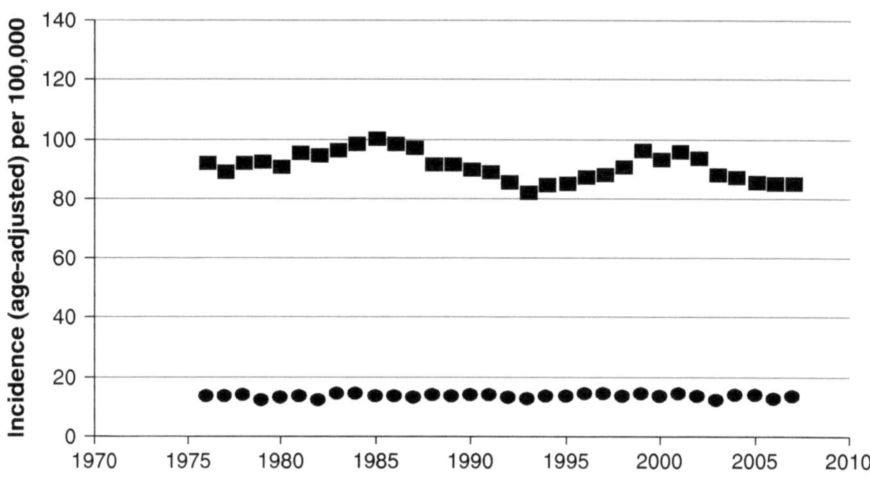

Fig. 20.8 Incidence rates of advanced breast cancer 1973–2007 for women aged 40–69 in US SEER 9 older cancer registries (Autier et al. 2011a; Esserman et al. 2009)

(Autier et al. 2011a; Esserman et al. 2009). US SEER data showed no decline over time in advanced breast cancer, even for distant breast cancer (Fig. 20.8). In the southeast region of the Netherlands where very detailed and complete data existed on breast cancer characteristics, no decline in the incidence of advanced breast cancer from 1989 to 2007 was found (Nederend et al. 2012).

In the United Kingdom, cancer registry data of Scotland, Northern Ireland, and the West Midlands showed no decline of the incidence of advanced breast cancer after screening introduction in 1989 (Autier et al. 2011a ; Autier and Boniol 2012).

In a study that mimicked the Nordic study on cervical cancer screening (Läärä et al. 1987), trends in breast cancer mortality within three pairs of European countries (the Netherlands and Belgium, Northern Ireland and Ireland, Sweden and Norway) were examined. In each pair, there was similar prevalence of risk factors for breast cancer death, access to treatment, and expenditures for health, but by year 1993, nationwide screening was in place in the first country of each pair, while screening was implemented 10 to 12 years later in the second country of the pair (Autier et al. 2011b). As shown in for the Sweden-Norway pair (Fig. 20.9), equivalent reductions in breast cancer mortality were observed from 1989 to 2007 in each country pair. These results agreed with the observation that breast cancer mortality reductions in high-income countries are unrelated to the temporal introduction of screening mammography (Autier et al. 2010; Bleyer 2011).

For screening methods other than mammography, one randomized trial in India that used breast clinical examination (BCE) did not report decreased rates of advanced cancer in women allocated to the BCE group, suggesting that this method is not likely to reduce the risk of breast cancer death (Sankaranarayanan et al. 2011).

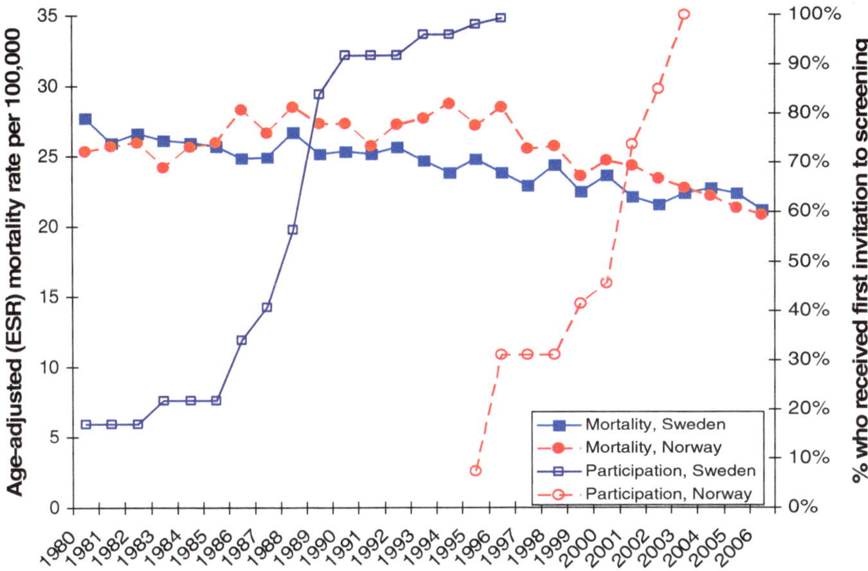

Fig. 20.9 Proportions of first invitation to mammography screening of women in eligible age groups and breast cancer mortality trends in Sweden and Norway

20.3.4 Prostate Cancer

Several randomized trials in Europe and in the USA have evaluated the ability of screening using measurements of serum prostate-specific antigen (PSA) to decrease prostate cancer mortality. Meta-analysis of results of these trials does not provide evidence that PSA screening decreases prostate cancer mortality, while there is evidence of substantial harmful effects associated with that screening (Boyle and Brawley 2009; Djulbegovic et al. 2010; Miller 2012).

In trials on PSA prostate cancer screening, more than 95 % of cancers were classified as clinical stage 2 in the US trial (Andriole et al. 2009) which is not informative. In the European Randomized Study of Screening for Prostate Cancer (ERSPC), PSA screening was associated with a 20 % reduction in the rate of patients diagnosed with distant metastases and a 21 % reduction in the risk of prostate cancer death (Schröder et al. 2012). However, there was no relationship between relative risks of death and of advanced cancer (Fig. 20.10) (Autier et al. 2012). This lack of correlation contrasts with aforementioned results of trials on cervical, colorectal, and breast screening, suggesting that causes other than PSA screening could be involved in mortality reductions observed in the ERSPC trial.

In the USA, where PSA screening has been highly prevalent since 1986, the annual age-adjusted incidence of clinical distant (stage 4) prostate cancers at diagnosis decreased from 28.1 in 1988 to 12.3 per 100 000 in 2003, representing an average 6.4 % annual decline (Cetin et al. 2010). This downward trend in incidence was

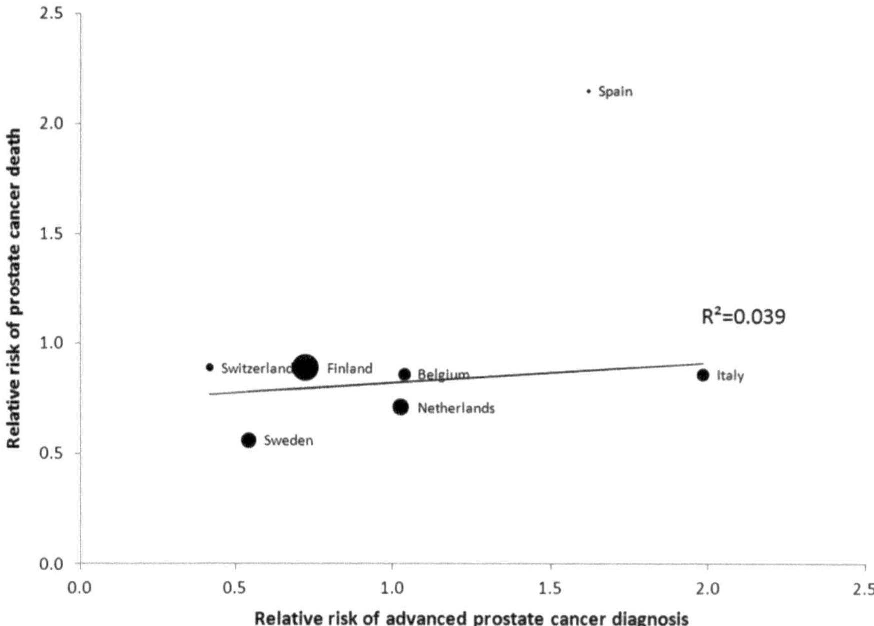

Fig. 20.10 Change in relative risks (RR) of death from prostate cancer according to relative risks of advanced prostate cancer diagnosis in ERSPC participating centers (Autier et al. 2012). The regression line was weighted on the inverse of the variance of the relative risk of death from prostate cancer. Dot sizes are proportional to center-specific weights

steeper in stage 4 patients with evidence of distant metastases at diagnosis, from 18.4 in 1988 to 6.7 per 100 000 in 2003, representing an average annual drop of 8.0 %.

There is thus an apparent contradiction between results of randomized trials and incidence trends of stage 4 prostate cancers in the USA. Of note, most published data on prostate cancer incidence trends by stage in the USA and in Europe focus on stage 4 cancers or lump together the "regional" and "distant" cancers. The few published data providing more details on incidence by clinical stage shed some light on this contradiction. In the Netherlands, the incidence of organ-confined cancer steeply increased after introduction of PSA screening in the early 1990s. Downward trends in stage 4 cancer starting in 1994 were noticeable, but at the same time trends in stage 3 cancers increased (Fig. 20.11) (Cremers et al. 2010). In Tyrol (Austria), where a regional screening program with PSA has been in place since 1988 (Bartsch et al. 2008), decreases in metastatic (M1) cancers after screening introduction were inversely correlated by an increasing incidence of T3–T4 M0 cancers (advanced cancers with no evidence of metastasis in distant organ at time of diagnosis). These data suggest that PSA screening allowed the detection of men with a prostate cancer that was no longer organ confined but that had not yet evolved into a clinical metastatic cancer (i.e., T3M0 and T4M0 cancers). Radiotherapy or initiation of hormone deprivation therapy at that moment may have delayed the development of clinical metastatic cancer. Because of competing causes of death, the "statistical

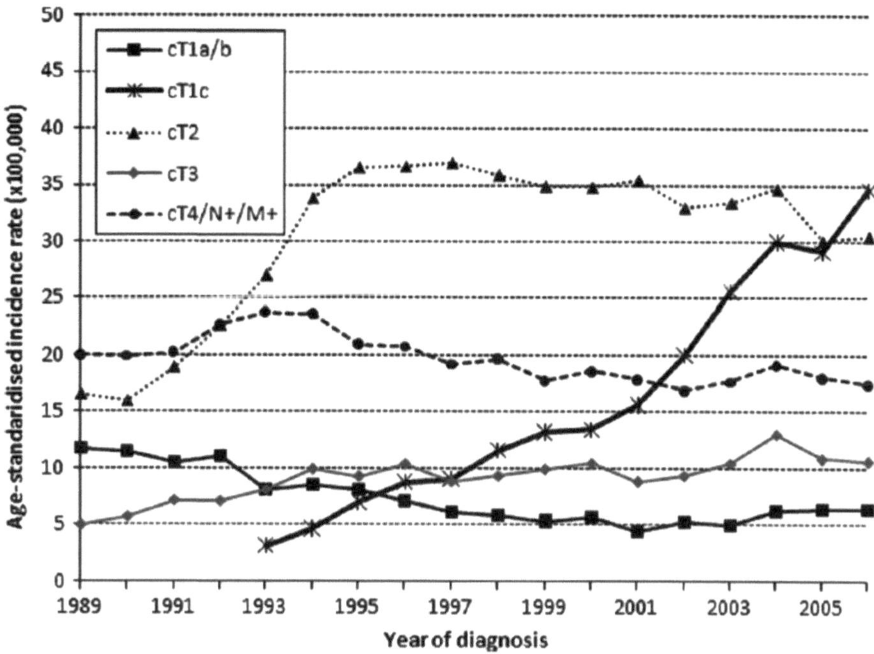

Fig. 20.11 Age-standardized incidence rates per 100,000 person-years (European Standard Population) for prostate cancer in the Netherlands 1989–2006, stratified by clinical stage (Cremers et al. 2010)

outcome" would have been a drop in deaths attributed to prostate cancer. This time shift induced by PSA testing of the moment an already advanced prostate cancer is diagnosed, which allows earlier initiation of radiotherapy or hormone deprivation treatment, fits well with the observation that in many countries, prostate cancer mortality started to decrease at the same time PSA screening was introduced (Bouchardy et al. 2008). The growth of most prostate cancers is believed to be slow, probably of the order of 10 to 20 years. If PSA screening had succeeded in preventing progression to stage 4 prostate cancers, thanks to detecting them when at an early stage (e.g., stage 1), then a significant lag time would have been needed for observing a change in prostate cancer mortality rates after PSA screening introduction.

20.4 Discussion

For cervical, colorectal, and breast cancer, results of randomized trials are quite consistent with an impact of screening on the risk of cancer death mediated through earlier detection of cancer that otherwise would have been more advanced, less curable, and often life threatening. The correlations between risk of advanced cancer and of cancer death are quite convincing given the diversity of designs (e.g., cluster randomization, left-to-nature control group) and screening methods used.

The translation of trial results (efficacy) to general populations (effectiveness) has been observed for cervical and colorectal cancers, two cancers whose early detection is essentially based on the identification and removal of precursor lesions.

For breast cancer, the translation of results from trials to general population screening seems to be weak or absent, and a controversy is still ongoing on whether general population breast screening is effective or not. The reasons underlying the discrepancy between randomized trials and general populations may be linked to the numerous criticisms of the Swedish trials on mammography screening that were probably not optimally designed (Gøtzsche and Olsen 2000; Twombly 2007).

Prostate cancer-screening trials did not yield results consistent with a benefit from PSA screening. However, some lines of data suggest that the benefits of screening may be linked to earlier initiation of radiotherapy or hormone deprivation treatment in men with locally advanced cancer. In any case, the harmful effects of PSA screening should deter men from participating in such screening (Boyle and Brawley 2009; USPSTF 2011; Heidenreich et al. 2012).

Screening for other cancers without a known precursor lesion (not examined in this work) seems poorly effective while being harmful, for instance, screening for neuroblastoma (that has been discontinued), for cutaneous melanoma, for thyroid cancer, and for stomach cancer.

20.4.1 A Frequent Mistake

The lower proportion of advanced breast cancer or a lower average size of invasive cancers after introduction of screening is frequently taken as evidence for screening efficiency. This reasoning is erroneous because the increase of the number of slow-growing or indolent screen-detected cancers will spuriously lead to reductions in the proportion of advanced (or of big) cancers, even if actual incidence rates of advanced cancer did not decrease (IARC 2002).

20.4.2 Advantages of Monitoring the Incidence of Advanced Cancer

A main advantage of using advanced cancer incidence as the surrogate for screening effectiveness is its independence from treatments. The availability of effective treatment is steadily increasing for a number of cancers that are or may be subject to screening, for instance, breast, cervical, and colorectal cancer. Improved treatments will thus contribute to reductions in cancer mortality. In breast cancer, introduction of screening in many high-income countries has coincided with greater use and introduction of effective treatments. It has proven extremely difficult to disentangle the respective roles of screening and of treatment in the dramatic decreases in breast cancer mortality that took place in North America and in many European countries over the last 20 years. Hence, monitoring of incidence of advanced cancer may serve as surrogate indicator for cancer mortality that would provide a reliable indication of the contribution of screening to reductions in cancer mortality.

20.4.3 Limitations of Monitoring the Incidence of Advanced Cancer

Numerous data have been published on cancer incidence in areas where population-based cancer registries are established. However, few data on advanced cancer incidence have been published. This paucity stems from a lack of cancer registries having complete and reliable collection of data on cancer stage.

The assessment of cancer extension can be done clinically or during the histological examination of tissues removed during biopsy or surgery. The former assessment is denoted the clinical staging (i.e., the cT stage) and the latter the pathological staging (i.e., the pT stage). Clinical staging is less accurate than pathology staging. For instance, large proportions of prostate cancer known to be present because of positive biopsy are not treated with radical prostatectomy, and thus, no histopathology of the whole gland is available (the cancer was left untreated or treated by tele- or brachytherapy or by hormone deprivation therapy). The clinical staging of prostate cancer is prone to errors, because, for instance, the clinical assessment of extraprostatic extension of cancer (i.e., the difference between cT1 and cT2 prostate cancer) is difficult.

Ways by which cancer extension is assessed vary between countries and medical institutions, depending on the practice of clinicians and histopathologists. In addition, changes in diagnosis and staging method influence staging, for instance, the introduction of sentinel node biopsy.

As a consequence of variability in staging, monitoring of advanced cancer incidence should rest on clinical or histopathological parameters most likely to remain more or less constant over time. In invasive breast cancer, the most robust parameter is the (largest) size of the tumor, with the threshold of less than or equal or more than 20 mm being the delineation between early and advanced cancer. For stabilizing time variations in staging practice, cancers registered in the US SEER data are classified as "local cancer," "regional cancer," "distant cancer," or "unstaged cancer" (Shambough et al. 1992). When cancer classification is mainly clinical and prone to errors (e.g., for prostate cancer), the reliability of the "local" and "regional" categories is questionable.

Changes in the prevalence of risk factors for cancer death are likely to affect the incidence of advanced cancers. However, environmental and lifestyle risk factors involved in the occurrence of advanced cancer are still largely unknown.

20.5 Conclusions

A growing body of data indicates that cancer screening when precursor lesions exist is effective, whereas cancer screening when no precursor lesion exists may be weakly or not effective and entails significant harm (e.g., false-positive tests, overdiagnosis, and overtreatment). These findings from multiple sources of data having different meaning (e.g., randomized trials, monitoring of advanced cancer, screening prevalence, variability in cancer mortality changes) may inform on the effectiveness and public health relevance of cancer-screening methods.

References

AJCC. American Joint Committee on Cancer. *AJCC Cancer Staging Manual*. 6th ed. New York, NY: Springer, 2002, pp 171–180.

Andriole GL, Grubb RL, Buys SS, Chia D, Church TR, Fouad MN et al. Mortality results from a randomized prostate–cancer screening trial. *N Engl J Med.* 2009; 360:1310–1319.

Autier P, Héry C, Haukka J, Boniol M, Byrnes G. Advanced breast cancer and breast cancer mortality in randomized controlled trials on mammography screening. *J Clin Oncol* 2009; 27: 5919–5923.

Autier P, Boniol M, LaVecchia C, Vatten L, Gavin A, Héry C et al. Disparities in breast cancer mortality trends between thirty European countries: retrospective trend analysis of WHO mortality database. *BMJ* 2010; 341: c3620.

Autier P, Boniol M, Middleton R, Doré JF, Héry C, Zheng T et al. Advanced breast cancer incidence following population-based mammographic screening. *Ann Oncol* 2011a; 22: 1726–1735.

Autier P, Boniol M, Gavin A, Vatten L. Breast cancer mortality in neighbouring European countries with different levels of screening but similar access to treatment: trend analysis of WHO mortality database. *BMJ* 2011b; 343: d4411.

Autier P, Boniol M. The incidence of advanced breast cancer in the West Midlands, United Kingdom. *Eur J Cancer Prev* 2012; 21: 217–221.

Autier P, Boniol M, Perrin P. Re: Prostate cancer mortality at 11-year follow-up by F Schroeder and Colleagues. *New Eng J Med* 2012 (in press).

Bartsch G, Horninger W, Klocker H, Pelzer A, Bektic J, Oberaigner W et al. Tyrol Prostate Cancer Demonstration Project: early detection, treatment, outcome, incidence and mortality. *BJU Int* 2008; 101: 809–816.

Bleyer A. US breast cancer mortality is consistent with European Data. *BMJ* 2011; 343: d5630.

Bouchardy C, Fioretta G, Rapiti E, Verkooijen HM, Rapin CH, Schmidlin F, et al. Recent trends in prostate cancer mortality show a continuous decrease in several countries. *Int J Cancer* 2008; 123: 421–429.

Boyle P, Brawley OW. Prostate cancer: current evidence weighs against population screening. *CA Cancer J Clin.* 2009; 59:220–224.

Cetin K, Beebe-Dimmer JL, Fryzek JP, Markus R, Carducci MA. Recent time trends in the epidemiology of stage IV prostate cancer in the United States: Analysis of data from the Surveillance, Epidemiology, and End Results Program. *Urology* 2010; 75: 1396–1405.

Djulbegovic M, Beyth RJ, Neuberger MM, Stoffs TL, Vieweg J, Djulbegovic B, et al. Screening for prostate cancer: systematic review and meta-analysis of randomised controlled trials. *BMJ.* 2010;341:c4543.

Cremers RGHM, Karim-Kos HE, Houterman S, Verhoeven RHA, Schröder FH, van der Kwast TH et al. Prostate cancer: Trends in incidence, survival and mortality in the Netherlands, 1989–2006. *Eur J Cancer* 2010; 46:2077–2087.

Edwards BK, Ward E, Kohler BA, Eheman C, Zauber AG, Anderson RN et al. Annual report to the nation on the status of cancer, 1975–2006, featuring colorectal cancer trends and impact of interventions (risk factors, screening, and treatment) to reduce future rates. *Cancer* 2010; 116:544–573.

Engholm G, Ferlay J, Christensen N, Bray F, Gjerstorff ML, Klint A et al. NORDCAN-a Nordic tool for cancer information, planning, quality control and research. *Acta Oncol* 2010; 49: 725–736. (www-dep.iarc.fr/nordcan).

Gøtzsche PC, Olsen O. Is screening for breast cancer with mammography justifiable? *Lancet* 2000; 355:129–134.
Esserman L, Shieh Y, Thompson I. Rethinking screening for breast cancer and prostate cancer. *JAMA* 2009; 302:1685–1692.
Hardcastle JD, Chamberlain JO, Robinson MHE, Moss SM, Amar SS, Balfour TW et al. Randomised controlled trial of faecal-occult-blood screening for colorectal cancer. *Lancet* 1996; 348:1472–1477.
Heidenreich A, Bolla M, Joniau S, van der Kwast T, Matveev V, Mason MD et al. *Guidelines on prostate cancer*. European Association of Urology 2012 (www.uroweb.org)
International Agency for Research on Cancer: *IARC/WHO handbooks of cancer prevention vol. 7: Breast Cancer Screening*. IARC Press, Lyon, 2002.
International Agency for Research on Cancer. *IARC/WHO handbooks of cancer prevention vol.10: cervix cancer screening*, vol. 10. IARC Press, Lyon, 2005.
Jemal A, Siegel R, Xu J, Ward E. Cancer Statistics, 2010. *CA Cancer J Clin* 2010; 60:277–300
Kronborg O, Fenger C, Olsen J, Jorgensen OD, Sondergaard O. Randomised study of screening for colorectal cancer with faecal-occult-blood test. *Lancet* 1996; 38:1467–1471.
Läärä E, Day NE, Hakama M. Trends in mortality from cervical cancer in the Nordic countries: association with organized screening programmes. *Lancet* 1987; i: 1247–1249.
Mandel JS, Church TR, Ederer F, Bond JH. Colorectal cancer mortality: effectiveness of biennial screening for fecal occult blood. *J Natl Cancer Inst* 1999; 91: 434–437.
Miller AB. New data on prostate cancer mortality after PSA screening. *New Engl J Med* 2012; 366: 1047–1048.
Nederend J, Duijm LE, Voogd AC, Groenewoud JH, Jansen FH, Louwman MW. Trends in incidence and detection of advanced breast cancer at biennial screening mammography in The Netherlands: a population based study. *Breast Cancer Research* 2012; 14: R10.
Sankaranarayanan R, Esmy PO, Rajkumar R, Muwonge R, Swaminathan R, Shanthakumari S et al. Effect of visual screening on cervical cancer incidence and mortality in Tamil Nadu, India: a cluster-randomised trial. *Lancet*. 2007; 370:398–406.
Sankaranarayanan R, Nene BM, Shastri SS, Jayant K, Muwonge R, Budukh AM et al. HPV screening for cervical cancer in rural India. *N Engl J Med*. 2009; 360:1385–1394.
Sankaranarayanan R, Ramadas K, Thara S, Muwonge R, Prabhakar J, Augustine P, et al. Clinical breast examination: preliminary results from a cluster randomized controlled trial in India. *J Natl Cancer Inst* 2011; 103:1476–1480.
Schröder FH, Hugosson J, Roobol MJ, Tammela TLJ, Ciatto S, Nelen V, et al. Prostate cancer mortality at 11-year follow-up. *New Engl J Med* 2012; 366:981–990.
Segnan N, Amarolli P, Bonelli L, Risio M, Sciallero S, Zappa M, et al. Once-only sigmoidoscopy in colorectal cancer screening: follow-up findings of the Italian Randomized Controlled Trial – SCORE. *J Natl Cancer Inst* 2011; 103:1310–1322.
Shambough E, Gloecker Ries L, Young J, Kruse M, Platz C, Ryan R. *SEER Extent of Disease - 1988: Codes and Coding Instructions*. National Institutes of Health: Washington DC, 1992.
Sigurdsson K, Sigvaldason H: Effectiveness of cervical cancer screening in Iceland, 1964–2002: a study on trends in incidence and mortality and the effect of risk factors. *Acta Obstet Gynecol Scand* 2006, 85:343–349.
Stock C, Haug U, Brenner H. Population-based prevalence estimates of history of colonoscopy or sigmoidoscopy: review and analysis of recent trends. *Gastrointest Endosc* 2010; 71:366–381.
Stock C, Brenner H. Utilization of lower gastrointestinal endoscopy and fecal occult blood test in 11 European countries: evidence from the Survey of Health, Aging and Retirement in Europe (SHARE). *Endoscopy* 2010; 42: 546–556.
Twombly R. American researchers question effect of Scandinavian mammography debate. *J Natl Cancer Inst* 2007; 99:1216–1217.
UICC. International Union Against Cancer (UICC), *TNM Classification of Malignant Tumours (6th edition)*, Wiley-Liss, New York, 2002.
U.S. Preventive Services Task Force. *Screening for prostate cancer: draft recommendation statement*. Rockville, MD: October 7, 2011 (http://www.uspreventiveservicestaskforce .org/draftrec3.htm).

Chapter 21
Using Mathematical Models to Inform Public Policy for Cancer Prevention and Screening

Natasha K. Stout, Michelle C. Dunn, J. Dik F. Habbema, David T. Levy, and Eric J. Feuer

21.1 Introduction

Randomized clinical trials and observational studies are the main types of studies for evaluating the effectiveness of cancer screening and prevention policies. Even after summarizing all available information from clinical trials and observational studies, key questions about generalizability may remain as trials and observational studies typically only include groups with specific characteristics (e.g., age, cancer risk), under specific conditions (e.g., screening frequency, type of intervention), and for a limited follow-up time. For example, until recently trials of colon cancer screening have included strategies only using guaiac-based fecal occult blood testing (FOBT) at short intervals and have not included other screening tests or longer intervals. Policymakers are generally interested in a longer sequence of screens than can be accomplished in a trial (e.g., annual screening from age 50 to 70), with follow-up over the entire remaining life rather than a fixed period. Mathematical modeling can address research questions and situations which have not been studied by these other methods. It is a complementary method that is particularly useful for

N.K. Stout (✉)
Department of Population Medicine,
Harvard Medical School and Harvard Pilgrim Health Care Institute,
133 Brookline Avenue, 6th Floor, Boston, MA 02215, USA
e-mail: natasha_stout@hms.harvard.edu

M.C. Dunn • E.J. Feuer
Surveillance Research Program Division of Cancer Control and Population Sciences,
National Cancer Institute, Bethesda, MD, USA

J.D.F. Habbema
Department of Public Health,
Erasmus MC University Medical Center Rotterdam, The Netherlands

D.T. Levy
Pacific Institute for Research and Evaluation, University of Baltimore, Baltimore, MD, USA

A.B. Miller (ed.), *Epidemiologic Studies in Cancer Prevention and Screening*, Statistics for Biology and Health 79, DOI 10.1007/978-1-4614-5586-8_21,

policy design and evaluation. For example, to inform colorectal cancer screening policies, modeling analyses have examined screening strategies using multiple screening tests including colonoscopy across a range of screening intervals over the entire life course.

Modeling can help connect disparate islands of direct evidence, providing a unified view of all the evidence. By design mathematical models can synthesize information from multiple studies to estimate multiple outcomes (e.g., cancer detection rates, reduction in mortality) relevant to policymakers. In doing so, models help fill evidence gaps left when new data collection is limited by ethical, financial, and/or time constraints. Models allow policymakers to ask and evaluate a range of questions and hypothetical scenarios including projections into the future. Further, models may also serve to hypothesis-generate and provide insight into unknowns about cancer natural history.

The use of models to aid policy evolved in the 1980s from modeling evaluations of diagnostic tests used to inform clinical decision making at the patient bedside. An early example in the policy arena extended trial evidence of breast cancer screening. Since long-term outcomes were not yet available from breast cancer trials, models were used to project potential benefits and risks of screening women in their 40s—a question that is still policy relevant today (Eddy 1989). This type of analysis was taken a step further by the *MISCAN* modeling group, who filled gaps in observational evidence for cervical cancer screening. They examined questions regarding the design and implementation of population-wide screening programs in the Netherlands (Habbema et al. 1984, 1985). The breadth of applications as well as model complexity has since expanded especially with increasing computing power.

Modeling has continued to gain prominence in the cancer policy arena to address a wide range of population-level policy questions about screening and prevention. Today many policy models exist for most major forms of cancer (Knudsen et al. 2007; Rutter et al. 2011; Stout et al. 2009). Spurring some of the recent growth in modeling has been the Cancer Intervention and Surveillance Modeling Network (CISNET) (www.cisnet.cancer.gov) funded by the US National Cancer Institute (NCI). CISNET is a consortium of modelers currently working in breast, prostate, colorectal, lung, and esophagus cancers. The group was formed in 2000 to improve understanding of the population impact of cancer control interventions on incidence, mortality, and related measures. Unlike many early cancer models, which were mostly focused on a single application, CISNET models are designed to study a range of health-care applications across the cancer control spectrum. A defining feature of CISNET is the comparative modeling approach, where multiple independent models address central questions in a collaborative fashion using shared inputs and common output templates. Comparing results across models helps evaluate the impact of model structure uncertainty on results and conclusions. When results are consistent across models developed under different assumptions, the robustness of the results adds credibility in formulating policy decisions; when results differ, the differences may highlight areas for further study. The collaborative approach is beneficial for both the modelers, who learn from each other, and the models, which will improve from the continuous peer review.

In the following sections, we first provide an overview of the mechanics of mathematical models and then describe a series of model applications organized by usage, from prospectively informing programs, guidelines, and policies in Section 3 to retrospectively evaluating programs and practice in Section 4. We have primarily drawn from our own experiences as modelers and CISNET members and acknowledge that the examples presented here are the tip of the iceberg. The chapter is not a systematic review, but instead the selected examples are meant to illustrate for model consumers the depth and breadth of model analyses as well as the current and potential contributions models can make to cancer policy worldwide. We conclude the chapter with remarks for readers who consider the use of models for a policy problem.

21.2 Mechanics of Modeling

Mathematical models, often referred to as computer simulation models, approximate the process of disease within a population. The natural history from initiation and growth through clinical detection and survival is typically simulated at an individual person level. The life courses of many simulated individuals are then aggregated to create a population. Superimposed are the dynamic processes of prevention, screening, and treatment.

Because the underlying preclinical biology of cancers is largely unknown, model builders must make assumptions about the structure of the disease process based on theories and available, often indirect, evidence. Disease progression may be modeled through a series of discrete disease states or in a continuous manner. For example, tumors may be approximated by a mass that grows in size according to a growth trajectory or by progression through cancer stages such as the progression from adenoma to carcinoma in colorectal cancer (Fig. 21.1). The disease process is approximated by discrete health states (boxes) beginning with "no lesion" and progressing (solid arrows) into adenomas of different sizes through to cancer and death. Dashed arrows illustrate processes that modify the transitions. For example, risk factors may modify the development and progression of a lesion while screening may halt the progression.

In the colorectal cancer example, the benefits of screening in terms of prevention of cancer and cancer mortality reductions are derived from detection earlier in the disease pathway. While a simplification of reality, heterogeneity of tumors within a population can be approximated by a population-level distribution over rates of progression or growth as well as by varying assumptions about tumor prognosis and response to treatment. These types of assumptions are what differentiate models from each other and can lead to differences in model outcomes across models (Clarke et al. 2006; Cronin et al. 2006). For example, a comparison of three colorectal cancer models reveals that model assumptions regarding the progression time from adenoma to carcinoma for colorectal cancer affect model conclusions regarding the effectiveness of screening tests (Kuntz et al. 2011; van Ballegooijen et al. 2011).

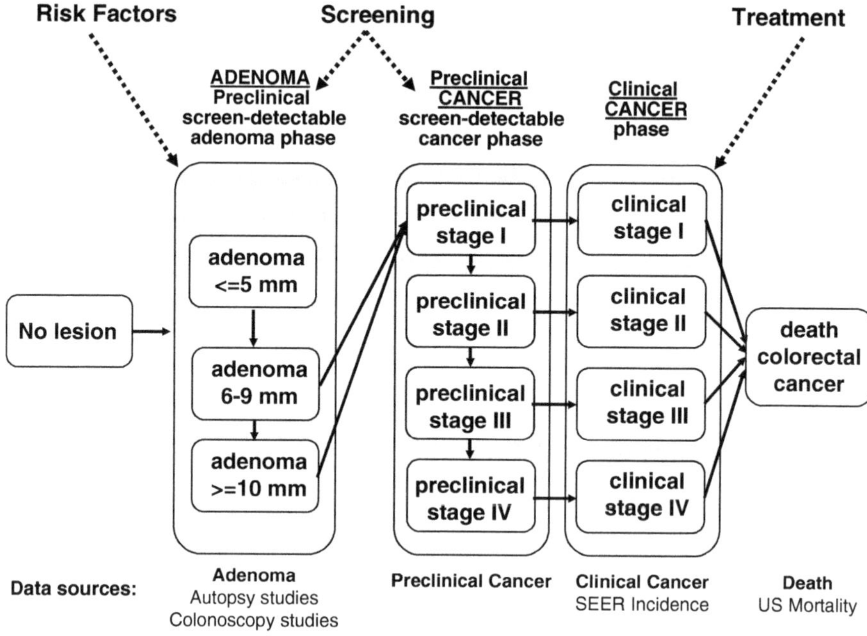

Fig. 21.1 Example schematic for a mathematical model of colorectal cancer

Assumptions and design choices about disease and the effects of interventions make modeling an art as much as a science, and models often earn the reputation as being "black boxes" (Boer et al. 2004). For this reason, evaluation of model performance is important to establish the credibility of model results to policymakers and other consumers. A modeler tries to inform the inner workings of the black box using clinical observations based on the unobserved natural history of the disease (e.g., autopsy studies, screening studies, population-based cancer registry data). A first step in this process is the estimation and/or calibration of model input parameters such that model outputs replicate observed data. Once calibrated, model outputs are further evaluated against independent data as available. In addition to evaluating assumptions, the credibility of a model is established by accounting for the uncertainty that may arise from observed data, model parameters, and model structure in model outputs and conclusions. These processes are an ongoing activity for the life of the model. As illustrated in the example from three colorectal cancer models above, models can be appropriately calibrated and validated but still produce differing results (Kuntz et al. 2011; van Ballegooijen et al. 2011).

The audience and the questions of interest help determine the level of detail included in a model. For policy evaluation, computer experiments are conducted by comparing model outputs resulting from varying model assumptions about the use and effectiveness of alternative screening and prevention strategies.

21.3 Modeling to Aid Policy Design

For the design and implementation of population-based screening and prevention strategies, policymakers need information about short- and long-term effects on population health as well as resource requirements. When policy decisions need to be made, especially for new technologies and interventions, long-term outcomes may not be readily available. Using available evidence, models can project outcomes necessary for making decisions, as illustrated in the following examples.

21.3.1 Designing Large-Scale Public Health Programs

Considerations in the design of public health programs may include implementation, capacity, budgetary limits, as well as issues of equity and equality. Modeling analyses can be designed to provide policymakers with necessary information to examine these considerations.

While randomized trials to evaluate the efficacy of cervical cancer screening programs have only been conducted in developing countries (see chapters by Burton, Broutet, and Bosch, this volume), inferences that routine screening with the Papanicolaou test, or “Pap smear,” does reduce cervical cancer mortality have been drawn from observational data over the past half century (Hakama, this volume). How to best use the available tests for screening and prevention (e.g., how frequently to screen, at what ages, and with which tests) has not been directly answered with trial or observational data. Modeling analyses have been conducted to address these questions.

For example, in the Netherlands, modeling studies have been used extensively in the design of their population-wide National Cervical Screening Program funded by the Ministry of Health. Following a 1970s pilot study of cervical cancer screening conducted in three regions, a nationwide screening program was introduced in the mid-1980s (Evaluation Committee on Early Detection of Cervical Cancer 1984; Habbema et al. 1985). This program covered the screening schedule used in the pilot regions: seven screenings, starting at age 35 and repeating at three-year intervals until age 53. At that time, a formal Health Technology Assessment (HTA) was undertaken, using the *MISCAN-cervix* model, which synthesized the internationally available evidence for a detailed effectiveness and cost-effectiveness analysis study. Conclusions from this study and from later additional modeling studies informed subsequent changes in the program (van Ballegooijen et al. 1993). First and foremost, the cost-effectiveness analysis showed that the current age range was too narrow and that the interval between screens could be lengthened. A few years later, the minister decided to implement a new schedule of seven screenings with a screening interval of five years, starting at age 30 and stopping at age 60. This new schedule was in accordance with the results of the modeling studies (National Health Insurance Council 1993).

Despite the guidelines, many women were screened more frequently and at younger ages. Another important finding from the HTA was that the addition of these more frequent or "opportunistic" screening exams on top of the recommended screens was not cost-effective. The Ministry of Health decided that opportunistic smears would no longer be reimbursed. The number of opportunistic smears in women younger than age 30 dropped by 75% (Bos et al. 2002; Rebolj et al. 2007).

Other policy decisions based on the HTA results aimed at increasing the uptake of screening, decreasing the very high proportion of borderline Pap smears requiring follow-up, better monitoring of women requiring follow-up, and reducing the number of smears which were repeated because of insufficient quality (National Health Insurance Council 1993).

With the availability of technologies to detect human papillomaviruses (HPV), the potential costs of cervical cancer control may escalate unless these technologies are used in a thoughtful way. As with many similar decisions, the Ministry asked for the advice of the Health Council of the Netherlands, akin to the US Institute of Medicine. In 2011, the Health Council released a report recommending that the Pap smear be replaced by an HPV-DNA test. Informed by two modeling studies that were commissioned by the council, the recommended number of screening tests in a woman's lifetime was reduced from seven when using the Pap smear to five with the HPV-DNA test at ages 30, 35, 40, 50, and 60. Triage strategies using the Pap smear to address the lower specificity of the HPV-DNA test were also discussed in the report (Health Council of the Netherlands 2011). As of early 2012, the Ministry of Health has yet to implement the recommendations. Modeling studies also informed an earlier report which advised HPV vaccination of 12-year-old girls (Health Council of the Netherlands 2008).

Thus the development of cervical cancer policy and practice in the Netherlands, as implemented by screening guidelines and revisions, followed a cycle of pilot studies and modeling; implementation of regional, population-based screening programs; surveillance; and model-based evaluation studies. As a result of these interactions, the Dutch Health Council asks for modeling studies to inform policy decisions on an array of health topics increasingly often.

Screening and prevention strategies implemented in high-income countries may not be feasible in settings with limited resources. Also, resources may not be available to conduct setting-specific clinical trials or to gather evidence on which to base policies. In this case, modeling may be the only solution for evaluating policies in a quantitative and systematic manner. Because policies are tailored to country-specific population health needs and resource levels, any modeling analysis informing policy must also be tailored. One example is a modeling analysis examining cervical cancer screening programs in the low-income countries of India, Kenya, Peru, South Africa, and Thailand (Goldie et al. 2005). This modeling analysis, done in conjunction with policymakers and potential funders of the screening programs, considered country-specific availability and costs of infrastructure and health-care providers, as well as travel time for women to attend screening and follow-up. Affordability, as measured by the cost-effectiveness of a screening policy, was tailored to each country's gross domestic product and per capita spending. Whereas modeling analyses for high-income country settings show that screening at regular intervals using Pap smears or HPV-DNA testing is affordable, in the resource-limited settings, recommended strategies employed only a few screens using tests which allow for immediate treatment (such as visual inspection). These strategies have the advantage in resource-limited settings of not relying on laboratory facilities or requiring multiple visits by the woman. The modeling framework used in this analysis allowed for explicit incorporation of relevant site-specific issues such as the locations and availability of laboratories and care providers.

21.3.2 Guideline Development

Since information needs for guideline development are similar to those for the design of public health programs, modeling analyses can likewise supplement existing evidence and illustrate potential benefits and harms across a range of policies under consideration. Unlike program policymakers who usually also allocate funding for policies, guideline decision makers usually do not consider cost explicitly, and therefore, their criteria for decision making may differ as well.

To illustrate, one example is the recent use of modeling by the US Preventive Services Task Force, a federally appointed group of experts who develop clinical recommendations for primary care settings. The task force has solicited evidence from models to help inform their screening and prevention recommendations for colorectal, breast, and cervical cancers (Kulasingam et al. 2011; Mandelblatt et al. 2009; Zauber et al. 2008). With an awareness of gaps in the current evidence base, the task force requested specific model analyses to address questions to inform their deliberations about proposed recommendations. We highlight the example of breast cancer screening.

In 2007, the US Preventive Services Task Force began the process of updating their breast cancer screening recommendations. To guide their decision making, the task force commissioned an extensive literature review focusing on new evidence regarding screening women in their 40s and older (Nelson et al. 2009). In addition, the task force solicited observational data on real-world outcomes of screening mammography in the USA from the NCI-funded Breast Cancer Surveillance Consortium (BCSC) and modeling evidence from the CISNET Breast Cancer Working Group.

Guided by the task force, the CISNET Breast Cancer Working Group, comprised of six independent modeling teams, conducted specific analyses regarding annual versus biennial screening across a range of starting and stopping ages (Mandelblatt et al. 2009). The analyses were designed to address in gaps in evidence about screening intervals and age ranges, questions which could not be fully answered by current clinical trial data and observational studies. Practical and ethical considerations limit the feasibility of a new study leaving modeling to fill in the gaps. To reflect the "real-world" practice, the models used information collected by the BCSC to inform the performance of mammography.

The six models each simulated a range of outcomes for 20 screening scenarios to illustrate trade-offs in benefits and risks. Metrics of benefits included long-term projections of expected mortality reductions and life years gained for each screening scenario compared with no screening, while metrics of harms included risk of a false-positive mammography and biopsy in the short term and risk of overdiagnosis in the long term. Results across the six models were qualitatively and quantitatively consistent regarding the magnitude of benefits and risks, and this consistency provided robustness and credibility to model results. Furthermore, the magnitude of benefit of mammography at reducing breast cancer mortality in general was consistent with evidence from randomized controlled trials. When focusing on screening frequency, models showed that the benefits in terms of mortality reductions were largely preserved with biennial compared with annual screening. In addition, potential harms such as the risk of a false-positive test result and biopsy were substantially reduced. When focusing on the age to begin screening, a key issue for the task force, model results were dependent on the choice of outcome measure for the benefits.

Considering modeling evidence in conjunction with the systematic review about net benefits of screening, the task force made several updates in their mammography screening guidelines (US Preventive Services Task Force 2009). Their recommendations were for routine biennial screening of women ages 50 through 79 and for women in their 40s; decisions about routine screening should be a personal one. The latter recommendation about women ages 40–49 reflected the recognition that while there were mortality benefits from screening in that age range, there were also not insubstantial harms, and therefore, a general recommendation for all women may not be appropriate.

These guidelines were publicly announced in the midst of a contentious policy debate regarding health reform legislation in the USA. In this political context, the guidelines were interpreted by opponents of the legislation as an example of government rationing of care. In particular, the perception of health-care rationing was exacerbated by the initial wording of the specific recommendation for personal choice rather than routine use of mammography for women 40–49. This became a touchstone even though prior recommendations from the task force had also encouraged personal choice for this age group. Although the wording of the recommendation was subsequently revised, the recommendation of personal choice remained despite the political objection.

21.3.3 Target and Goal Setting

Modeling has a distinct advantage over other methods for informing the design of public health targets and goals. By posing unlimited "counterfactual-type" analyses, models can provide quantitative information about the long-term effects of alternate ways of achieving public health goals. Further modeling can not only assist in setting targets and evaluating progress in achieving targets but also in linking upstream targets (e.g., obesity rates, smoking rates) to downstream targets (e.g., cancer mortality rates). We illustrate this with two examples from the USA.

As a method for improving and monitoring public health, each decade the US Federal Government develops a series of health goals, the "Healthy People" goals (www.healthypeople.gov). These goals, numbering in the hundreds, range from setting targets for improving health behaviors to reducing disease burden and disparities. Each is developed through multiyear processes involving expert consensus. Recently modeling was used to evaluate the feasibility of achieving the Healthy People 2010 goals for colorectal cancer prevention (Vogelaar et al. 2006). A series of analyses with two models of colorectal cancer examined the projected impacts of achieving the Healthy People goals for eight risk factors, screening use, and treatment use on colorectal cancer mortality versus continuing on current trends in these areas. An interactive website was developed as a planning tool for policy-makers (www.cisnet.cancer.gov/projections/colorectal/).

Another example of modeling to inform cancer prevention targets is in tobacco control for the state of Kentucky. Across all metrics, the state of Kentucky ranks among the worst for tobacco control. Over one quarter of all adults and 15% of youths in the state of Kentucky are smokers. Disparities are widespread and these rates nearly double for adults with less than a high school education. Citizens of the state experience some of the highest lung cancer mortality rates in the United States. The Healthy People 2010 goal was to reduce adult smoking prevalence to 12% (Levy et al. 2005). While Kentucky has the potential to reduce smoking rates, setting policy in the state is politically challenging because tobacco production is important to the local economy.

To understand how Kentucky might meet the Healthy People 2010 goal, policy-makers used the *SimSmoke* Tobacco Control Policy simulation model (Levy et al. 2008b). The model considers the effect of six different types of tobacco control policies on smoking prevalence and smoking-attributable deaths: cigarette tax increases, smoke-free air laws, media campaigns, marketing restrictions, health warnings, cessation treatment policies, and youth access restrictions. The model can be used to illustrate the impact of different policies and how multiple policies can be used in combination to address these issues. Using readily available data on population, smoking rates, and public policies in Kentucky, modelers in conjunction with academics, special interests groups, and members of the state health planning staff tailored the model. Results were validated against the period 1993–2007 and found to predict well the observed slow decline in smoking rates.

The model showed that tobacco control policies can have a large impact on smoking rates and save lives in Kentucky. Higher cigarette taxes and smoke-free air laws each reduced smoking prevalence by about 10% in relative terms. Media campaigns and cessation treatment policies each reduced smoking prevalence by more than 5%. To meet the *Healthy People 2010* goal of a 12% smoking prevalence, states such as Kentucky would have needed to implement a combined set of the strong tobacco control policies. In Kentucky, with a set of policies suggested by the *Healthy People 2010* goals, smoking prevalence is projected to fall to about 19% by 2011, 26% below the status quo level of 25.5%, and to about 14% by 2026, with over 17,000 smoking-attributable deaths avoided. While some policies (e.g., higher tax rate) have been implemented, the state is still unfortunately far from their goals.

In addition to the state of Kentucky, the SimSmoke model has been applied to over 30 nations and 5 states. For nations, such as Thailand (Levy et al. 2008a) and South Korea (Levy et al. 2010), and states, such as Arizona (Levy et al. 2007b) and California (Levy et al. 2007a), which have had active tobacco control policies, the model has been used to show the effects of past policies on smoking rates and the consequent reduction in smoking-attributable deaths. The model has also been used to project future smoking rates and deaths averted as a result of implementing stronger policies, such as those required under WHO's Framework Convention for Tobacco Control. The basic structure of the model in this example is now being applied to other cancer risk factors such as alcohol and obesity.

21.3.4 Designing Limited-Scale Programs for Health Promotion

An ongoing modeling analysis initiated by the US Centers for Disease Control and Prevention (CDC) illustrates the use of modeling for the design of a limited-scale health promotion program (Personal communication: NT Van Ravesteyn 2012). The CDC-funded National Breast and Cervical Cancer Early Detection Program (NBCCEDP) has been providing cancer screening for underserved populations in the USA since 1991 (http://www.cdc.gov/cancer/nbccedp/about.htm). The program operates under a fixed budget with a goal of covering the cost of routine breast and cervical cancer screening for as many eligible underserved women as possible. For breast cancer screening, the program has been providing routine mammography for women ages 40 to 65 using plain-film technology. The rapid adoption of digital mammography in the USA posed a coverage dilemma for the program. Digital mammography has been shown to perform better than plain-film mammography for a subset of women with dense breasts but is more costly (Tosteson et al. 2008). Once complete, the modeling analysis will provide estimates of the number of women served and the overall health benefit if the CDC program were to cover the use of digital mammography for screening. By estimating long-term health benefits, modeling can systematically address these questions in a timely fashion.

21.3.5 Defining Reimbursement Policies

Modeling is well suited to help policymakers such as payers who face budgetary constraints examine whether a new or emerging technology should be adopted and covered and at what price or level of reimbursement. When the performance characteristics of a new technology are not yet known, modeling can be used to determine a threshold performance level based on existing technologies for which the new technology may be adopted. On the other hand, when the performance characteristics of the new technology are known, a modeling analysis can help determine the particular threshold price at which a new technology is similarly affordable as an existing one. For example, this approach was employed by the US Centers for Medicare and Medicaid (CMS) to inform coverage and reimbursement policies for three new screening tests for colorectal cancer with known performance characteristics: computerized tomographic colonography (CTC or "virtual colonoscopy"), stool-based DNA testing, and the fecal immunochemical test (FIT) (Zauber et al. 2007, 2009). CMS currently reimburses for the routine use of FOBT, sigmoidoscopy, and colonoscopy for screening. The modeling analysis found that the threshold reimbursements for CTC and stool-based DNA testing would need to be lower than that of colonoscopy and/or of proposed manufacturer prices. Of the three, only the FIT test was accepted as a covered test by CMS at close to the threshold reimbursement level suggested by model results. Based on other considerations about the two tests including the risk of incidental findings seen with CTC imaging as well as the threshold modeling analysis, CMS concluded that CTC and stool-based DNA testing not be covered at this time.

21.4 Modeling to Aid Policy Evaluation

Once cancer control programs have been designed, guidelines issued, and reimbursement polices set, models can evaluate cancer prevention strategies as used in real-world settings to ensure that resources are allocated efficiently to improve population health. For this purpose, models can be designed to examine the policy impact on the full population over a given time period by incorporating secular trends in risk factors, prevention activities, screening tests, and treatment patterns, as needed. By approximating real-world behavior in participation and performance over time, models with secular trends more accurately capture the true population-based impact (Dewilde and Anderson 2004). Similar to the target and goal setting analyses described in Sect. 3.3, model analyses can compare the implemented policy with "counterfactual" policies and ask questions such as how well did the policy perform compared with other possible policies and how might the implemented policy be improved.

21.4.1 Evaluation of Public Health Programs

Models can be used to evaluate population-wide public health programs by examining efforts to improve program participation and by quantifying the effects of program modifications such as changing age boundaries, frequency, type of test, or prevention alternatives. For example, in the Netherlands, a modeling analysis examined whether to extend the upper age limit of 70 years for their ongoing breast cancer screening program. Modeling helped fill gaps in evidence, as magnitude of the benefits and risks of screening in older women is not directly answerable with existing data. Both the natural history of breast cancer and the efficacy of mammography for breast cancer screening in older women have uncertainty, and a new trial to examine the efficacy in older women is not feasible in part because of the large sample sizes needed (Boer et al. 1995). To account for this uncertainty, two opposing scenarios about the benefits of mammography were considered: optimistic and pessimistic. When quality-of-life effects from overtreatment are accounted for, the benefits are maintained when screening women in their 80s and 90s under the optimistic scenario. In contrast, the pessimistic scenario shows declining benefits from screening past age 80. Considering costs as well as health effects favors ending screening at age 75. As a result, it was concluded that a limited extension screening women at older ages was warranted in the Netherlands. However, screening at ages greater than 75 was not recommended because of the increasingly more unfavorable balance between health benefits from early detection and the risk of overdiagnosis and overtreatment of breast cancer that occurs as competing cause mortality increases with age (Boer et al. 1995).

21.4.2 Evaluation of Clinical Practice

With no organized screening program and with a range of guidelines and insurance coverage policies on screening, mammography use in the USA is not uniform. Consequently, evaluation of the downstream effects of screening on incidence and mortality is difficult. However, in the absence of formal programs, models can be used to assess progress in real-world cancer control activities as illustrated by the following examples.

In 2000 a Cochrane meta-analysis of mammography trials indicated that, after eliminating trials that were considered flawed, the remaining trials showed no benefit (Gotzsche and Olsen 2000). This finding threw the mammography screening research community into disarray, as there were unlikely to be new trials of mammography. However, from 1989 to 2000 US breast cancer mortality fell 24% for women aged 30 to 79. Since the dissemination of screening mammography and adjuvant therapies for breast cancer occurred approximately at the same time, modeling was needed to separate the contributions of each to the mortality decline. To investigate, an analysis with seven independent models using common inputs on utilization patterns of mammography and adjuvant therapy was conducted (Berry et al. 2005). This analysis was one of the first that used multiple models to address the same research question and control for experimental conditions by sharing key inputs. All models agreed on three points: both screening and treatment reduced breast cancer mortality, the observed reduction in breast cancer mortality could not be attributed to either factor alone, and each contributed about equally to the decline. Figure 21.2 illustrates the range of results for screening and adjuvant treatment across the models.

The estimated percent reductions in the breast cancer mortality rate attributable to screening and adjuvant treatment for each model (designated by letter) illustrate the range across models as well as the consistency of results. The contour plot indicating

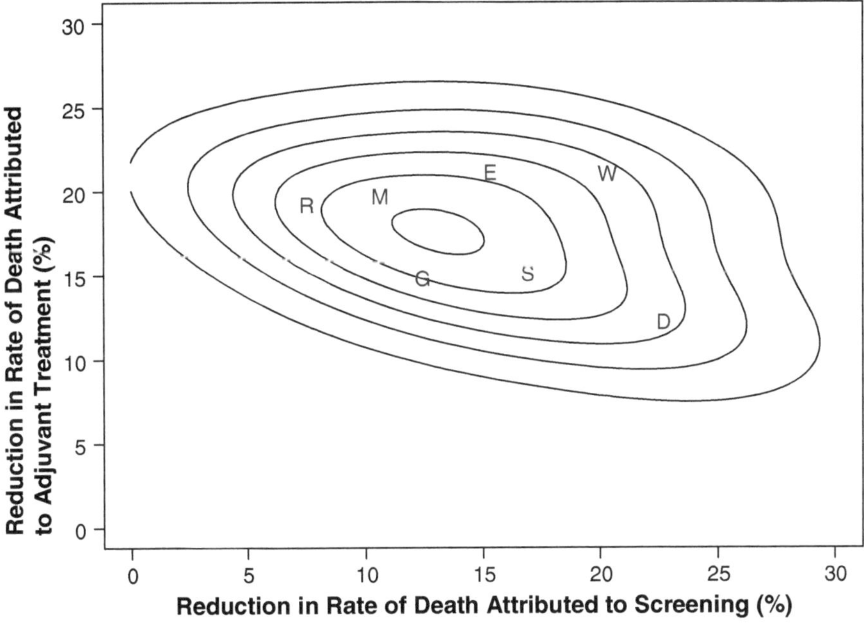

Fig. 21.2 Results from a comparative modeling analysis with seven models

the joint likelihood of the percent reductions (rings indicate increasing probability with the peak in the center) illustrates one way to summarize results from multiple models (Reprint of Fig. 3a, Berry et al. 2005).

The narrower range of the results for treatment compared with mammography reflects the fact that the underlying evidence regarding treatment efficacy is more consistent. While typically results based on observational data are validated using controlled trials, this example used observational data, combined in a novel way using seven different models, to help confirm mammography benefits when randomized controlled trial results alone could not settle the debate. These results yielded high public attention, garnering a front-page article and editorial in the New York Times, and were discussed in a book on the history of cancer research (Mukherjee 2010).

A subsequent modeling analysis focused on evaluating how screening had been used in the USA. The analysis compared the health benefits and monetary costs of actual and alternative mammography screening practices in the USA from 1990 to 2000 (Stout et al. 2006). Because the model used was population-based, this analysis was able to examine the full budgetary impact of screening policies. The analysis indicated that past mammography practice had improved the health of the US population but came at a cost. However, as illustrated in Fig. 21.3, alternative screening strategies including less frequent screening but increased participation could have resulted in greater health benefits for a lower overall cost than mammography as it had been actually practiced.

The figure shows model estimates for the costs and health effects of screening mammography as actually practiced (star), no screening (diamond), and 66

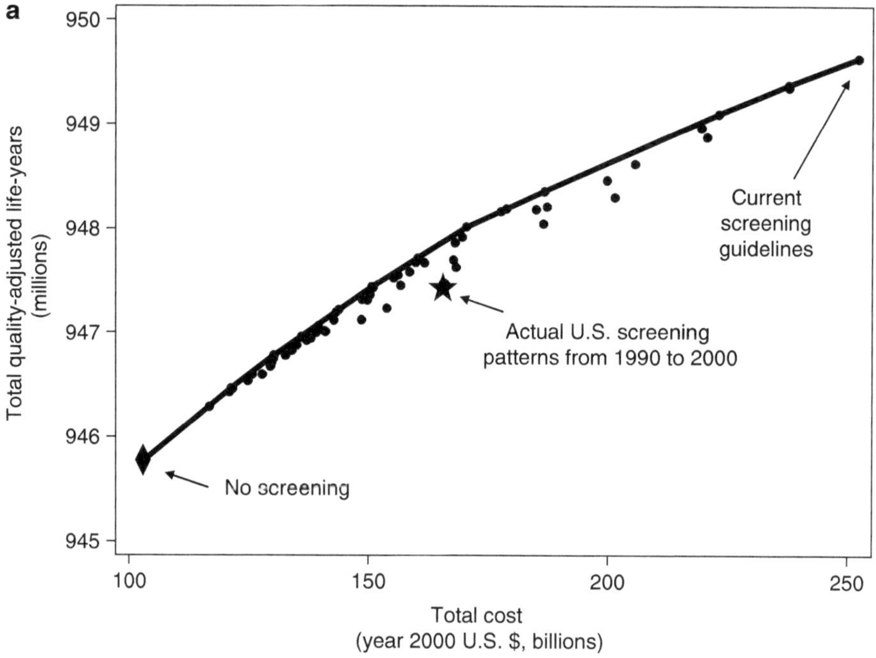

Fig. 21.3 One example of retrospective policy evaluation

alternative screening strategies (dots). Screening strategies located above and to the left of the star represent those that lead to better health for similar or lower cost than the actual use of mammography. The dot labeled "current screening guidelines" represents the policy of annual screening for ages 40–84 as recommended in the USA at the time of the analysis. This strategy would lead to the greatest health effects but is also the most costly (Reprint of Fig. 1, Stout et al. 2006).

Thus as a society, mammography was saving lives, but not in a very efficient way. When small, yet common, potential harms, such as anxiety associated with a false-positive mammogram, are included, conclusions drawn from the analysis may be affected as the overall population health gains are reduced especially when screening occurs more frequently as had been recommended by the guidelines during that time period. This type of modeling approach has also been used to compare the performance of cervical screening guidelines internationally as illustrated in Fig. 21.4.

This figure shows model estimates for cervical cancer screening strategies as practiced by a range of countries. The numbers on the curve refer to the number of screening in a lifetime for a particular strategy. Similar to the US analysis, this illustrates both how country-specific guidelines (open boxes with abbreviated country names) perform in terms of health and cost and how they could be improved (Reprint of Fig. 3, van den Akker-van Marle et al. 2002).

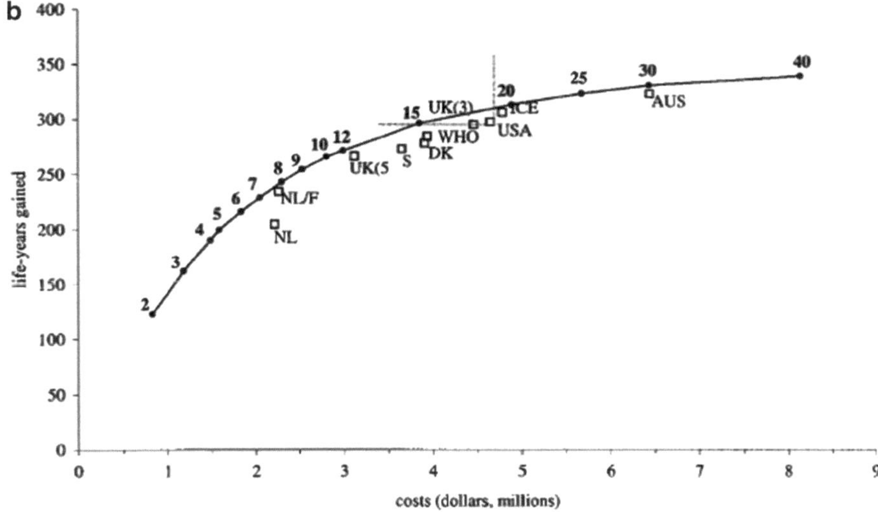

Fig. 21.4 A second example of retrospective policy evaluation

21.5 Collaborating with Modelers

Mathematical modeling is increasingly being used to aid the prospective design of programs and guidelines as well as the retrospective evaluation of existing cancer control efforts. While not substitutes for data, models can be invaluable tools in the synthesis of existing evidence and in the extrapolation and projection of multiple outcomes for multiple policy alternatives. Furthermore, these methods can often be used in situations where other study methods are infeasible.

Mathematical modeling is, however, only a tool. It can provide up-front information regarding potential outcomes for a particular policy problem, but models do not provide answers. For model results to be most relevant for and accepted by clinicians, health-care leaders, and policymakers requires active collaboration between modelers and policymakers at all phases of a model analysis. Modeling is a highly interdisciplinary field by nature, and direct interaction with policymakers would be welcomed. To foster such collaboration, we close with a few practical points for policymakers regarding the modeling process.

As with any study, the design and execution of a model analysis take time. Because the construction and thorough validation of the models underlying an analysis also take a considerable amount of time, often working with an established modeling team may be more efficient. Approaching modelers early in the development of policy design or evaluation efforts is key for both modelers and policymakers. The initial steps for policymakers and modelers in formulating an analysis include specifying the policy alternatives under consideration, defining the scope of the study, assessing if structural changes are needed to the model, identifying additional data to customize the model, and delineating outcomes of interest. The modeling process is often iterative as insight into the policy problem may be gained at any point. An analysis may need to be refined and/or expanded depending on model results and their interpretation as well as the needs of the policymaker.

References

Berry DA, Cronin KA, Plevritis SK, Fryback DG, Clarke L Zelen M et al for the Cancer Intervention and Surveillance Modeling Network (CISNET) Collaborators. Effect of screening and adjuvant treatment on mortality from breast cancer. *N Eng J Med* 2005; 353:1784-1792.

Boer R, de Koning HJ, van Oortmarssen GJ, van der Maas PJ. In search of the best upper age limit for breast cancer screening. *Eur J Cancer* 1995a; 31:2040-2043.

Boer R, Plevritis S, Clarke L. Diversity of model approaches for breast cancer screening: A review of model assumptions by the Cancer Intervention and Surveillance Modeling Network (CISNET) breast cancer groups. *Stat Methods Med Res* 2004; 13:525-538.

Bos AB, van Ballegooijen M, van Oortmarssen GJ, Habbema JDF. Women who participate in spontaneous screening are not at higher risk for cervical cancer than women who attend programme screening. *Eur J Cancer* 2002; 38:827-831.

Clarke LD, Plevritis SK, Boer R, Cronin KA Feuer EJ. A comparative review of CISNET breast models used to analyze U.S. breast cancer incidence and mortality trends. *J Natl Cancer Inst Monogr 2006*; 36:96-105.

Cronin KA, Feuer EJ, Clarke LD, Plevritis SK. Impact of adjuvant therapy and mammography on U.S. mortality from 1975 to 2000: Comparison of mortality results from the CISNET breast cancer base case analysis. *J Natl Cancer Inst Monogr* 2006; 36:112-121.

Dewilde S, Anderson R. The cost-effectiveness of screening programs using single and multiple birth cohort simulations: A comparison using a model of cervical cancer. *Med Decis Making* 2004; 24:486-492.

Eddy DM. Screening for breast cancer. *Ann Intern Med* 1989;111:389-399.

Evaluation Committee on Early Detection of Cervical Cancer. *Report about the second round of the mass screening program in the pilot regions Nijmegen, Rotterdam and Utrecht* (In Dutch). Ministerie VOMIL, Leidschendam, 1984.

Goldie SJ, Gaffikin L, Goldhaber-Fiebert JD, Gordillo-Tobar A, Levin C, Mahe C et al. Cost-effectiveness of cervical-cancer screening in five developing countries. *N Engl J Med* 2005; 353:2158-2168.

Gotzsche PC, Olsen O. Is screening for breast cancer with mammography justifiable? *Lancet* 2000; 355:129-134.

Habbema JDF, van Oortmarssen GJ, Lubbe JTN, van der Maas PJ. The miscan simulation program for the evaluation of screening for disease. *Comput Methods Programs Biomed* 1984; 20:79-93.

Habbema JDF, van Oortmarssen GJ, Lubbe JTN, van der Maas PJ. Model building on the basis of Dutch cervical cancer screening data. *Maturitas* 1985; 7:11-20.

Health Council of the Netherlands. *Vaccination for cervical cancer.* Health Council, The Hague, The Netherlands, 2008.

Health Council of the Netherlands. *Screening for cervical cancer*. Health Council, The Hague, The Netherlands, 2011.

Knudsen AB, McMahon PM, Gazelle GS. Use of modeling to evaluate the cost-effectiveness of cancer screening programs. *J Clin Oncol* 2007; 25:203-208.

Kulasingam SL, Havrilesky L, Ghebre R, Myers ER. *Screening for cervical cancer: A decision analysis for the U.S. Preventive Services Task Force*. Agency for Healthcare Research and Quality, Rockville, MD, 2011.

Kuntz KM, Lansdorp-Vogelaar I, Rutter CM, Knudsen AB, van Ballegooijen M, Savarino JE et al. A systematic comparison of microsimulation models of colorectal cancer. *Med Decis Making* 2011; 31:530-539.

Levy DT, Benjakul S, Ross H, Ritthiphakdee B. The role of tobacco control policies in reducing smoking and deaths in a middle income nation: Results from the Thailand SimSmoke simulation model. *Tob Control* 2008a;17:53-59.

Levy DT, Cho SI, Kim YM, Park S, Suh MK, Kam S. SimSmoke model evaluation of the effect of tobacco control policies in Korea: The unknown success story. *Am J Publ Hlth* 2010; 100:1267-1273.

Levy DT, Hyland A, Higbee C, Remer L, Compton C. The role of public policies in reducing smoking prevalence in California: Results from the California tobacco policy simulation model. *Health Policy* 2007a;82:167-185.

Levy DT, Nikolayev L, Mumford E, Compton C. The Healthy People 2010 smoking prevalence and tobacco control objectives: Results from the SimSmoke tobacco control policy simulation model (United States). *Cancer Causes Control* 2005;16:359-371.

Levy DT, Ross H, Powell L, Bauer JE, Lee HR. The role of public policies in reducing smoking prevalence and deaths caused by smoking in Arizona: Results from the Arizona tobacco policy simulation model. *J Public Health Manag Pract* 2007b; 13:59-67.

Levy DT, Tworek C, Hahn EJ, Davis RE. The Kentucky SimSmoke tobacco policy simulation model: Reaching Healthy People 2010 goals through policy change. *South Med J* 2008b; 101:503-507.

Mandelblatt JS, Cronin KA, Bailey S, Berry DA, de Koning HJ, Draisma G et al. Effects of mammography screening under different screening schedules: Model estimates of potential benefits and harms. *Ann Intern Med* 2009;151:738-747.

Mukherjee S. *The emperor of all maladies: A biography of cancer.* Scribner, New York, 2010.

National Health Insurance Council. *Principles for the restructuring of the organised cervical cancer screening programme-final decision* (In Dutch). ZiekenfondsRaad, Amstelveen, The Netherlands, 1993.

Nelson HD, Tyne K, Naik A, Bougatsos C, Chan BK, Humphrey L. Screening for breast cancer: An update for the U.S. Preventive Services Task Force. *Ann Intern Med* 2009; 151:727-737.

Rebolj M, van Ballegooijen M, Berkers LM, Habbema JDF. Monitoring a national cancer prevention program: Successful changes in cervical cancer screening in the Netherlands. *Int J Cancer* 2007;120:806-812.

Rutter CM, Knudsen AB, Pandharipande PV. Computer disease simulation models: Integrating evidence for health policy. *Acad Radiol* 2011:18:1077-1086.

Stout NK, Knudsen AB, Kong CY, McMahon PM, Gazelle GS. Calibration methods used in cancer simulation models and suggested reporting guidelines. *Pharmacoeconomics* 2009; 27:533-545.

Stout NK, Rosenberg MA, Trentham-Dietz A, Smith MA, Robinson SM, Fryback DG. Retrospective cost-effectiveness analysis of screening mammography. *J Natl Cancer Inst* 2006; 98:774-782.

Tosteson ANA, Stout NK, Fryback DG, Acharyya S, Herman B, Hannah L et al. Cost-effectiveness of digital mammography breast cancer screening: Results from ACRIN DMIST. *Ann Intern Med* 2008; 148:1-10.

US Preventive Services Task Force. Screening for breast cancer: U.S. Preventive Services Task Force recommendation statement. *Ann Intern Med* 2009; 151:716-726.

van Ballegooijen M, Boer R, van Oortmarssen GJ, Koopmanschap MA, Lubbe JTN, Habbema JDF. *Cervical cancer screening programme: Age ranges and intervals. An updated cost-effectiveness analysis* (In Dutch). . Department of Public Health, Erasmus University, Rotterdam, 1993.

van Ballegooijen M, Rutter CM, Knudsen AB, Zauber AG, Savarino JE, Lansdorp-Vogelaar I et al. Clarifying differences in natural history between models of screening: The case of colorectal cancer. *Med Decis Making* 2011; 31:540-549.

van den Akker-van Marle ME, van Ballegooijen M, van Oortmarssen GJ, Boer R, Habbema JDF. Cost-Effectiveness of Cervical Cancer Screening: Comparison of Screening Policies. *J Natl Cancer Inst* 2002;94:193-204.

Vogelaar I, van Ballegooijen M, Schrag D, Boer R, Winawer SJ, Habbema JDF et al. How much can current interventions reduce colorectal cancer mortality in the U.S.? *Cancer* 2006; 107:1624-1633.

Zauber AG, Knudsen AB, Rutter CM, Lansdorp-Vogelaar I, Savarino JE, van Ballegooijen M, Kuntz KM. Cost-effectiveness of CT colonography to screen for colorectal cancer, Technology Assessment Report. Agency for Healthcare Research and Quality, Rockville, MD, 2009. (Available at: http://www.cms.gov/determinationprocess/downloads/id58TA.pdf)

Zauber AG, Lansdorp-Vogelaar I, Knudsen AB, Wilschut J, van Ballegooijen M, Kuntz KM. Evaluating test strategies for colorectal cancer screening: A decision analysis for the U.S. Preventive Services Task Force. *Ann Intern Med* 2008; 149:659-669.

Zauber AG, Lansdorp-Vogelaar I, Wilschut J, Knudsen AB, van Ballegooijen M, Kuntz KM. Cost-effectiveness of DNA stool testing to screen for colorectal cancer, Technology Assessment Report. Agency for Healthcare Research and Quality, Rockville, MD, 2007. (Available at: http://www.cms.gov/determinationprocess/downloads/id52TA.pdf)

Chapter 22
Role of the Oncologist in Cancer Prevention

William Hryniuk

22.1 Introduction

More than 40% of individuals will develop cancer in their lifetime, and cancer is now the number one cause of death. Although newer treatments are more effective, they are also increasingly expensive. Meanwhile, it is becoming evident that one-third of all cancers can be prevented by application of existing knowledge (UICC 2010). As a result of these trends, there has been a paradigm shift of emphasis: from cancer treatment to cancer prevention.

Physicians specializing in the treatment of cancer patients (surgical oncologists, radiation oncologists, medical oncologists, and hematologists) have been caught up in this paradigm shift. Their efforts are resulting in steady improvement in cancer survival as they select the optimal treatment path for each patient from a widening array of options: new surgical and radiation techniques, an avalanche of new systemic agents, and a rapidly expanding genetic database which is revolutionizing the approach to targeted therapy—the era of personalized medicine. Following on their success, oncologists are now being entreated to expand their role to encompass cancer prevention.

W. Hryniuk (✉)
CAREpath, 123 Edward Street, Suite 502, Toronto, ON M5G 1E, Canada
e-mail: whryniuk@carepath.ca

A.B. Miller (ed.), *Epidemiologic Studies in Cancer Prevention and Screening*,
Statistics for Biology and Health 79, DOI 10.1007/978-1-4614-5586-8_22,

22.2 Calls for Expanding the Roles of Oncologists in Cancer Prevention

22.2.1 *The "Teachable Moment"*

Oncologists' clinical expertise, research experience, and relationship with their patients create a unique opportunity to provide advice and guidance toward lifestyle changes that would reduce cancer recurrence in cancer survivors. During this "teachable moment," they might induce greater changes in behavior in their patients than other health-care providers, particularly during repeated follow-up visits (Ganz 2005). As a demonstration of its commitment to cancer prevention, the American Society of Clinical Oncology has established a standing Cancer Prevention Committee and encouraged its membership to take a leadership role in risk assessment and cancer prevention in cancer survivors by integrating these aspects into clinical practice (Zon et al. 2008).

22.2.2 *Survivors "Lost in Transition"*

Oncologists are also being confronted by the findings of the Institute of Medicine's (IOM) landmark study, "Lost in Transition" (Institute of Medicine 2005). The results highlighted the plight of cancer patients who, having completed initial treatment, are still left with a range of significant residual problems related not only to the risk of cancer recurrence but also to the need for rehabilitation. Thus, the IOM emphasized the need for better coordination between specialists and primary care providers to prevent recurrence of cancer (including second primaries) and provide increased surveillance for earlier detection as well as to:

- Assess medical and psychosocial late effects
- Intervene in the consequences of cancer and its treatment including medical problems such as lymphedema and sexual dysfunction
- Reduce symptoms, including pain and fatigue
- Address psychological distress in cancer survivors and their caregivers
- Advise on concerns related to employment, insurance, and disability

22.2.3 *Treatment-Induced Second Primaries*

Because of more effective treatments, cancer survivors are living longer. However, they are also developing second primaries at other sites. The increasing emergence of second primaries is of considerable concern since they are caused, at least in part, by treatment of the initial cancer. Such malignancies comprise up to 16% of all cancers (Travis et al. 2006) and are a particular problem among survivors of pediatric cancers (Meadows et al. 2009). Specific examples include:

- Breast cancer in young women treated with radiotherapy for Hodgkin's disease (Bhatia et al. 1996)
- Uterine corpus cancer in women treated with tamoxifen for breast cancer (Bernstein et al. 1999)
- Leukemia in women treated with platinum compounds for ovarian cancer (Travis et al. 1999)
- Leukemia in women receiving dose-intensive chemotherapy for breast cancer (Levine et al. 1998)
- Skin cancer in patients receiving the anti-melanoma drug vemurafenib (Weeraratna 2012)

In addition, a variety of malignancies can occur in:

- Patients treated with radiation for testicular cancer (Travis et al. 2005), cervical cancer (Behtash et al. 2002), and prostate cancer (Brenner et al. 2000)
- Women treated for papillary thyroid cancer (Canchola et al. 2006)
- Patients treated for myeloma (Thomas et al. 2012)
- Patients treated for chronic lymphocytic leukemia (Royle et al. 2011)

22.3 Definition(s) of Cancer Prevention

Before suggesting how oncologists' practice could be redirected toward cancer prevention, it is necessary to first define the term. Surprisingly, there seems to be no agreement among oncologists about exactly what is meant by cancer prevention. The European Society of Medical Oncology (ESMO) has taken the position that cancer prevention is "The reduction of cancer mortality via reduction in the incidence of cancer achieved by lifestyle or dietary modifications, identifying the individuals with genetic predisposition and screening them and by chemoprevention" (Baselga and Senn 2008).

Expanding on this definition, ESMO recognized the traditional three levels of cancer prevention:

Primary prevention: reduction in incidence by controlling or avoiding exposure to risk factors or by increasing an individuals' resistance to these factors by immunization or chemoprevention

Secondary prevention: detection of cancer at an early stage by screening when treatment is more effective, leading to a higher rate of cure and a reduced frequency of more serious consequences of disease

Tertiary prevention: prevention of locoregional relapse and/or metastatic disease after primary (initial) treatment by surgery or radiation

On the other hand, the American Society of Clinical Oncology (ASCO) Committee on Cancer Prevention has adopted a somewhat different definition:

"A reduction in the risk of developing clinically evident cancer, whether first or second primary cancer, or of developing intraepithelial neoplasia (IEN), a frequent cancer precursor" (Lippman et al. 2004).

The ASCO committee declined to further subclassify prevention into the three traditional levels recognized by ESMO.

22.4 Need for Rehabilitation

The situation is further complicated by the fact that when the term "*tertiary prevention*" is applied to diseases other than cancer, the definition has been focused on rehabilitation as "Methods to reduce the negative impact of extent of disease by restoring function and reducing disease related complications" (Wikipedia 2012). While rehabilitation of cancer survivors has attracted considerable attention, including that of the IOM, it has not been included in cancer agencies' definitions of tertiary cancer prevention but there are exceptions (Alberts and Hess 2008).

In this chapter, we address the issues facing oncologists, describe the roles they presently play in cancer prevention, suggest possible additional roles, and propose how they might be engaged more fully in a practical manner. For discussion purposes, the chapter is organized around the ESMO definition of cancer prevention (Baselga and Senn 2008).

22.5 Present Roles of Oncologists in Cancer Prevention

22.5.1 Primary and Secondary Prevention

22.5.1.1 Societal (Public) Roles

Practicing oncologists are engaged as volunteers advocating for cancer prevention in the public arena. They contribute to and participate in awareness campaigns, serve as members in community partnerships, and work with coalitions to advance tobacco control, espouse healthy eating and exercise habits, and counsel avoidance of exposure to excess sunlight and occupational and environmental carcinogens. However, their efforts have been limited, are largely one-off, and remain unorganized.

22.5.1.2 Professional (Medical) Roles

Oncologists also engage in primary and secondary prevention as part of their professional duties such as:

- Surgery to remove organs and tissues at high risk of developing cancer (Bertagnolli 2005)

- Radiation to ablate ovarian function in patients unsuitable for surgery
- Participation in clinical trials testing alternative methods of cancer treatments which might result in fewer secondary malignancies (Meyer et al. 2012)
- Participation in clinical trials testing the effectiveness of chemoprevention agents in high-risk individuals (Zon et al. 2008)
- Service on committees overseeing screening programs
- Encouragement of patients with genetically transmitted risk for cancer to encourage first-degree relatives to undergo genetic counseling (Guillem et al. 2006; Garber and Offit 2005)
- Encouragement of patients and their families to adopt healthy lifestyles

22.5.2 Tertiary Prevention

Oncologists efforts are also directed at preventing locoregional relapse and/or metastatic disease by:

- Radiating tissue beds and node-bearing areas after surgery to reduce local recurrence
- Administering adjuvant systemic therapy to eliminate distant micrometastases after surgical or radiation removal/ablation has eradicated the primary cancer
- Designing and conducting clinical trials testing local and systemic adjuvant treatments

22.6 Possible Additional Roles of Oncologists in Cancer Prevention

22.6.1 Primary and Secondary Prevention

22.6.1.1 Societal (Public) Roles

Oncologists' efforts could have a greater impact if they focused on targeted areas:

- Greater participation in public campaigns advocating prevention and screening
- Lobbying governments to introduce policies which foster cancer prevention
- Encouraging granting agencies to increase funds for cancer prevention research
- Lobbying for improved reimbursement for cancer prevention by oncologists

However, to maximize their impact on the public at large, it will be necessary for oncologists' professional societies and cancer agencies to include cancer prevention as a priority, provide resources to support activities in the targeted areas, and deputize representatives to liaise with volunteer cancer groups in combining efforts to achieve the stated goals.

22.6.1.2 Professional Roles

Based on their special medical and research expertise, oncologists could, with relatively little effort and time expenditure, contribute to primary and secondary cancer prevention simply by providing advice in four important areas which have been relatively neglected:

- Identification of high-risk individuals using presently available screening tools (New NCI Risk Website, Harvard School of Public Health[1], Central Pennsylvania Medical Oncology Group, Mayo Clinic[2])
- Design of trials to alter lifestyle in high-risk individuals
- Encouragement and support of primary care physicians in the administration of chemoprevention agents to high-risk individuals (Zon et al. 2008)
- Education of students and trainees about the importance of cancer prevention

Although these activities would incur opportunity costs to oncologists (time and effort deflected from their primary mission of treating cancer), large returns might accrue for minimal effort. One area of cancer prevention that oncologists can hardly avoid is prevention of recurrence in cancer survivors.

22.6.2 Prevention of Cancer Recurrence in Cancer Survivors

The American Cancer Society has adopted the premise that risk factors which lead to development of the initial cancer are probably the same as those predisposing to its recurrence or the development of a second primary. The society has therefore recommended that reduction of risk factors in cancer survivors should be a priority (Doyle et al. 2006). As noted earlier, the IOM has also placed a top priority on the prevention of recurrent and new cancers among cancer survivors. Since oncologists have a unique opportunity to alter the behavior of their patients through the "teachable moment" and since the treatments they administer can lead to development of second primaries, the largest contribution they might make to cancer prevention, in addition to testing less carcinogenic therapies, would be to counsel their own patients on how to reduce risk through behavioral change (Straus 2012).

Such counseling would require identification of risk factors unique to each patient through administration of detailed questionnaires (including the Gail model for survivors whose primary cancer was other than breast) (Chen et al. 2006), followed by appropriate advice based on questionnaire results (Demark-Wahnefried et al. 2006).

Specific areas in which behavioral changes could make a difference include:

- Cessation of smoking in patients with head and neck cancer (Chen et al. 2011)
- Top of Form

[1] http://www.yourdiseaserisk.harvard.edu

[2] http://www.mayoclinic.com/health/cancer-prevention/CA00024

- Lowering dietary fat in ER-negative breast cancer survivors (Chlebowski et al. 2006)
- Dietary change in colon cancer survivors (Meyerhardt et al. 2007; Zell et al. 2007)
- Weight reduction in obese breast cancer survivors (Djuric et al. 2002; Ewertz et al. 2011) after screening for mood disorders (Djuric et al. 2002; Jenkins et al. 2003)
- Increasing physical activity in all survivors (Knols et al 2005; Meyerhardt et al. 2006a; Meyerhardt et al. 2006b; Zell 2011)
- Reducing alcohol consumption in breast cancer survivors (Kwan et al. 2010)
- Psychological interventions in breast cancer survivors (Andersen et al. 2008)

As well, oncologists could ensure their patients enroll in screening schedules to detect second primaries and encourage them to accept chemoprevention agents when appropriate.

22.7 Barriers to an Expanded Role for Oncologists

Oncologists have not been quick to respond to calls for involvement in additional activities related to cancer prevention (Chlebowski et al. 1992; Ganz et al. 2006). Their reluctance is understandable not only because of the opportunity costs but also because of significant barriers to dispersion of their efforts.

A major barrier has been oncologists' discomfort with becoming involved in areas in which they lack expertise. Forty-three percent of respondents in the 2004 ASCO survey said they needed more information on what was involved in cancer prevention (Ganz et al. 2006). To address this gap, ASCO has developed a range of educational offerings. One of the first was the *ASCO Curriculum: Cancer Genetics & Genetic Susceptibility Testing*, which set forth a policy for genetic testing for cancer susceptibility (Zon et al 2008). As well, the Cancer Prevention Track has been initiated at the ASCO Annual Meeting. It remains to be seen if these resources will increase oncologists' involvement in cancer prevention.

Another barrier is lack of sufficient reimbursement for prevention activities. In the 2004 survey of ASCO members, 65% of respondents pinpointed this deficiency (Ganz et al. 2006). Reimbursement schedules in the USA for counseling services have since been improved [(a) Centers for Medicare and Medicaid Services, Zon et al 2006]. Again, it remains to be seen if improved reimbursement will significantly increase oncologists' involvement in cancer prevention since few claims for these services were reported initially [(b) Centers for Medicare and Medicaid Services claims data].

Lack of role clarity is a significant barrier. Screening and prevention for average risk individuals are usually provided by primary care providers (see Katz, this volume). While the oncologist might provide prevention services to cancer survivors at increased risk for second cancers (ASCO Policy Statement 2009), experience has shown that maximum benefit of preventive care is achieved when follow-up is provided by a medical oncologist working in close collaboration with a primary care provider (Earle et al. 2003; Earle and Neville 2004). And therein lies the problem: the discontinuity of care provided to cancer survivors.

22.8 Prerequisites for Expanding Oncologists' Role in Cancer Prevention

Greater involvement by oncologists in cancer prevention would require them to assume a leadership role in overcoming barriers to collaboration and coordination with primary care providers. The roles of the two groups have to be specified, lines of communication arranged, and steps taken to enable the respective parties to carry out their roles. The barriers to achieving these ends and the methods for overcoming them have been well summarized in a report prepared for the Canadian Association of Provincial Cancer Agencies "Supporting the Role of Primary Care in Cancer Follow-up" (Chomik 2010). There was general agreement not only on the need for precise description of roles and for tools to stay connected with each other but also for:

- Provision of widely accepted prevention and screening guidelines
- Further education and training
- Access to resources
- Assurance that patients would remain satisfied with greater primary care provider involvement
- Adequate compensation for both groups

These steps are necessary but not sufficient. An additional step is active engagement of oncologists with specialists of other disciplines who can identify proven strategies for effecting behavioral change (Earle et al. 2003; Earle and Neville 2004).

Notwithstanding the importance of the many opportunities presented to oncologists for greater involvement in cancer prevention, given the obstacles to achieving this end, it remains to determine in practical terms how they could contribute while still attending to their primary duty of providing optimal treatment. Addressing these barriers in a practical manner could be effected by taking advantage of the proposal by the Institute of Medicine: produce a "survivorship care plan."

22.9 The Survivorship Care Plan (SCP)

To meet the objectives outlined in their report, the IOM described a survivorship care plan (SCP) which would be prepared for each cancer patient upon completion of initial therapy. Such an SCP would cover:

- Cancer type, treatments received, and their potential consequences
- The timing and content of recommended follow-up
- Recommendations regarding preventive practices and how to maintain health and well-being
- Information on legal protections regarding employment and access to health insurance
- Availability of psychosocial services in the community

Following these lines, there has been considerable interest in developing an SCP (Ganz and Hahn 2008; Horning 2008; Lewis et al. 2009; Faul et al. 2010; Salz et al. 2012) which would:

- Detail the patient's cancer and treatment history (Gilbert et al. 2008; Miller 2008; Ristovski-Slijepcevic 2008)
- Be organized around a set of widely known clinical practice guidelines (Earle 2006; Gilbert et al. 2008)
- Identify health priorities including psychosocial concerns and lifestyle practices (Earle 2006; Gilbert et al. 2008; Ristovski- Slijepcevic 2008)
- Address employment, insurance, and economic issues (Earle 2006)
- Identify which providers will be responsible for which roles (Earle 2006; Gilbert et al. 2008)
- Specify recommended tests and their frequency to monitor for recurrence, second malignancies, ongoing toxicities, and late effects (Faul et al. 2010)
- Provide contact information for each specialist (Miller 2008)
- Be modified according to concerns and needs of the individual patient
- Be shared among the patient, the primary care provider, and members of the patient's support network (Gilbert et al. 2008; Miller 2008)

22.9.1 Results from a Randomized Trial Testing the Effectiveness of an SCP

Not surprisingly, in the present era of evidence-based medicine, one version of an SCP has already been studied in a randomized trial to determine if it could improve outcomes compared to usual practice of having the oncologist send a discharge letter to the primary care provider (Grunfeld et al. 2011). The specific objectives were to assess whether the SCP could better reduce patients' perceived level of psychological distress, improve health-related quality of life, produce more satisfaction, and improve continuity/coordination of care. The test SCP was generated after receiving input from the oncologist, the primary care provider, and patients. It included a personalized summary of treatment, follow-up guidelines, and a kit describing supportive care resources. The SCP was transmitted to the patient by an oncology nurse during a 30-min educational session. Surprisingly, the results of the trial showed no differences in any of the outcome measures between the SCP and the oncologist's discharge letter.

However, closer examination of the trial revealed it was restricted to only breast cancer survivors and 36% of candidates offered the study declined to participate. It also did not address the main objectives of a primary care provider as envisaged by the IOM: There were no patient-specific recommendations for healthy living to prevent cancer recurrence or second primaries, no recommendations for early detection and prevention of the late consequences of the cancer or its treatment, nor any recommendations addressing concerns related to employment, insurance, or disability. Thus, the results cannot yet be taken as evidence negating the possible utility of an SCP as recommended by the IOM. As one observer put it, "The study will not be believed by unshakeable SCP fans" (Smith and Snyder 2011). Notwithstanding the negative results, they do emphasize the importance of subjecting the concept of an SCP to rigorous scientific study. Thus, it still remains to determine if an SCP would achieve the objectives originally laid out by the IOM.

22.9.2 The SCP as an Instrument for Involving Oncologists in Cancer Prevention

On the assumption that testing the effectiveness of an SCP as suggested by the IOM continues to be worthwhile, a trial of its utility could also serve as a means of engaging oncologists in cancer prevention. To do so would require, in addition to meeting the requirements for rehabilitation specified in the IOM report, two additional steps in the preparation of a test SCP: First, a detailed profile would be required of each patient's lifestyle and behavior in order to identify risky behaviors and indicate where corrective measures were best applied. Several comprehensive self-administered risk-assessment questionnaires referred to earlier could be used for this purpose. Secondly, appropriate corrective measures could be tailored to each patient based on questionnaire results and integrated into the test SCP.

22.9.3 SCP Generated by a Discharge Conference

The corrective measures required to reduce the risk of cancer recurrence in the individual case could be based on practical advice generated at a "discharge conference." The discharge conference would be led by the treating oncologist and attended by a panel of experts including nutritionists, physiotherapists, behavioral scientists, geneticists, social workers, and nurses. The oncologist would present to the panel the survivor's case history, indicate the immediate and possible late complications of therapy, estimate chances of recurrence of the original cancer and of a new primary, and provide results of the risk-assessment questionnaire. Panel members, focusing their expertise on the case at hand, would discuss and define the most effective and practical ways to reduce the risk factors identified by the questionnaire. These recommendations would be added to the SCP along with the other elements required by the IOM.

Such a multidisciplinary "discharge conference" would be analogous to the site-specific multidisciplinary "treatment conferences" now routinely held in which various subspecialty oncologists gather together and formulate a customized treatment plan for each patient admitted to the cancer center.

Organization of the analogous discharge conference would not only result in specifying risk reduction maneuvers tailored to the individual case; it would also engage oncologists at the point where they had the most interest: improving their patient's well-being. By presiding at the discharge conferences, oncologists would also learn about current concepts and methods for preventing cancer. With a better knowledge base and improved understanding, they might be motivated to take up challenges in the broader areas of cancer prevention. As a corollary, the other participating professionals, by becoming familiar with the details of cases presented by the oncologist, would get a better grasp of the individual variations encountered in practice.

22.9.4 SCP Generated by the Oncology Team

An alternative approach to the multidisciplinary discharge conference would be to have the SCP prepared by the original treatment team of oncology physician and oncology nurse. The nurse or her designate could administer and interpret the risk-assessment questionnaire, and the team would then identify interventions and advise on practical means for implementing them. The team would also formulate the other elements of the SCP, transmit them to the patient, and ensure the completed SCP was copied to all care providers (Miller 2008). Responsibility for this process would have to be accepted by the treatment team. It would require them to acquire more detailed knowledge of cancer prevention, knowledge which is not in their lexicon. It would also incur opportunity costs, diverting attention away from their primary role. While this approach for producing the SCP might be more economical of aggregate professional time compared to a discharge conference, by not engaging the combined expertise of more specialized disciplines, it probably would not produce equivalent results. It would, however, be more akin to "usual practice."

22.10 Importance of Evaluation of the Utility of the SCP

Either model for generating the SCP, discharge conference or oncology team approach, should be subjected to careful evaluation. To that end, advantage could be taken of a time-honored and integral component of oncologists' professional activity: personal involvement in clinical research. Outcomes from an SCP should be compared with usual practice or alternative models to evaluate its effectiveness in meeting the objectives specified by the IOM. If utility of the SCP were proven, oncologists would be more inclined to become involved in cancer prevention as part of their routine practice.

22.11 Conclusion

As oncologists have steadily improved their treatment of cancer, their success has evoked calls for them to become more involved with cancer prevention and rehabilitation. Although they have not been in the habit of thinking of themselves as a hub for cancer prevention, their concern for keeping patients staying cancer-free should be preeminent. To quote a past president of the American Society of Oncology, Dr George Sledge: "if we do not address causation, who will? and how?" (Sledge 2012).

ASCO has formed a Cancer Survivorship Committee which held its first meeting in 2011 and developed goals for the year as a necessary first step in the process. But it will take more than a committee to recruit oncologists into an active role in cancer prevention and more than oncologists to prevent cancer in survivors. The answer to "who will?" may require a variety of other disciplines. The answer to "how?" could be, by moving behind the stalking horse of clinical research, to entice oncologists to become involved in tests of the effectiveness of an SCP compared to "usual practice."

References

Alberts DS, Hess LM. *Fundamentals of Cancer Prevention.* Springer-Verlag Berlin Heidelberg, 2008; pp 6–7.

Andersen BL, Yang H-C, Farrar WB, Golden-Kreutz DM, Emery CF, Thornton LM. Psychologic intervention improves survival for breast cancer patients. A Randomized Clinical Trial. *Cancer* 2008; 113:3450–3458.

ASCO. Policy Statement Highlights Oncologist's Role in Providing Cancer Prevention Services *J Oncol Pract* 2009; 5: 10–12.

Baselga J, Senn H-J. The perspective and role of the medical oncologist in cancer prevention: A Position Paper by the European Society of Medical Oncology. *Annals of Oncology* 2008; 19:1033–1035.

Behtash N, Tehranian A, Ardalan FA, Hanjani P. Uterine Papillary Serous Carcinoma after Pelvic Radiation Therapy for Cancer of the Cervix. *J Obst & Gynecol* 2002; 22:96–97.

Bernstein L, Deapen D, Cerhan JR, Schwartz SM, Liff J, McGann-Maloney E, et al. Tamoxifen Therapy for Breast Cancer and Endometrial Cancer Risk. *J Natl Cancer Inst* 1999; 91:1654–1662.

Bertagnolli MM. Surgical Prevention of Cancer. *J Clin Oncol* 2005; 23:324–332.

Bhatia S, Robison LL, Oberlin O, Greenberg M, Bunin G, Fossati-Bellani F, et al. Breast Cancer and Other Second Neoplasms after Childhood Hodgkin's Disease. *N Engl J Med* 1996; 334:745–751.

Brenner DJ, Curtis R, Hall EJ, Ron E. Second Malignancies in Prostate Carcinoma Patients after Radiotherapy Compared with Surgery. *Cancer* 2000; 88:398–406.

Canchola AJ, Horn-Ross PL, Purdie DM. Risk of Second Primary Malignancies in Women with Papillary Thyroid Cancer. *Am J Epidemiol* 2006; 163:521–527.

Centers for Medicare and Medicaid Services (a): National coverage determination for smoking and tobacco-use cessation counseling http://www.cms.hhs.gov/mcd

Centers for Medicare and Medicaid Services (b): claims data. http://www.cms.hhs.gov/mcd

Central Pennsylvania Medical Oncology Group: Cancer risk assessment. http://www.hmc.psu.edu/ cpog/risk/index.htm & Fox Chase Cancer Center: What are your cancer risks? www.fccc.edu/cancer/risk-quiz.html

Chen AM, Chen LM, Vaughan MA, Sreeraman R, Farwell DG, Luu Q et al. http://www.redjournal.org/article/S0360-3016(09)03526-3/abstract - article-footnote-1Tobacco Smoking During Radiation Therapy for Head-and-Neck Cancer Is Associated With Unfavorable Outcome. *Intl J Radn Oncol Biology Physics* 2011; 79:414–419.

Chen J, Pee D, Ayyagari R, Graubard B, Schairer C, Byrne C, Benichou J. Projecting Absolute Invasive Breast Cancer Risk in White Women With a Model That Includes Mammographic Density. *J Natl Cancer Inst* 2006; 98:1215–1226.

Chlebowski RT, Blackburn GL, Thomson CA, Nixon DW, Shapiro A, Hoy MK, et al. Dietary Fat Reduction and Breast Cancer Outcome: Interim Efficacy Results from the Women's Intervention Nutrition Study. *J Natl Cancer Inst* 2006; 98:1767–1776.

Chlebowski RT, Sayre J, Frank-Stromborg M, Lillington LB. Current Attitudes and Practice of American Society of Clinical Oncology-Member Clinical Oncologists Regarding Cancer Prevention and Control. *J Clin Oncol* 1992; 10:165–168.

Chomik TA Consulting & Research Ltd. http://www.capca.ca/wpcontent/uploads/CAPCA.SupportingPrimaryCareinCancerFollowup.Report.Oct31..10.Final.pdf, 2010

Demark-Wahnefried W, Pinto BM, Gritz ER. Promoting Health and Physical Function Among Cancer Survivors: Potential for Prevention and Questions that Remain. *J Clin Oncol* 2006; 24:5125–5131.

Djuric Z, DiLaura N, Jenkins I, Mood D, Jen C, Bradley E, Hryniuk W. Combining Weight Loss Counseling with the Weight Watchers Plan for Obese Breast Cancer Survivors. *Obesity Research* 2002; 10:657–665.

Doyle C, Kushi LH, Byers T, for the 2006 Nutrition, Physical Activity and Cancer Survivorship Advisory Committee: Nutrition and Physical Activity During and after Cancer Treatment: an American Cancer Society Guide for Informed Choices. *CA Cancer J Clin* 2006; 56:323–353.

Earle CC, Burstein HJ, Winer EP, et al. Quality of Non-breast Cancer Health Maintenance Among Elderly Breast Cancer Survivors. *J Clin Oncol* 2003; 21:1447–1451.

Earle CC, Neville BA. Under-use of Necessary Care Among Cancer Survivors. *Cancer* 2004; 101:1712–1719.

Earle CC. Failing to plan is planning to fail: Improving the Quality of Care with Survivorship Care Plans. *J Clin Oncol* 2006; 24:5112–5116.

Ewertz M, Jensen M, Gunnarsdottir KA, Hojris I, Jakobsen EH, Nielsen D, et al. Effect of Obesity on Prognosis after Early Stage Breast Cancer. *J Clin Oncol* 2011; 29:25–31.

Faul L, Shibata D, Townsend I, Jacobsen, P. Improving Survivorship Care for Patients with Colorectal Cancer. *Cancer Control* 2010; 17:35–43.

Ganz PA. Teachable Moment for Oncologists: Cancer Survivors, 10 Million Strong and Growing! *J Clin Oncol* 2005; 23:5458–5460.

Ganz PA, Kwan L, Somerfield MR, Albert D, Garber JE, Offit K. The Role of Prevention in Oncology Practice: Results From a 2004 Survey of American Society of Clinical Oncology Members. *J Clin Oncol* 2006; 24:2948–2957.

Ganz PA, Hahn EE. Implementing a Survivorship Care Plan for Patients with Breast Cancer. *J Clin Oncol* 2008; 26:759–767.

Garber JE, Offit K. Hereditary Cancer Predisposition Syndromes. *J Clin Oncol* 2005; 23:276–292.

Gilbert S, Miller D, Hollenbeck B, Montie J, Wei, J. Cancer Survivorship: Challenges and Changing Paradigms. *J Urol* 2008; 179:431–438.

Grunfeld, E, Julian JA, Pond G, Maunsell E, Coyle D, Folkes A, et al. Evaluating Survivorship Care Plans: Results of a Randomized Clinical Trial of Patients with Breast Cancer. *J Clin Oncol* 2011; 29:4755–4762

Guillem JG, Wood WC, Moley J, Berchuck A, Karlan BY, Mutch DJ et al. ASCO/SSO Review of Current Role of Risk-Reducing Surgery in Common Hereditary Cancer Syndromes. *J Clin Oncol* 2006; 24:4642–4660.

Horning SJ. Follow-up of Adult Cancer Survivors: New Paradigms for Survivorship Care Planning. *Hematol/Oncol Clinics of North America* 2008; 22:201–210.

Institute of Medicine. *From Cancer Patient to Cancer Survivor: Lost in Transition* http://books.nap.edu/openbook.php?record_id=11468, 2005

Jenkins I, Djuric Z, Darga L, DiLaura N, Hryniuk W. Influence of Psychiatric Diagnosis on Weight Loss Maintenance in Obese Breast Cancer Survivors. *Obesity Research* 2003; 11:1369–1375.

Knols R, Aaronson NK, Uebelhart D, Fransen J, Aufdemkampe G. Physical Exercise in Cancer Patients during and after Medical Treatment: A Systematic Review of Randomized and Controlled Clinical Trials. *J Clin Oncol* 2005; 23:3830–3842.

Kwan ML, Kushi LH, Weltzien E, Tam EK, Castillo A, Sweeney C, et al. Alcohol Consumption and Breast Cancer Recurrence and Survival Among Women With Early-Stage Breast Cancer: The Life After Cancer Epidemiology Study. *J Clin Oncol* 2010; 29:4410–4416.

Levine MN, Bramwell VH, Pritchard KI, Norris BD, Shepherd LE, Abu-Zahra H, et al. Randomized Trial of Intensive Cyclophosphamide, Epirubicin, and Fluorouracil Chemotherapy Compared

With Cyclophosphamide, Methotrexate, and Fluorouracil in Premenopausal Women With Node-Positive Breast Cancer. *J Clin Oncol* 1998; 16:2651–2658.

Lewis R, Neal R, Hendry, M, France, B, Williams, N, Russell, D, et al. Patients' and Healthcare Professionals' Views of Cancer Follow-up: Systematic Review. *Br J Gen Practice* 2009; 59:e248–259.

Lippman SM, Levin B, Brenner DE, Gordon GB, Aldige CR, Kramer BS, et al. Cancer Prevention and the American Society of Clinical Oncology. *J Clin Oncol* 2004; 22:3848–3851.

Meadows AT, Freidman DL, Neglia JP, Mertens AC, Donaldson SS, Stovall M, et al. Second Neoplasms in Survivors of Childhood Cancer: Findings from the Childhood Cancer Survivor Study Cohort. *J Clin Oncol* 2009; 27:2356–2362.

Meyer RM, Gospodarowicz MK, Connors JM, Pearcey RG, Wells WA, Winter JN, et al. ABVD Alone versus Radiation-Based Therapy in Limited-Stage Hodgkin's Lymphoma. *N Eng J Med* 2012; 366:399–408.

Meyerhardt JA, Giovannucci EL, Holmes MD, Chan AT, Chan JA, Colditz GA et al. Physical Activity and Survival after Colorectal Cancer Diagnosis. *J Clin Oncol* 2006a; 24:3527–3534.

Meyerhardt JA, Heseltine D, Niedzwiecki D, Hollis D, Saltz LB, Mayer RJ, et al. Impact of Physical Activity on Cancer Recurrence and Survival in Patients with Stage III Colon Cancer: Findings from CALGB 89–803. *J Clin Oncol* 2006b; 24:3535–3541.

Meyerhardt JA, Niedzwiecki D, Hollis D, Saltz LB, Hu FB, Mayer RJ, et al. Association of Dietary Patterns with Cancer Recurrence and Survival in Patients with Stage III Colon Cancer. *JAMA* 298:754–764.

Miller R. Implementing a Surviving Care Plan for Patients with Breast Cancer. *Clin J Oncol Nursing* 2008; 12:479–487.

New NCI Risk Website Aims at Consumers. *J Natl Cancer Inst* 2006; 98:1596–1598.

Ristovski-Slijepcevic, S. Environmental Scan of Cancer Survivorship in Canada: Conceptualization, Practice, and Research. Vancouver, BC: Canadian Partnership Against Cancer; BC Cancer Agency, 2008

Royle JA, Baade PD, Joske D, Girschik J, Fritschi L. Second cancer Incidence and Cancer Mortality Among Chronic Lymphocytic Leukemia Patients: a Population-based Study. *Br J Cancer* 2011; 105:1076–1081.

Salz T, Oeffinger KC, McCabe MS, Layne TM, Bach PB et al. Survivorship Care Plans in Research and Practice. *Ca Cancer J for Clinician*, in press, 2012

Sledge G. *ASCO Connection*, January 2012; p12

Smith TJ, Snyder C. Is It Time for (Survivorship Care) Plan B? *J Clin Oncol* 2011; 29:4740–4742.

Straus DJ. Chemotherapy Alone for Early-Stage Hodgkin's Lymphoma. *N Eng J Med* 2012; 366:399–408.

Thomas A, Malankody S, Korde N, Kristinsson SY. Second Malignancies Following Multiple Myeloma: from 1960s to 2010s. Blood 2012; published on line before print Feb 6

Travis LB, Holowaty EJ, Bergfeldt K, Lynch CF, Kohler BA, Wiklund T et al. Risk of Leukemia after Platinum-based Chemotherapy for Ovarian Cancer. *N Eng J Med* 1999; 340:351–357.

Travis LB, Fosså SD, SJ, McMaster ML, Lynch CF, Storm H. Second Cancers Among 40,576 Testicular Cancer Patients: Focus on Long-term Survivors. *J Natl Cancer Inst* 2005; 97:1354–1365.

Travis LB, Rabkin CS, Brown LM, Allan JM, Alter BP, Ambrosone CB et al. Cancer Survivorship-Genetic Susceptibility and Second Primary cancers: Research Strategies and Recommendations. *J Natl Cancer Inst* 2006; 98:15–25.

UICC. Office Press release, One Third of All Cancers are Preventable but Urgent Action is Still Needed: http://www.uicc.org/general-news/one-third-all-cancers-are-preventable-urgent-action-still-needed 2010

Weeraratna A. RAF Around the Edges-The Paradox of BRAF Inhibitors. *N Engl J Med* 2012; 366:271– 273.

Wikipedia. Definitions, Tertiary Prevention http://en.wikipedia.org/wiki/Medical_Subject_Headings, 2012

Zell JA, Ignatenko NA, Yerushalmi HF, Ziogas A, Besselsen DG, Gerner EW et al. Risk and Risk Reduction Involving Arginine Intake and Meat Consumption in Colorectal Tumorigenesis and Survival. *Intl J Cancer* 2007; 120:459–468.

Zell JA. Clinical Trials Update: Tertiary Prevention of Colorectal Cancer. *Carcinog.* 2011; 10:8.

Zon RT, Goss E, Vogel VG, Chlebowski RT, Jatoi I, Robson ME et al. American Society of Clinical Oncology Policy Statement: the Role of the Oncologist in Cancer Prevention and Risk Assessment. *J Clin Oncol* 2008; 27:986–993.

Zon RT, Towle E, Ndoping M, Levinson J, Colbert A, Williams C. Reimbursement for Preventive Counseling Services. *J Oncol Practice* 2006; 2:214–218.

Chapter 23
Integrating Prevention and Screening for Lung Cancer into Clinical Practice

William Hocking

23.1 Introduction

Cancer is responsible for approximately 25% of deaths annually in the United States. In 2011, it is estimated that lung cancer will account for 14% of new cancer diagnoses and 27% of cancer deaths, approximately 157,000 in the USA. Lung cancer is the leading cause of cancer mortality among men and women in the USA, resulting in as many deaths as breast, prostate, colorectal, and pancreatic cancers combined (Siegel et al. 2011). Trends in lung cancer incidence follow tobacco smoking trends. In the USA, smoking prevalence peaked at about 42% in the 1960s and by 2010 declined to approximately 19% (Centers for Disease Control and Prevention 2011a). Smoking rates by state are shown in Fig. 23.1.

Among women, this pattern lags about 10 years behind men. Lung cancer incidence began declining in the early 1980s, mortality rates began to decline in the 1990s for men, and these trends have continued (Siegel et al. 2011). In women, lung cancer incidence and mortality rates are just beginning to plateau (Siegel et al. 2011), and for the first time there has been a decline in both for the 2003–2007 interval (Kohler et al. 2011).

Globally, lung cancer is the leading cancer, with an estimated 1.6 million cases (13%) and 1.4 million deaths (18%) in 2008 (Jemal et al. 2011). Worldwide, lung cancer is the most common cancer and leading cause of cancer mortality in men, whereas among women it is the fourth most common cancer and second most common cause of cancer death. While lung cancer incidence and mortality generally track with tobacco smoking prevalence, an aberration occurs in China where there is a low frequency of tobacco use in women but a high burden of lung cancer that is probably related to indoor air pollution from cooking stoves.

W. Hocking, MD (✉)
Marshfield Center, 1000 N Oak Ave, Marshfield, WI 54449, USA
e-mail: hocking.william@marshfieldclinic.org

A.B. Miller (ed.), *Epidemiologic Studies in Cancer Prevention and Screening*, Statistics for Biology and Health 79, DOI 10.1007/978-1-4614-5586-8_23,

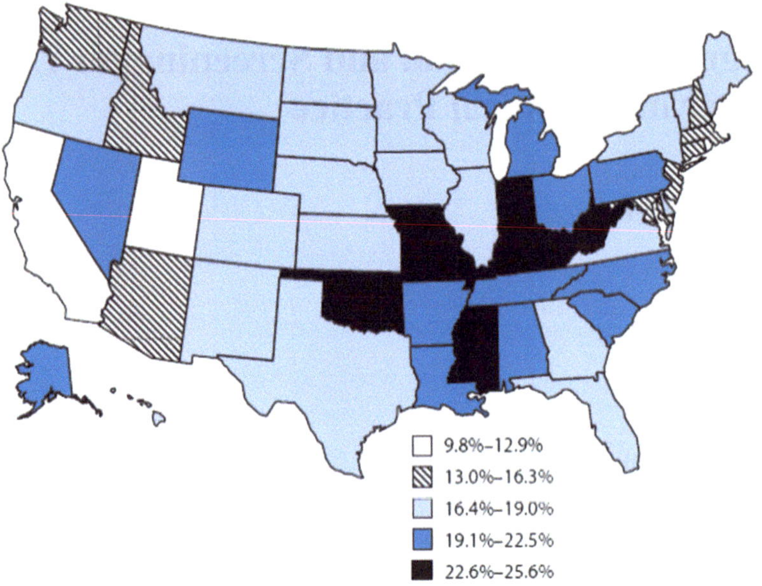

Fig. 23.1 Percentage of current cigarette smokers aged ≥18 years by state. Behavioral Risk Factor Surveillance System, United States, 2009 (Centers for Disease Control and Prevention 2010a)

Despite the strong association with tobacco use, globally about 15% of lung cancers among men and an estimated 50% among women (25% overall) are not associated with smoking. This places lung cancer among never-smokers as the seventh to eighth most common cause of cancer mortality worldwide (Jemal et al. 2011; Sun et al. 2007). Lung cancer incidence among never-smokers is higher in women than men (Wakelee et al. 2007). Lung cancer in never-smokers also exhibits other differences from cancer in smokers, including epidemiologic, biologic, histologic, and clinical features, as well as response to therapeutic agents (Wakelee et al. 2007; Toh et al. 2006). Furthermore, only 10–15% of smokers will develop lung cancer. Other factors, including individual susceptibility and other environmental exposures, are also important in determining the risk for lung cancer (Thun et al. 2002).

Lung cancer occurs more commonly in people of lower socioeconomic status, probably due to associations with lung cancer risk factors such as smoking, diet, occupation, and exposure to carcinogens (Alberg et al. 2005; Siegel et al. 2011). Lung cancer incidence and mortality are higher in African-American men than white men (Siegel et al. 2011).

23.2 Clinical Aspec ts of Lung Cancer

Lung cancer diagnosed at an early stage has a 5-year survival as high as 60–70% (Ginsberg and Rubinstein 1995; Goldstraw et al. 2007; Naruke et al. 1988) and perhaps as high as 85% when an asymptomatic lung cancer is diagnosed radiographically (International Early Lung Cancer Action Program Investigators 2006) and is amenable to surgical resection. However, lung cancer is usually diagnosed in a patient who presents with symptoms that reflect more advanced disease, and only about 15% of lung cancers are early stage at diagnosis (Siegel et al. 2011). While treatment for more advanced stages of lung cancer has recently improved, overall 5-year survival for lung cancer is about 16%.

As a result of these dismal outcomes for clinically diagnosed lung cancer, attention has focused on prevention and early detection through screening. The remainder of this chapter will review the evidence supporting these approaches to reducing the burden of lung cancer and discuss how these data may be applied in current clinical practice.

23.3 Overview of Lung Cancer Epidemiology

Developing effective prevention and early detection or screening strategies requires an understanding of the etiologic factors in lung cancer. Exposure to tobacco smoke is the major environmental risk factor for lung cancer, dwarfing the impact of other exposures. Nevertheless, there are other environmental exposures that also play a role in lung carcinogenesis and are important to consider in prevention strategies.

23.3.1 Tobacco

Exposure to tobacco smoke is the dominant cause for lung cancer and is estimated to be responsible for about 85–90% of lung cancers in the USA. Continuous smokers have a 20-fold increased risk compared to never-smokers. Risk is related to age, dose (number of cigarettes per day), and most strikingly to duration of smoking (Doll and Peto 1978). In the United States, adult smoking rates have gradually declined from a peak of 42% in 1965 to 19% in 2010 (Centers for Disease Control and Prevention 2011a), and approximately 25% of the population are former smokers (Centers for Disease Control and Prevention 2011b). Among women, the smoking rate has declined from about 34% in the 1960s to 17% in 2010, while in men the most recent smoking rate was 21.5% (Centers for Disease Control and Prevention 2011a). Globally there is a wide variation in smoking rates by country, ranging from 6% to 40% (Naurath and Jones 2007). Although lung cancer risk declines after smoking cessation, it does not return to the baseline risk of a never-smoker, and former smokers remain at an elevated lifelong risk for development of lung cancer (Doll et al. 2004; Crispo et al. 2004; Ebbert et al. 2003).

In addition to the direct impact of tobacco smoking, exposure to secondhand smoke (environmental tobacco smoke) is an important risk factor for lung cancer. Secondhand smoke has been designated a human carcinogen. In 1988–1989, secondhand smoke exposure in the USA was documented using the biomarker cotinine in 88% of nonsmokers (Pirkle et al. 2006). In 2007–2008, this level declined to 40.1% (Centers for Disease Control and Prevention 2010b), a substantial improvement related to efforts to increase smoke-free indoor air environments at work and home. However, a substantial minority of the US population remains at risk due to this exposure (Centers for Disease Control and Prevention 2010b).

23.3.2 Radon

Radon-222 is a gas formed by decay of uranium-238 that is found in the soil and rocks of the earth's crust. Radon was first recognized as a lung carcinogen among metal miners, and the risk of lung cancer correlates with exposure dose. Carcinogenesis is thought to be related to release of alpha particles by various decay progeny, resulting in direct DNA damage, as well as oxidative damage produced by reactive oxygen species (Alavanja 2002; Darby et al. 2001). Radon exposure in the general population occurs by the gas penetrating house foundations through cracks or other openings. For each 100 Becquerels (Bq) /m^3 (a measure of alpha disintegrations) increase in radon exposure, there is an estimated excess relative risk of lung cancer ranging from 8% to 21% in Europe and North America (Krewski et al. 2005; Turner et al. 2011). About 4–6% of US homes exceed the Environmental Protection Agency's level for mitigation of radon (148 Bq/m^3) (Lubin 2010). It has been estimated that radon may be responsible for 10–14% of the total lung cancer burden, making it the second leading cause of lung cancer.

23.3.3 Other Environmental Exposures

Air pollution (Pope et al. 2002; Turner et al. 2011) and exposure to asbestos, silica, arsenic, and other heavy metals (Steenland et al. 1996; Neuberger and Field 2003) are also associated with an increase in lung cancer risk. Household air pollution from indoor cook stoves is associated with lung cancer, particularly among women in developing countries (Zhang and Smith 2007).

The relationship of postmenopausal hormone replacement therapy (HRT) among women to lung cancer risk has been controversial, but there is some evidence that prolonged HRT may increase the risk of lung cancer (Baik et al. 2010; Slatore et al. 2010; Smith et al. 2009) and other evidence suggesting a protective effect (Rodriguez et al. 2008). There is also some evidence that HRT may have a negative impact on prognosis of lung cancer (Chlebowski et al. 2009).

23.3.4 Diet

The role of diet in lung cancer risk remains controversial. Theoretically, diets high in antioxidants might reduce oxidative damage to DNA caused by carcinogens contained in tobacco smoke. A number of large cohort studies have investigated the effects of various dietary constituents and lung cancer risk. There is evidence that diets high in consumption of red meat increase lung cancer risk (Lam et al. 2009a). Diets high in cruciferous vegetables are weakly associated with decreased risk of lung cancer (Lam et al. 2009b). High dietary fruit intake is associated with reduced lung cancer risk (Miller et al. 2004) as were vegetables in an update of that analysis (Linseisen et al. 2007). Diets high in β-cryptoxanthin, a carotenoid found in oranges, are associated with reduced lung cancer risk (Männistö et al. 2004). An analysis of dietary habits and lung cancer risk in the Nurses' Health Study and Health Professionals Follow-up Study demonstrated that higher fruit and vegetable consumption was associated with lower lung cancer risk in women but not men, although among never-smokers, both men and women were protected (Feskanich et al. 2000). In the National Institutes of Health-American Association for Retired People (NIH-AARP) diet and health study, total fruit and vegetable intake was unrelated to lung cancer risk, but high intake of certain specific groups of fruits and vegetables was associated with decreased lung cancer risk (Wright et al. 2008).

Serum levels of vitamin B6 and methionine correlate inversely with lung cancer risk, with a risk reduction in excess of 50% for participants with elevated levels of these nutrients in the European Prospective Investigation into Cancer and Nutrition (EPIC) cohort (Johansson et al. 2010). Isoflavones, phytoestrogens with weak estrogenic activity contained in soy products and chickpeas, have been associated with reduced lung cancer incidence. Studies of isoflavone dietary intake and plasma levels have shown an inverse relationship between isoflavones and lung cancer (Shiels et al. 2011; Yang et al. 2011). High levels of alcohol consumption, specifically liquor and beer, may be associated with increased lung cancer risk in smokers (Korte et al. 2002; Chao 2007), but in nonsmokers, alcohol does not appear to be a risk factor (Thun et al. 2009). Red wine consumption is associated with a protective effect (Chao et al. 2008).

23.4 Host Factors and Lung Cancer

23.4.1 Family History and Genetics

A family history of lung cancer among first-degree relatives is associated with an approximately twofold increased risk of developing lung cancer (Brennan et al. 2011; Matakidou et al. 2005; Tokuhata and Lilienfeld 1963). The risk is higher when the relative's cancer occurs at an early age (<50 years) (Jonsson et al. 2004; Matakidou et al. 2005) and appears to be greater among African-Americans (Coté et al. 2005). Families carrying p53 germ-line mutations also have an elevated risk of lung cancer (Hwang et al. 2003).

Several genetic loci have been associated with lung cancer risk. Linkage studies have identified a locus at 6q23–25 containing the *RGS17* gene that may be a lung cancer susceptibility gene (Bailey-Wilson et al. 2004; You et al. 2009). Glutathione S transferase is important in detoxification of carcinogens in tobacco smoke, and the glutathione S transferase M1 *(GSTM1)* null genotype has been associated with a slightly increased risk of lung cancer (Benhamou et al. 2002), as well as bladder cancer, another tobacco-associated cancer. A single nucleotide polymorphism (SNP) associated with the promoter region for cyclin A2 has been associated with lung as well as colorectal and hepatocellular carcinomas (Kim et al. 2011). The *CHEK2 1157 T* mutation is associated with breast, colon, and prostate cancers, but a significantly decreased risk of lung cancer (Brennan et al. 2007).

Genome-wide association studies (GWAS) have recently identified three additional lung cancer susceptibility loci. The 15q25 locus contains six coding regions, including three cholinergic nicotine-receptor genes (Amos et al. 2008; Hung et al. 2008). While the nicotine-receptor genes are associated with smoking intensity, there also is a direct biological effect of these receptors on lung cancer susceptibility. The 5p15 locus has been associated specifically with risk for adenocarcinomas of the lung (Landi et al. 2009). The gene located at 5p15 considered most likely associated with this effect is *TERT*, the telomerase reverse transcriptase necessary for telomere maintenance (Brennan et al. 2011). Another locus at 6p21.33, the HLA coding region, is associated with lung cancer risk (Wang et al. 2008).

23.4.2 Chronic Lung Disease and Inflammation

Chronic obstructive pulmonary disease (COPD) is associated with an increased risk of lung cancer, but this association is potentially confounded by the role of tobacco smoking (Mayne et al. 1999; Samet et al. 1986; Skillrud et al. 1986). In a lung cancer case-control study, the risk of developing lung cancer was about twofold for participants with COPD, emphysema, or chronic bronchitis, after adjustment for smoking and other risk factors (Koshiol et al. 2009). Furthermore, COPD has been associated with lung cancer mortality in a population of never-smokers (Turner et al. 2007). Homozygous alpha1-antitrypsin deficiency (ATD) is associated with the early onset of emphysema, whereas heterozygous carriers usually do not exhibit clinically apparent lung disease. However, alpha1-ATD carriers do have an elevated risk of lung cancer (Yang et al. 2008).

An increased lung cancer risk is associated with the presence of pulmonary scarring on chest radiography (Yu et al. 2008). Lung cancer risk is elevated following tuberculosis (Engels et al. 2008; Shiels et al. 2011) and pneumonias caused by other organisms. Elevated inflammatory markers such as C-reactive protein (CRP) (Chaturvedi et al. 2010) and circulating interleukins 6 and 8 (Pine et al. 2011) are also associated with increased risk of lung cancer.

A systematic review and meta-analysis demonstrated a lung cancer relative risk of 1.80 for COPD, chronic bronchitis, or emphysema combined, as well as 1.43 and 1.76 for a prior history of pneumonia and tuberculosis, respectively (Brenner et al.

2011). Thus, chronic inflammation of the lung may be the common factor in the elevated lung cancer risk associated with these conditions.

23.5 Identification of High-Risk Populations

The major population of interest for prevention efforts is tobacco smokers—current and former. However, since lung cancer among never-smokers accounts for an estimated 400,000 cases of lung cancer worldwide annually, identification of other high-risk populations who might benefit from either targeted prevention efforts or screening is potentially useful in reducing lung cancer mortality. In addition, only approximately 5–18% of smokers develop lung cancer (Mattson et al. 1987), so identifying higher-risk smokers would also be useful in directing both prevention and screening strategies, as the Gail model has done for breast cancer (Gail et al. 1989).

A risk prediction model for lung cancer would be useful for physicians and patients in weighing the relative risks and benefits of either a prevention or screening strategy. Identifying higher-risk populations would also improve the ability to investigate new prevention or screening approaches. Models that identify a small proportion of the population with a high risk of developing lung cancer would be most useful.

There have been several attempts to develop lung cancer risk prediction models (Cassidy et al. 2007). Age and smoking history are usually incorporated in these models but are insufficient to define the highest risk population. In the Bach model, based on data from the randomized, placebo-controlled prevention Carotene and Retinol Efficacy Trial (CARET) (Omenn et al. 1994), additional factors included duration of abstinence, duration of smoking, smoking intensity, study arm (study drug or placebo), sex, and asbestos exposure. Application of this model to a subset of the Mayo Clinic low-dose computed tomography (CT) screening trial demonstrated a wide range of predicted 10-year lung cancer risk from <1.0% to 15%. In addition, about 50% of lung cancers were predicted to occur in the highest risk quartile, suggesting the model could be used to select a very-high-risk cohort for prevention or early detection interventions (Bach et al. 2003).

Two risk prediction models, based on the randomized, controlled Prostate, Lung, Colorectal, and Ovarian (PLCO) Cancer Screening Trial, incorporated a number of variables including socioeconomic status, body mass index (BMI), family history of lung cancer, COPD, and recent chest radiograph, in addition to age and smoking history (Tammemagi et al. 2011). One model was for the general population and the second for ever-smokers. This model performed well across genders and in both whites and nonwhites. A predictive nomogram from this model is shown in Fig. 23.2.

The nomogram can be used as follows. For each individual predictor listed in the left column, identify the individual's value on the line to the right, draw a perpendicular line to the top points' line, and obtain the point value. Carry this out for each predictor

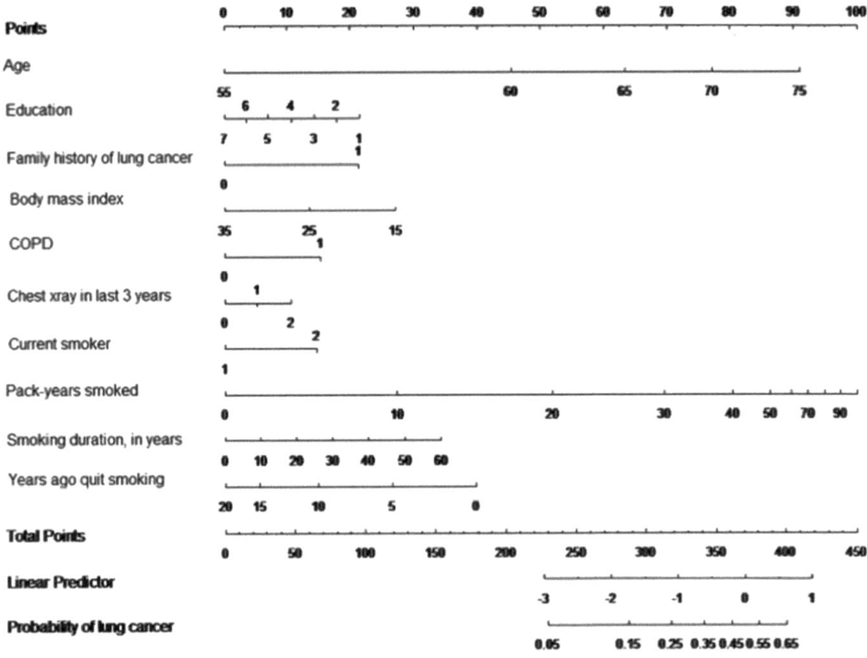

Fig. 23.2 Lung cancer risk prediction nomogram for estimating 9-year probability of lung cancer in former or current smokers

and add the points' values to get the total points. Draw a perpendicular line down from the total points' line to the probability of lung cancer line to obtain the probability of lung cancer value for the individual.

For example, an individual whose age is 65 years (63 points), who has a high school education, (14 points), a family history of lung cancer (21 points), a BMI of 25 (13 points), COPD (14 points), chest radiographs on two occasions in the past three years (10 points), who is a current smoker (14 points) with a 50-pack-year smoking history (85 points) and who smoked for a duration of 50 years (28 points), and has a quit time of 0 (is a current smoker) (37 points) has total points of 299, which by a perpendicular line connects down to a nine-year probability of lung cancer of 0.18% or 18 %.

Nomogram Predictors

Education: 1=less than eight years, 2=8–11 years, 3=12 years or completed high school, 4=after high school training, 5=some college, 6=college graduate, and 7=postgraduate.

For family history of lung cancer and COPD (chronic obstructive pulmonary disease), 1 represents that a past history is present.

Body mass index is weight in kilograms divided by height in meters squared.

Chest X-ray (in last three years): 0=none, 1=on one occasion, and 2=on two or more occasions.

Current smoker: 2 = yes, 1 = no.

Pack-years smoked are the average number of packages smoked per day times the number of years smoked.

Several lung cancer risk models have been described based on a case-control study of lung cancers at the University of Texas MD Anderson Cancer Center (Spitz et al. 2007). A model for never-smokers incorporated exposure to environmental tobacco smoke and family history of lung cancer; a former smoker model included emphysema, absence of hay fever, dust exposure, and family history; the current smoker model included asbestos exposure and family history.

In the future, identification of biological and genetic markers that can be combined with demographic and epidemiologic variables should result in further improvements in lung cancer risk prediction (Dunn et al. 2010).

23.6 Lung Cancer Prevention in Clinical Practice

Lung cancer prevention efforts in clinical practice currently involve control of tobacco use (Kelley and McCrory 2003). Chemoprevention trials to date have not demonstrated the efficacy of any agents in reducing lung cancer incidence or mortality (Kelley and McCrory 2003; Caraballoso et al. 2003). However, because former smokers remain at an elevated lifetime risk of lung cancer, identifying effective chemoprophylactic agents remains an attractive strategy.

23.6.1 Tobacco Cessation

Control of tobacco use is the most important element in lung cancer prevention worldwide. As tobacco use has declined over the last five decades in the USA, lung cancer incidence has followed, but unfortunately, there has been a plateau in adult smoking rates at about 20% in the last 5 years (Dube et al. 2009). From a public health perspective, continued focus on tobacco cessation remains an essential component of efforts to reduce lung cancer mortality.

About 70% of smokers indicate a desire to stop smoking, and there is no other single intervention that will positively impact the health of patients more than helping them succeed. Advice by the physician or another clinician has been shown to significantly increase long-term abstinence rates.

The Agency for Healthcare Research and Quality (AHRQ) published a clinical practice guideline and a quick reference tool for clinicians that provides a very useful framework for incorporating smoking control efforts into practice (PHS Guideline Update Panel, et al. 2008; U.S. Department of Health and Human Services 2009; Fiore and Baker 2011). As pointed out in this guideline, tobacco use is a chronic disease, effective treatments exist, but achieving success may require repeated interventions. Clinicians and health care systems should develop a systematic

Table 23.1 The 5 "As" of tobacco cessation therapy

Ask—systematically identify tobacco users at every visit
Advise—strongly urge tobacco users to quit
Assess—determine the willingness to make a quit attempt
Assist—aid the patient in quitting (counseling and medication)
Arrange—ensure follow-up contact

approach to assessment of tobacco use and intervention for tobacco users. The AHRQ guideline outlines a "5 As" model for managing tobacco dependence in clinical practice (Table 23.1). The assessment phase allows categorizing patients into three groups: (1) those willing to quit now, (2) those unwilling to quit now, and (3) those who have recently quit. Each group requires a different focus.

Tobacco use status should be incorporated into the vital signs, and preferably the electronic medical record, and updated at each encounter. However, incorporating smoking status into the vital signs alone does not result in improved cessation rates (Piper et al. 2003) and should be combined with promptings to discuss cessation (McCullough et al. 2009; Seale et al. 2010). All tobacco users should be strongly encouraged to stop, and those interested in quitting should be assisted in developing their quit plan and offered supportive counseling and appropriate medications. Combined counseling and pharmacologic therapy has been shown to be more effective than either modality alone. A variety of medications are FDA approved for treatment of tobacco dependence (Ebbert et al. 2007) (Table 23.2).

Smokers who currently express an unwillingness to quit should be counseled in an attempt to increase their motivation to eliminate their tobacco dependence. Recent quitters should be assessed for relapse risk and offered supportive counseling and, if necessary, medication. All three groups should have follow-up in the office or by telephone. While smoking cessation should be the goal of intervention, reduction in smoking intensity has been shown to reduce the risk of lung cancer (Godtfredsen et al. 2005).

23.6.2 Chemoprevention

Based on epidemiologic evidence that diets high in vegetable and fruit content might be protective for lung cancer, several large randomized, controlled trials were conducted in the 1980s–1990s to determine if antioxidant vitamin supplements could reduce lung cancer incidence and mortality. The α-tocopherol, β-carotene (ATBC) Lung Cancer Prevention Study compared the effects of these two agents on lung cancer incidence in Finnish male smokers. There was no effect observed for α-tocopherol, but the group receiving β-carotene experienced an 18% increase in risk of lung cancer (Alpha-Tocopherol Beta Carotene Cancer Prevention Study Group 1994). In the β-Carotene and Retinol Efficacy Trial (CARET), the combination of these two agents was compared with placebo. The intervention arm demonstrated

Table 23.2 Pharmacotherapies for treatment of tobacco dependence

	Medication	Precautions/comments	Dosing
First line	Bupropion hydrochloride	Seizure disorder, eating disorder	150 mg daily for 3 days, then twice daily; start 1–2 weeks prior to quit date; continue at least 12 weeks, up to 6 months
	Varenicline	Renal disease; may cause depression, sleep disturbance; nausea common	0.5 mg daily for 3 days, 0.5 mg twice daily for 4 days, then 1 mg twice daily; start 1 week prior to quit date; continue 12–24 weeks
	Nicotine gum (OTC) 2 or 4 mg	May cause dry mouth, dyspepsia; caution in people with dental disease	≤ 20 CPD—2 mg up to 24 per day >20 CPD—4 mg up to 24 per day
	Nicotine patch (OTC) 24 h systems—21, 14, 7 mg/24 h 16 h systems—15 mg/16 h	Ease of use, skin reactions	21 mg/h for 4 weeks, 14 mg/h for 2 weeks, 7 mg/h for 2 weeks
	Nicotine nasal spray	Rapid delivery, flexible dosing; nasal and eye irritation	1 spray each nostril up to 5 per hour or 40 per day
	Nicotine inhaler	Flexible dosing, well tolerated	6–16 cartridges per day
	Nicotine lozenge (OTC) 2 or 4 mg	Ease of use; heartburn, nausea common	<20 CPD—2 mg >20 CPD—4 mg Use 1–2 lozenges every 1–2 h
Second line	Nortriptyline	Many potential side effects	Initial 25 mg daily, increase to 75–100 mg as needed, start 10–28 days prior to quit date, continue 12 weeks
	Clonidine	Many potential side effects	0.10 mg orally twice daily or 0.10-mg patch daily, start 3 days prior to quit date, continue 3–10 weeks

OTC = available over the counter; CPD = cigarettes per day

a 28% increase in lung cancer incidence, a 46% increase in lung cancer mortality, and a 17% increase in all-cause mortality (Omenn et al. 1996). Recent reviews and meta-analyses of trials utilizing vitamin A and retinoids (Fritz et al. 2011) or β-carotene (Gallicchio et al. 2008) for prevention of lung cancer concluded that there is no demonstrated benefit of these compounds and that β-carotene may be detrimental, particularly in high-risk individuals. Furthermore, in a large cohort study of vitamin and supplement use in Washington State, the use of supplements containing β-carotene, retinol, or lutein was associated with higher risk of lung cancers (Satia et al. 2009).

Epidemiologic studies have suggested an inverse relationship between dietary selenium and lung cancer risk (van den Brandt et al. 1993) (Zhuo et al. 2004). In general, trials of selenium supplementation have not demonstrated a reduction in cancer incidence (Dennert et al. 2011). In the Nutritional Prevention of Cancer (NPC) Trial, subjects with nonmelanoma skin cancers were randomized to receive selenium supplements or placebo and were followed for the development of various cancers over 13 years (Clark et al. 1996). Selenium supplementation reduced the total and prostate cancer incidence (Duffield-Lillico et al. 2002). Overall lung cancer incidence was not decreased in the group receiving selenium supplementation; however, in the subjects with the lowest baseline plasma selenium levels, there appeared to be a significant reduction in lung cancer risk (Reid et al. 2002).

Despite the biologic and epidemiologic evidence that vitamins and micronutrients may play a role in carcinogenesis, there is little evidence for benefit of supplements from randomized trials, and increasingly there is the suggestion that supplements may prove harmful, as demonstrated for β-carotene in the ATBC and CARET trials, and in the Selenium and Vitamin E Prevention Trial (SELECT), which showed a 17% increased risk of prostate cancer in subjects receiving vitamin E supplements (Klein et al. 2011).

A number of specific molecular pathways that are involved in the pathogenesis of lung cancer are now being studied as potential chemoprevention and therapeutic targets (Hirsch and Lippman 2005). A prime candidate is the prostaglandin-arachidonic acid pathway. Use of aspirin and other nonsteroidal anti-inflammatory agents (NSAIDs) has been associated with a reduction in lung cancer risk (Khuder et al. 2005; Slatore et al. 2009; Van Dyke et al. 2008), but this effect has not been consistently demonstrated (Hayes et al. 2006). Celecoxib, an inhibitor of cyclooxygenase-2 (COX-2), has been shown to decrease markers of proliferation and inflammation in the bronchial epithelium of former smokers, and the decline in proliferative biomarker was associated with a decrease in the size of pulmonary nodules (Mao et al. 2011).

Another interesting target is the family of peroxisome proliferator-activated receptors (PPARs). These nuclear receptors are ligand-activated transcription regulators involved in control of a variety of cellular functions, including differentiation and apoptosis, and they interact with arachidonic acid metabolic pathways (Hirsch and Lippman 2005). Thiazolidinediones are PPARγ ligands used to treat diabetes mellitus. In a retrospective study, a 33% statistically significant reduction in lung cancer was observed in patients receiving one of these agents, compared to other agents for treatment of diabetes (Govindarajan et al. 2007).

23.6.3 Prevention in Clinical Practice: Summary

The mainstay of prevention continues to be tobacco avoidance and cessation measures. No randomized controlled trials of dietary interventions have been shown to reduce lung cancer risk. Based on the epidemiologic evidence, it is reasonable to recommend a diet low in red meat and high in fresh fruit, cruciferous vegetables, and soy products. Alcohol should be used in moderation, but moderate red wine intake may have a protective effect. There is no evidence to support the recommendation of vitamin, mineral, or trace element supplementation for reduction of lung cancer risk, and there is the possibility of harm with these supplements. At the present time, chemoprevention remains an area of active investigation, but there are no agents with established clinical effectiveness.

23.7 Lung Cancer Screening

While lung cancer prevention through avoidance of tobacco use is a very important strategy for reducing the lung cancer burden, it is not sufficient as the sole approach for a number of reasons. First, even with effective tobacco control programs, there remains a large pool of former smokers who will remain at increased risk for lung cancer. Furthermore, it has been difficult to achieve abstinence rates above 80%, and in many parts of the world, tobacco control efforts are poorly organized and limited in scope. As a result, there will be a large pool of smokers and former smokers who remain at risk in the foreseeable future. In addition, 15–25% of lung cancers occur in never-smokers.

23.7.1 Lung Cancer Screening Modalities

Lung cancer screening studies have focused primarily on radiographic screening with either chest radiograph (CXR) or chest computed tomography (CT) scans or sputum cytology. However, several other modalities have potential for lung cancer screening, particularly development of biomarkers.

23.7.1.1 Sputum Cytology

Cytologic analysis of sputum for the presence of malignant cells is a simple, commonly available, and relatively inexpensive technique used in the diagnosis of pulmonary neoplasms and could potentially contribute to screening for lung cancer. This approach might be particularly effective in detection of more centrally located tumors located in the proximal bronchial tree.

In the early 1970s, the National Cancer Institute (NCI) sponsored the "NCI Cooperative Early Lung Cancer Group," including Mayo Clinic, Memorial Sloan-Kettering Cancer Center (MSKCC), and Johns Hopkins. This resulted in three randomized trials carried out at these institutions to study the effect of CXR and sputum cytology on early detection and mortality from lung cancer (Berlin et al. 1984). Eligibility for these trials required males, age 45 or older, and smoking of one or more packs per day. The MSKCC and Hopkins trials (Melamed et al. 1984; Tockman et al. 1985) compared annual CXR to CXR and sputum cytology. While these studies demonstrated that 43% of squamous cancers were detected exclusively by sputum cytology, no reduction in lung cancer mortality could be demonstrated (Melamed et al. 1984; Tockman et al. 1985; Tockman 1986).

A more recent analysis of combined data from the MSKCC and Hopkins trials with a mean follow-up of 7.2 years suggested that there may be an approximate 10% mortality reduction attributed to screening with sputum cytology (Doria-Rose et al. 2009). This benefit occurred in the heaviest smokers and was the result of fewer deaths from squamous and large cell cancers. These trials were limited to male smokers, so conclusions about women and never-smokers cannot be drawn.

23.7.1.2 Chest Radiography (CXR)

Interest in screening for lung cancer with CXR dates to the 1960s when several trials compared CXR to routine care (Brett 1968; Brett 1969; Friedman et al. 1986). No lung cancer mortality reduction was demonstrated.

While the MSKCC and Hopkins trials in the NCI Cooperative Early Lung Cancer Group evaluated the role of sputum cytology, the Mayo Lung Project (MLP) studied the role of CXR in screening for lung cancer (Berlin et al. 1984). In the MLP, all subjects underwent an initial screen with CXR and sputum cytology before randomization into screened and control groups. The screened group was to receive CXR and sputum cytology every 4 months, and the control group was *advised* to have an annual CXR and sputum cytology. The screened group had an excess of lung cancers, a higher rate of resectability, and improved 5-year survival rate. However, the overall and lung cancer-specific mortality rates were no different between the screened and control groups (Fontana et al. 1986). The MLP has undergone extensive reanalysis to try to understand these findings. Follow-up has now extended an additional 16 years and demonstrates a persistent excess of cases in the screened arm, despite the cessation of screening after 3 years. This finding lends strong support to the presence of overdiagnosis in the MLP (Marcus et al. 2006).

Overdiagnosis is the identification of cancers through screening that would not have otherwise been discovered during the lifetime of the subject due either to indolent clinical behavior or the presence of competing causes of mortality or both (Welch and Black 2010). While overdiagnosis is a well-established phenomenon in screening for breast and prostate cancers, the concept of indolent lung cancer has been considered untenable by many clinicians.

In a Czech randomized screening trial, a similar finding of a persistent excess of lung cancers in the screened group was reported (Kubik et al. 2000). In these CXR screening trials, overdiagnosis of lung cancer is estimated to exceed 20% of screen-detected lung cancers.

Screening with CXR and more recently with low-dose chest computed tomography (LDCT) detects a higher proportion of adenocarcinomas, and many of these tumors have a doubling time >400 days (Hasegawa et al. 2000; Lindell et al. 2007) which is consistent with indolent clinical behavior. The occurrence of overdiagnosis of lung cancer is also supported by necropsy series demonstrating clinically unrecognized lung cancers unrelated to the cause of death (McFarlane et al. 1986). Thus, there is now convincing evidence that overdiagnosis does occur when screening for lung cancer.

The early trials of CXR screening were limited by small sample size and the occurrence of a high frequency of screening (contamination) in the control groups, raising concern that a small but clinically important benefit from CXR screening might have been missed. In 1993, the NCI initiated the Prostate, Lung, Colorectal, and Ovarian (PLCO) Cancer Screening Trial (Prorok et al. 2000) to determine whether screening programs reduce mortality in these cancers. PLCO was powered to detect a 10% reduction in lung cancer mortality.

PLCO enrolled 154,901 participants; 77,445 were randomized to the screening arm and received four annual CXRs. The lung component of PLCO differed from prior lung cancer screening trials in several important respects, including the inclusion of women and never-smokers, the absence of scheduled CXR screening in the control group, and the large sample size (Hocking et al. 2010). Screenings were conducted at ten centers across the United States with a compliance rate of 86% and contamination in the control group of only 11%. Overall, 7.5% of screens were positive, and the positive predictive value was 1.7%. Through 13 years of follow-up, lung cancer incidence was 20.1 per 10,000 person-years, with 1213 lung cancer deaths in the screened group and 19.2 and 1230, respectively, in the control group. Thus, there was no evidence of a reduction in mortality with CXR screening (Oken et al. 2011). Overdiagnosis, defined as the excess of lung cancers in the screened group compared with the usual care group, is estimated to account for approximately 6% of the lung cancers in the screened group.

The PLCO trial is the largest randomized screening trial ever conducted on CXR screening and provides strong evidence that screening for lung cancer with CXR does not result in a reduction in lung cancer mortality with long-term follow-up, the primary goal of any screening program.

23.7.1.3 Low-Dose Computed Tomography (LDCT)

Continuous advances in multidetector CT now permit high-resolution imaging of the chest in a single breath hold. Low-radiation-dose CT can be performed without loss of image quality (Nadich et al. 1990). In the 1990s, several groups began

Table 23.3 National Lung Screening Trial eligibility and exclusions

Eligibility	Age 55–74 years
	≥30 pack-years smoking history
	Former smokers quit ≤15 years
Exclusions	Previous lung cancer diagnosis
	Chest CT within 18 months
	Hemoptysis
	Unexplained weight loss >15 lbs

single-arm trials evaluating LDCT screening for lung cancer in high-risk populations. The Early Lung Cancer Action Project (ELCAP) began in 1992 and compared the performance of a baseline CXR and LDCT in the same patients (Henschke et al. 1999). The ELCAP demonstrated that LDCT compared with CXR detected noncalcified nodules in 23% vs. 7% and lung cancers in 2.7% vs. 0.7%, respectively. Of the cancers detected by LDCT, 85% were stage I, and 96% were resectable. ELCAP was subsequently expanded to a collaboration among investigators in several countries, known as International-ELCAP (I-ELCAP). In a baseline and subsequent annual screening program, I-ELCAP reported that 85% of cancers were stage I and estimated the 10-year survival of all cancers detected to be 80%, 88% for stage I cancers (International Early Lung Cancer Action Program Investigators 2006). Several other groups have reported results of observational, single-arm LDCT screening programs (Diederich et al. 2004; Sobue et al. 2002; Sone et al. 2001; Swensen et al. 2005; Menezes et al. 2010; Pastorino et al. 2003; Toyoda et al. 2008; Wilson et al. 2008).

While the results from ELCAP, I-ELCAP, and other observational studies provide useful information about the performance of LDCT screening and on the surface appear to show a benefit of screening, lessons from earlier screening trials have demonstrated that survival rates are improved by early detection, even if there is no reduction in mortality rate, and the only approach that can conclusively determine the benefit of a screening program is a randomized controlled trial (Welch et al. 2007).

In 2002, the NCI initiated the National Lung Screening Trial (NLST), a randomized study comparing annual LDCT to CXR screening over 3 years, powered to detect a 20% mortality reduction (National Lung Screening Trial Research Team 2011a). The decision to use a CXR control group was based on the PLCO, which was ongoing at that time, in the event that a mortality benefit was demonstrated from CXR screening (Church and National Lung Screening Trial Executive Committee 2003). Screening was conducted at 33 sites in the United States. The eligibility and exclusion criteria for NLST are shown in Table 23.3.

The NLST randomized 53,454 participants from 2002 to 2004, and screening was completed in 2007 for the entire group. By October 2010, with a median follow-up of 6.5 years, there were 247 deaths from lung cancer in the LDCT group and 309 in the CXR group, representing a 20% reduction in lung cancer mortality in the LDCT arm (National Lung Screening Trial Research Team 2011b). This is the first demonstration that any screening modality reduces deaths from lung cancer and represents a milestone in lung cancer management. In addition, all-cause mortality was reduced by 6.7% in the LDCT group, suggesting that the effects of screening were not otherwise deleterious.

In the NLST, 6.9% of CXR and 24.2% of LDCT were considered positive, but 94.5% and 96.4%, respectively, were false positives, similar to findings from other lung cancer radiographic screening trials. Thus, of all screening examinations, 23.3% of LDCTs and 6.5% of CXRs were false positives.

In both groups, the diagnostic evaluation after a positive screening test was most commonly further imaging tests. An invasive diagnostic procedure (percutaneous needle biopsy, bronchoscopy, mediastinoscopy, thoracoscopy, or thoracotomy) occurred in 9.6% of the screen positives in the LDCT group and in 12.8% of the CXR group. One or more complications after further diagnostic testing occurred in 1.4% and 1.6% of the participants in the LDCT and CXR groups, respectively. In the LDCT group, major complications occurred in 0.06% of those without a subsequent cancer diagnosis and 11.2% in those diagnosed with lung cancer, compared with 0.02% and 8.2% in the CXR group. Complications from lung cancer screening programs often relate to percutaneous biopsy of lung nodules. In a retrospective review of 15,865 patients who underwent needle transthoracic needle biopsy, pneumothorax occurred in 15.0% (6.6% requiring chest tube) but only 1.0% experienced hemorrhage (Wiener et al. 2011). In the LDCT arm, there were 16 deaths (10 in participants with lung cancer) within 60 days of an invasive diagnostic procedure, out of 18,146 positive screens (0.09%) and in the CXR arm, there were 10 deaths (all had lung cancer) out of 5043 positive screens (0.20%).

At the time of NLST reporting, there were 645 lung cancers per 100,000 person-years in the LDCT group and 572 in the CXR group, representing an excess of 13% in the LDCT arm, which may reflect overdiagnosis. Longer follow-up will be necessary to clarify the amount of overdiagnosis in NLST.

Aside from the immediate complications of the diagnostic evaluation resulting from a positive screen and the impact of overdiagnosis, exposure to radiation through repeated radiographic procedures is the other major concern with screening for lung cancer (Huppmann et al. 2010). While the risk of radiation exposure depends on the characteristics of the population being screened as well as the screening program, it has been estimated that LDCT screening annually for smokers and former smokers beginning at age 50 could add 0.5–5.5% additional risk of lung cancer (Brenner 2004).

There are several smaller randomized trials of LDCT screening for lung cancer ongoing in Europe (Pastorino et al. 2003), including the Dutch-Belgian (NELSON) (van Iersel et al. 2007), Danish (DLCST) (Pedersen et al. 2009), DANTE (Infante et al. 2009), Italian (ITALUNG) (Pegna et al. 2009), and German (LUSI) (Becker and Kauczor 2008) trials and the United Kingdom trial (UKLS) scheduled to start in 2012. These studies will provide additional data on mortality reduction, overdiagnosis, cost-effectiveness, and the effect of different screening intervals and durations.

23.7.1.4 Biomarkers

Biomarkers have been defined as an objectively measured feature that is an indicator of normal biologic processes, pathogenic processes, or the pharmacologic response to a therapeutic intervention (Biomarkers Definitions Working Group 2001). Biomarkers may be molecular, biochemical, physiologic, anatomic, or histologic features (Dunn et al. 2010).

In lung cancer, biomarkers are being evaluated in blood, sputum, and exhaled breath. In the blood, one promising approach is the identification of unique patterns of serum proteins in patients with early lung cancer (Han et al. 2008; Yildiz et al. 2007). One panel of serum biomarkers including carcinoembryonic antigen (CEA), retinol-binding protein, α1-antitrypsin, and squamous cell carcinoma antigen correctly classified 71.4% of patients with cancer and 66.6% of those without cancer in a validation study (Patz et al. 2007). Another panel of six blood biomarkers correctly classified 95% of cases, and the receiver-operating curve (ROC) area under the curve (AUC) was 0.979 (Farlow et al. 2010a). Using electrospray ionization mass spectrometry, early stage lung cancer patients were distinguished from controls with a sensitivity of 0.84, specificity 0.71, and an AUC 0.87 (Hocker et al. 2011).

Tumors provoke a humoral immune response, and antibodies directed to tumor antigens can be detected in serum prior to the development of symptoms (Qiu et al. 2008) as well as in early stage lung cancers (Chapman et al. 2008; Leidinger et al. 2010). Single autoantibodies have low sensitivity due to tumor heterogeneity, but a panel of antibodies has much greater sensitivity for detection of lung cancers (Lam et al. 2011). Several autoantibody panels have been reported for lung cancer detection (Lam et al. 2011; Farlow et al. 2010b; Leidinger et al. 2010). A panel of three autoantibodies (annexin I, 14-3-3theta, LAMR1) yielded a receiver-operating curve AUC of 0.73 in detection of presymptomatic lung cancer (Qiu et al. 2008).

A panel of autoantibodies to six tumor-related antigens (p53, NY-ESO-1, CAGE, GBU4-5, Annexin 1, SOX2) has demonstrated a sensitivity of 31–43% (overall about 40%) and specificity of 84–89% and was positive in both early and late stage lung cancers (Boyle et al. 2011; Lam et al. 2011; Murray et al. 2010). This assay is now being marketed by Oncimmune as *EARLY*CDT™ and shows promise as an early detection test in high-risk populations.

Another approach to lung cancer biomarkers is the detection of aberrant nucleic acid patterns. A variety of abnormalities in DNA and RNA can be detected, including oncogene mutations, mutations of tumor suppressor genes (p53), promoter hypermethylation, and microsatellite abnormalities (Ziegler et al. 2002; Bremnes et al. 2005). Mutations in circulating DNA can be detected in a majority of lung cancer patients, even in early stage patients, but at this time not with the sensitivity to provide an early detection test (Andriani et al. 2004). Plasma-free DNA levels are elevated in lung cancer patients, compared to normal controls (Sozzi et al. 2003; Paci et al. 2009), but in a study of plasma DNA levels in patients undergoing LDCT screening, this test was not able to discriminate lung cancer patients from those without cancer (Sozzi et al. 2009). It may be that release of DNA into the blood from lung cancer is a relatively late event that would reduce the utility in detecting small early cancers, but more study is required.

Specific genetic markers can be detected in sputum of lung cancer patients (Li et al. 2007), and a panel of six genes was shown to have higher sensitivity than sputum cytology for detection of stage I or II non-small-cell lung cancer (NSCLC) (81.4% vs. 41.9%) with high specificity (96.2% vs. 100%, respectively) (Jiang et al. 2010). The use of fluorescence in situ hybridization (FISH) testing for specific genetic targets (Varella-Garcia et al. 2010) and detection of aberrant microRNA (miRNA) patterns in sputum (Xie et al. 2010) also show promise for early detection. In a small study of stage I NSCLC patients, combining sputum FISH analysis with CT scanning was shown to improve the accuracy of diagnoses, particularly for central tumors (Jiang et al. 2009). Sputum studies are more sensitive to centrally located and squamous cancers.

Aberrant DNA methylation occurs in lung cancer, affecting genes that are relevant to the process of carcinogenesis, such as the p16 tumor suppressor gene (Belinsky et al. 1998; Lamy et al. 2002). This change can be detected in circulating DNA (Tsou et al. 2002) as well as in sputum (Palmisano et al. 2000) and bronchial lavage (Kim et al. 2004; Topaloglu et al. 2004) specimens. The pattern of serum DNA methylation in a panel of genes has been used to distinguish patients with lung cancer from controls without cancer (Begum et al. 2011). Preliminary data show that this approach may be useful in distinguishing patients with lung cancer from those with a false-positive finding on LDCT lung screen (Ostrow et al. 2010). A panel of genes in sputum has also been shown to increase the prediction of lung cancer but with a sensitivity and specificity of only 64% (Belinsky et al. 2006).

MicroRNAs (miRNAs) are noncoding RNAs involved in regulation of gene expression (Bartel 2004) and are commonly aberrantly regulated in cancer (Croce 2009). MiRNA abnormalities are present in lung cancer (Lin et al. 2010), and patterns of miRNA can distinguish histologic subtypes of lung cancer and may be useful as prognostic and predictive markers (Fanini et al. 2011). Aberrant miRNA patterns in the blood can be detected in early stage NSCLC, and specific patterns have been shown to perform well in predicting the presence of early lung cancer with receiver-operating curve AUCs of 0.75 (Foss et al. 2011) and 0.926 (Shen et al. 2011). A panel of 34 miRNAs tested in participants in the Italian COSMOS LDCT screening trial demonstrated a sensitivity of 71%, a specificity of 90%, and an AUC of 0.89 (Bianchi et al. 2011). Altered miRNA patterns in sputum samples may also be useful in the early detection of squamous lung cancers (Xing et al. 2010). There are distinct gene expression profiles in the peripheral blood of patients with NSCLC that can be detected in early stage cancers and may also have potential for early detection (Showe et al. 2009; Zander et al. 2011).

Another approach to biomarker discovery in lung cancer among smokers is examination of tobacco-specific carcinogens. One of the most potent carcinogens in tobacco smoke is 4-(methylnitrosamino)-1-(3-pyridyl)-1-butanone (NNK), which is metabolized to 4-(methylnitrosamino)-1-(3-pyridyl)-1-butanol (NNAL), that can be measured in both serum and urine (Church et al. 2009; Yuan et al. 2009). Elevated levels of serum NNAL (Church et al. 2009) and urinary NNAL (Yuan et al. 2009) are associated with an increased risk of subsequent lung cancer. This finding has implications both for identification of high-risk populations among smokers and potentially for development of chemoprevention agents.

An interesting approach to detection of lung cancer is through the analysis of exhaled breath (Amann et al. 2011; Chan et al. 2009; Mazzone 2008). Exhaled breath contains both volatile organic compounds (VOC) that can be measured and characterized by gas chromatography and mass spectroscopy and nonvolatile compounds that can be analyzed in exhaled breath condensates. Lung cancer patients have distinct patterns of VOC in exhaled breath that can be used to distinguish them from patients without cancer (Phillips et al. 1999). A variety of sensor systems are being studied that have the potential for clinical application (Machado et al. 2005; Mazzone et al. 2007). A model using a colorimetric sensor array combined with clinical parameters showed an AUC 0.811, sensitivity 70%, and specificity 86% in distinguishing NSCLC from controls (Mazzone et al. 2012). Recently, gold nanoparticle sensors have been used to detect lung cancer (Peng et al. 2009) and distinguish lung cancer histologies (Barash et al. 2011). An example of exhaled breath condensate is the measurement of several angiogenic markers, which in a preliminary study, showed excellent discrimination of lung cancer patients from healthy individuals and patients with chronic lung disease (Gessner et al. 2010).

23.7.2 Lung Cancer Screening in Clinical Practice

Until late 2010, there was little to support screening for lung cancer in clinical practice (Manser et al. 2004). The most recent United States Public Health Service Preventive Services Task Force guideline, published in 2004, concludes that current data do not support screening for lung cancer by any modality but indicates that the data are also insufficient to conclude that screening is not effective (Humphrey et al. 2004; U.S. Preventive Services Task Force 2004).

Publication of the NLST results has changed the landscape. There is now definitive evidence that LDCT screening can reduce mortality from lung cancer (National Lung Screening Trial Research Team 2011b). The National Comprehensive Cancer Network (NCCN) published a lung cancer screening guideline for the first time (NCCN Clinical Practice Guidelines in Oncology 2012). This guideline recommends screening individuals who meet the NLST eligibility criteria but also suggest screening for patients who meet all three of the following criteria: 50 years or older with 20 or more pack-years smoking history and one additional lung cancer risk factor. The NCCN guideline recommends annual LDCT screening until age 74, although there are no data on the benefit or risks of a screening program of this duration. Other public health groups are reviewing the data and will likely issue lung cancer screening recommendations in the near future. These guidelines will evolve as data from cost-effectiveness analyses, modeling studies, and the results of ongoing randomized lung cancer screening trials become available.

Table 23.4 Lung cancer screening: unanswered questions

Who should be screened?
People who meet the NLST eligibility criteria
Other risk groups (e.g., <30 pack-years smoking, family history of lung cancer, occupational exposure, radon exposure)
What is the most effective approach to diagnostic evaluation after a positive LDCT screen?
How often should LDCT screens be performed?
How long should LDCT screening continue?
What is the optimal interval for LDCT screening?
What are the most effective criteria for a positive LDCT?
What is the extent of overdiagnosis with LDCT screening?
What is the cost-effectiveness of LDCT screening?
What effect does LDCT screening have on quality of life?
What is the health risk of radiation exposure from LDCT screening?
How can LDCT be combined with biomarker studiers to improve screening performance?

The International Association for the Study of Lung Cancer (IASLC) conducted a workshop on lung cancer screening in 2011 after publication of the NLST results. The IASLC is focusing on the development of guidelines and recommendations for (1) identification of high-risk individuals for screening, (2) developing national screening programs, (3) evaluation of "indeterminate" pulmonary nodules discovered on LDCT, (4) pathology reporting for nodules discovered by screening, (5) surgical and therapeutic interventions for nodules identified by screening, and (6) integration of smoking cessation practices into lung cancer screening programs (Field et al. 2012).

While the NLST results are paradigm changing, many questions remain unanswered (Table 23.4).

Although funding for large randomized trials to resolve all of these issues may not be available, cost-effectiveness analyses and modeling studies will help to provide some of the answers. Cost issues are important in the United States and Western Europe, but in many areas of the world, LDCT is simply not available for mass screening of high-risk populations. It is imperative that the benefit of screening does not compromise continued vigorous tobacco control efforts globally. Most third-party payers have not approved coverage for LDCT lung cancer screening in late 2011, although one large insurer, WellPoint, has decided to cover LDCT for patients who meet the NLST eligibility criteria (Matthews 2011).

For the clinician, the NLST results provide a rationale to consider lung cancer screening in high-risk patients who meet the NLST eligibility guidelines. In addition, other risk groups, such as those defined in the NCCN guideline, may benefit from screening, although more research in this area is needed. It is important that patients being offered LDCT screening are informed about the potential risks as well as benefits of screening (Table 23.5).

When considering screening, it is imperative that the diagnostic resources to follow-up or further evaluate abnormalities discovered on the screening LDCT are available. Guidelines for follow-up and management of small pulmonary nodules

Table 23.5 Potential pros and cons of LDCT lung cancer screening

Pros	Cons
Reduced lung cancer mortality	False-positive LDCT, resulting in:
	Anxiety, stress
	Unnecessary testing
Teachable moment for smoking cessation	Overdiagnosis
	Morbidity and mortality from diagnostic testing
	Radiation exposure with increased risk of secondary malignancies
	False-negative examinations
	Cost to health care system

Table 23.6 Fleischner Society guidelines for management of pulmonary nodules (MacMahon et al. 2005)

Recommendations for follow-up and management of nodules smaller than 8 mm detected incidentally at nonscreening computed tomography (CT)

Nodule size (mm)a	Low-risk patient[b]	High-risk patient[c]
≤4	No follow-up needed[d]	Follow-up CT at 12 months; if unchanged, no further follow-up[e]
>4–6	Follow-up CT at 12 months; if unchanged, no further follow-up[e]	Initial follow-up CT at 6–12 months, then at 18–24 months if no change[e]
>6–8	Initial follow-up CT at 6–12 months, then at 18–24 months if no change[e]	Initial follow-up CT at 3–6 months, then at 9–12 and 24 months if no change[e]
>8	Follow-up CT at around 3, 9, and 24 months; dynamic contrast-enhanced CT, PET, and/or biopsy	Same as for low-risk patient

Note: Newly detected indeterminate nodule in persons 35 years of age or older

[a]Average of length and width

[b]Minimal or absent history of smoking and of other known risk factors

[c]History of smoking or of other known risk factors

[d]The risk of malignancy in this category (<1%) is substantially less than that in a baseline CT scan of an asymptomatic smoker

[e]Nonsolid (ground glass) or partly solid nodules may require longer follow-up to exclude indolent adenocarcinoma

from the Fleischner Society (Table 23.6) (MacMahon et al. 2005), and more recently a preliminary guideline for management of subsolid nodules (Godoy and Naidich 2009), provide a useful approach to clinical practice. The use of lung nodule volume and volume-doubling time may also be useful in management of these patients (van Klaveren et al. 2009).

Institutions that establish a formal program for LDCT screening for lung cancer should strongly consider linking the screening process to interventions aimed at smoking cessation. The screening process can serve as a "teachable moment" used to encourage and support smoking cessation (Taylor et al. 2007; Townsend et al. 2005). A recent cost-effectiveness analysis of LDCT screening projected that unless screening was associated with an increase in smoking cessation, the cost of screening was $126,000–$169,000 per quality-adjusted life year (QALY), substantially higher than screening costs for other cancers. If screening resulted in doubling of quit rates, the cost of screening was estimated to be $75,000 per QALY, more in line with other screening programs (Evans and Wolfson 2011; McMahon et al. 2011).

23.8 Conclusions

There is now clear evidence that screening for lung cancer with LDCT scans can reduce lung cancer mortality. While controversy over the risks and benefits of LDCT screening continues (Jett and Midthun 2011; Silvestri 2011), LDCT can be offered in the appropriate clinical settings to high-risk patients. Development of clinically validated biomarkers will improve the accuracy of screening and should further shift the risk benefit balance in favor of screening. An active area of investigation is the combination of radiographic and biomarker screening. Despite the proven benefit of LDCT screening, smoking cessation must remain a high priority and should be an integral component of any screening program.

Aside from tobacco use prevention and cessation, there are no clearly effective prevention strategies available. In the future, identification of agents that target pathways involved in lung carcinogenesis holds the potential to reduce lung cancer incidence and mortality. While most attention is focused on prevention and screening in current or former smokers, lung cancer among never-smokers is a major cause of mortality, and identification of high-risk populations of never-smokers who might benefit from these approaches should not be ignored.

References

Alberg AJ, Brock MV, Samet JM. Epidemiology of lung cancer: looking to the future. *J Clin Oncol* 2005; 23:3175-3185.

Alavanja MC. Biologic damage resulting from exposure to tobacco smoke and from radon: implication for preventive interventions. *Oncogene* 2002; 21:7365-7375.

Alpha-Tocopherol, Beta Carotene Cancer Prevention Study Group. The effect of vitamin E and beta carotene on the incidence of lung cancer and other cancers in male smokers. *N Engl J Med* 1994; 330:1029-1035.

Amann A, Corradi M, Mazzone P, Mutti A. Lung cancer biomarkers in exhaled breath. *Expert Rev Mol Diagn* 2011; 11:207-217.

Amos CI, Wu X, Broderick P, Gorlov IP, Gu J, Eisen T, et al. Genome-wide association scan of tag SNPs identifies a susceptibility locus for lung cancer at 15q25.1. *Nat Genet* 2008; 40:616-622.

Andriani F, Conte D, Mastrangelo T, Leon M, Ratcliffe C, Roz L, et al. Detecting lung cancer in plasma with the use of multiple genetic markers. *Int J Cancer* 204; 108:91-96.

Bach PB, Kattan MW, Thornquist MD, Kris MG, Tate RC, Barnett MJ, et al. Variations in lung cancer risk among smokers. *J Natl Cancer Inst* 2003; 95:470-478.

Baik CS, Strauss GM, Speizer FE, Feskanich D. Reproductive factors, hormone use, and risk for lung cancer in postmenopausal women, the Nurses' Health Study. *Cancer Epidemiol Biomarkers Prev* 2010; 19:2525-2533.

Bailey-Wilson JE, Amos CI, Pinney SM, Petersen GM, de Andrade M, Wiest JS, et al. A major lung cancer susceptibility locus maps to chromosome 6q23-25. *Am J Hum Genet* 2004; 75:460-474.

Barash O, Peled N, Tisch U, Bunn PA Jr, Hirsch FR, Haick H. Classification of lung cancer histology by gold nanoparticle sensors. *Nanomedicine* 2011;[Epub ahead of print].

Bartel DP. MicroRNAs: genomics, biogenesis, mechanism, and function. *Cell* 2004; 116:281-297.

Becker NDS, Kauczor HU. LUSI: the German component of the European trial on the efficacy of multi-slice CT for the early detection of lung cancer. *Onkologie* 2008; 31:320.

Begum S, Brait M, Dasgupta S, Ostrow KL, Zahurak M, Carvalho AL, et al. An epigenetic marker panel for detection of lung cancer using cell-free serum DNA. *Clin Cancer Res* 2011; 17:4494-4503.

Benhamou S, Lee WJ, Alexandrie A-K, Boffetta P, Couchardy C, Butkiewicz D, et al: Meta- and pooled analyses of the effects of glutathione S-transferase M1 polymorphisms and smoking on lung cancer risk. *Carcinogenesis* 2002; 23:1343-1350.

Belinsky SA, Liechty KC, Gentry FD, Wolf HJ, Rogers J, Vu K, et al. Promoter hypermethylation of multiple genes in sputum precedes lung cancer incidence in a high-risk cohort. *Cancer Res* 2006; 66:3338-3344.

Belinsky SA, Nikula KJ, Palmisano WA, Michels R, Saccomanno G, Gabrielson E, et al. Aberrant methylation of p16(INK4a) is an early event in lung cancer and a potential biomarker for early diagnosis. *Proc Natl Acad Sci U S A* 1998; 95:11891-11896.

Berlin NI, Buncher CR, Fontana RS, Frost JK, Melamed MR. The National Cancer Institute Cooperative Early Lung Cancer Detection Program. Results of the initial screen (prevalence). Early lung cancer detection: Introduction. *Am Rev Respir Dis* 1984; 130:545-549.

Bianchi F, Nicassio F, Marzi M, Belloni E, Dall'olio V, Bernard L, et al. A serum circulating miRNA diagnostic test to identify asymptomatic high-risk individuals with early stage lung cancer. *EMBO Mol Med* 2011; 3:495-503.

Biomarkers Definitions Working Group. Biomarkers and surrogate endpoints: preferred definitions and conceptual framework. *Clin Pharmacol Ther* 2001; 69:89-95.

Boyle P, Chapman CJ, Holdenrieder S, Murray A, Robertson C, Wood WC, et al. Clinical validation of an autoantibody test for lung cancer. *Ann Oncol* 2011; 22:383-389.

Bremnes RM, Sirera R, Camps C. Circulating tumour-derived DNA and RNA markers in blood: a tool for early detection, diagnostics, and follow-up? *Lung Cancer* 2005; 49:1-12.

Brennan P, Hainaut P, Boffetta P. Genetics of lung-cancer susceptibility. *Lancet Oncol* 2011; 12:399-408.

Brennan P, McKay J, Moore L, Zaridze D, Mukeria A, Szeszenia-Dabrowska N, et al. Uncommon CHEK2 mis-sense variant and reduced risk of tobacco-related cancers: case control study. *Hum Mol Genet* 2007; 16:1794-1801.

Brenner DJ. Radiation risks potentially associated with low-dose CT screening of adult smokers for lung cancer. *Radiology* 204; 231:440-445.

Brenner DR, McLaughlin JR, Hung RJ. Previous lung diseases and lung cancer risk: a systematic review and meta-analysis. *PLoS One* 2011; 31:e17479.

Brett GZ. The value of lung cancer detection by six-monthly chest radiographs. *Thorax* 1968; 23:414-420.

Brett GZ. Earlier diagnosis and survival in lung cancer. *Br Med J* 1969; 4:260-262.

Caraballoso M, Sacristan M, Serra C, Bonfill X. Drugs for preventing lung cancer in healthy people. *Cochrane Database of Syst Rev* 2003:CD002141.

Cassidy A, Duffy SW, Myles JP, Liloglou T, Field JK. Lung cancer risk prediction: a tool for early detection. *Int J Cancer* 2007; 120:1-6.

Centers for Disease Control and Prevention (CDC). Vital signs: current cigarette smoking among adults aged >or=18 years---United States, 2005-2010. *MMWR Morb Mortal Wkly Rep.* 2011a; 60:1207-12.

Centers for Disease Control and Prevention, Atlanta, GA. *Behavioral Risk Factor Surveillance System Survey.* 2011b. Available at: http://apps.nccd.cdc.gov/brfss.

Centers for Disease Control and Prevention (CDC). Vital signs: nonsmokers' exposure to seconhand smoke --- United States, 1999-2008. *MMWR Morb Mortal Wkly Rep.* 2010b; 59:1141-1146.

Chan HP, Lewis C, Thomas PS. Exhaled breath analysis: novel approach for early detection of lung cancer. *Lung Cancer* 2009; 63:164-168.

Chao C. Associations between beer, wine, and liquor consumption and lung cancer risk: a meta-analysis. *Cancer Epidemiol Biomarkers Prev* 2007; 16:2436-2447.

Chao C, Slezak JM, Caan BJ, Quinn VP. Alcoholic beverage intake and risk of lung cancer: the California Men's Health Study. *Cancer Epidemiol Biomarkers Prev* 2008; 17:2692-2699.

Chapman CJ, Murray A, McElveen JE, Sahin U, Luxemburger U, Türeci O, et al. Autoantibodies in lung cancer: possibilities for early detection and subsequent cure. *Thorax* 2008; 63:228-233.

Chaturvedi AK, Caporaso NE, Katki HA, Wong HL, Chatterjee N, Pine SR, et al. C-reactive protein and risk of lung cancer. *J Clin Oncol* 2010; 28:2719-2726.

Chlebowski RT, Schwartz AG, Wakelee H, Anderson GL, Stefanick ML, Manson JE, et al. Oestrogen plus progestin and lung cancer in postmenopausal women (Women's Health Initiative trial): a post-hoc analysis of a randomised controlled trial. *Lancet* 2009; 374:1243-1251.

Church TR, National Lung Screening Trial Executive Committee. Chest radiography as the comparison for spiral CT in the National Lung Screening Trial. *Acad Radiol* 2003; 10:713-715.

Church TR, Anderson KE, Caporaso NE, Geisser MS, Le CT, Zhang Y, et al. A prospectively measured serum biomarker for a tobacco-specific carcinogen and lung cancer in smokers. *Cancer Epidemiol Biomarkers Prev* 2009; 18:260-266.

Clark LC, Combs GF Jr, Turnbull BW, Slate EH, Chalker DK, Chow J, et al. Effects of selenium supplementation for cancer prevention in patients with carcinoma of the skin. A randomized controlled trial. Nutritional Prevention of Cancer Study Group. *JAMA* 1996; 276:1957-1963.

Coté ML, Kardia SL, Wenzlaff AS, Ruckdeschel JC, Schwartz AG. Risk of lung cancer among white and black relatives of individuals with early-onset lung cancer. *JAMA* 2005; 293:3036-3042.

Crispo A, Brennan P, Jöckel KH, Schaffrath-Rosario A, Wichmann HE, Nyberg F, et al. The cumulative risk of lung cancer among current, ex- and never-smokers in European men. *Br J Cancer* 2004; 91:1280-1286.

Croce CM. Causes and consequences of microRNA dysregulation in cancer. *Nat Rev Genet* 2009; 10:704-714.

Darby S, Hill D, Doll R. Radon: a likely carcinogen at all exposures. *Ann Oncol* 2001; 12:1341-1351.

Dennert G, Zwahlen M, Brinkman M, Vinceti M, Zeegers MP, Horneber M. Selenium for preventing cancer. *Cochrane Database Syst Rev* 2011:CD005195.

Diederich S, Thomas M, Semik M, Lenzen H, Roos N, Weber A, et al. Screening for early lung cancer with low-dose spiral computed tomography: results of annual follow-up examinations in asymptomatic smokers. *Eur Radiol* 2004; 14:691-702.

Doll R, Peto R. Cigarette smoking and bronchial carcinoma: dose and time relationships among regular smokers and lifelong non-smokers. *J Epidemiol Community Health* 1978; 32:303-313.

Doll R, Peto R, Boreham J, Sutherland I. Mortality in relation to smoking: 50 years' observations on male British doctors. *BMJ* 2004; 328:1519 doi:10.1136/bmj.38142.554479.AE

Doria-Rose VP, Marcus PM, Szabo E, Tockman MS, Melamed MR, Prorok PC. Randomized controlled trials of the efficacy of lung cancer screening by sputum cytology revisited: a combined mortality analysis from the Johns Hopkins Lung Project and the Memorial Sloan-Kettering Lung Study. *Cancer* 2009; 115:5007-5017.

Dube SR, Asman K, Malarcher A, Carabollo R. Cigarette Smoking Among Adults and Trends in Smoking Cessation United States, 2008. MMWR Weekly 2009; 58:1227–1232.

Duffield-Lillico AJ, Reid ME, Turnbull BW, Combs GF Jr, Slate EH, Fischbach LA, et al. Baseline characteristics and the effect of selenium supplementation on cancer incidence in a randomized clinical trial: a summary report of the Nutritional Prevention of Cancer Trial. *Cancer Epidemiol Biomarkers Prev* 2002; 11:630-639.

Dunn BK, Wagner PD, Anderson D, Greenwald P. Molecular markers for early detection. *Semin Oncol* 2010; 37:224-242.

Ebbert JO, Sood A, Hays JT, Dale LC, Hurt RD. Treating tobacco dependence: review of the best and lastest treatment options. *J Thorac Oncol* 2007; 2:249-256.

Ebbert JO, Yang P, Vachon CM, Vierkant RA, Cerhan JR, Folsom AR, et al. Lung cancer risk reduction after smoking cessation: observations from a prospective cohort of women. *J Clin Oncol* 2003; 21:921-926.

Engels EA. Inflammation in the development of lung cancer: epidemiological evidence. *Expert Rev Anticancer Ther* 2008; 8:605-615.

Evans WK, Wolfson MC. Computed tomography screening for lung cancer without a smoking cessation program--not a cost-effective idea. *J Thorac Oncol* 2011; 6:1781-1783.

Fanini F, Vannini I, Amadori D, Fabbri M. Clinical Implications of MicroRNAs in Lung Cancer. *Semin Oncol* 2011; 38:776-780.

Farlow EC, Patel K, Basu S, Lee BS, Kim AW, Coon JS, et al. Development of a multiplexed tumor-associated autoantibody-based blood test for the detection of non-small cell lung cancer. *Clin Cancer Res* 2010a; 16:3452-3462.

Farlow EC, Vercillo MS, Coon JS, Basu S, Kim AW, Faber LP, et al. A multi-analyte serum test for the detection of non-small cell lung cancer. *Br J Cancer* 2010b; 103:1221-1228.

Field JK, Smith RA, Aberle DR, Oudkerk M, Baldwin DR, Yankelevitz D, et al. International Association for the Study of Lung Cancer Computed Tomography Screening Workshop 2011 Report. *J Thorac Oncol* 2012; 7:10-19.

Fiore MC, Baker TB. Clinical practice. Treating smokers in the health care setting. *N Engl J Med* 2011; 365:1222-1231.

Fontana RS, Sanderson DR, Woolner LB, Taylor WF, Miller WE, Muhm JR. Lung cancer screening: the Mayo Program. *J Occup Med* 1986; 28:746-750.

Foss KM, Sima C, Ugolini D, Neri M, Allen KE, Weiss GJ. miR-1254 and miR574-5p. serum-based microRNA biomarkers for early-stage non-small cell lung cancer. *J Thorac Oncol* 2011; 6:482-488.

Friedman GD, Collen MF, Fireman BH. Multiphasic Health Checkup Evaluation: a 16-year follow-up. *J Chronic Dis* 1986; 39:452-463.

Fritz H, Kennedy D, Fergusson D, Fernandes R, Doucette S, Cooley K, et al. Vitamin A and retinoid derivatives for lung cancer: a systematic review and meta analysis. *PLoS One* 2011; 6:e21107.

Gail MH, Brinton LA, Byar DP, Corle DK, Green SB, Schairer C, et al. Projecting individualized probabilities of developing breast cancer for white females who are being examined annually. *J Natl Cancer Inst* 1989; 81:1879-1886.

Gallicchio L, Boyd K, Matanoski G, Tao XG, Chen L, Lam TK, et al. Carotenoids and the risk of developing lung cancer: a systematic review. *Am J Clin Nutr* 2008; 88:372-383.

Gessner C, Rechner B, Hammerschmidt S, Kuhn H, Hoheisel G, Sack U, et al. Angiogenic markers in breath condensate identify non-small cell lung cancer. *Lung Cancer* 2010; 68:177-184.

Ginsberg RJ, Rubinstein LV. Randomized trial of lobectomy versus limited resection for T1 N0 non-small cell lung cancer. Lung Cancer Study Group. *Ann Thorac Surg* 1995; 60:615-623.

Godoy MC, Naidich DP. Subsolid pulmonary nodules and the spectrum of peripheral adenocarcinomas of the lung: recommended interim guidelines for assessment and management. *Radiology* 2009; 253:606-622.

Godtfredsen NS, Prescott E, Osler M. Effect of smoking reduction on lung cancer risk. *JAMA* 2005; 294:1505-1510.

Goldstraw P, Crowley J, Chansky K, Giroux DJ, Groome PA, Rami-Porta R, et al. The IASLC Lung Cancer Staging Project: proposals for the revision of the TNM stage groupings in the forthcoming (seventh) edition of the TNM Classification of malignant tumours. *J Thorac Oncol* 2007; 2:706-714.

Govindarajan R, Ratnasinghe L, Simmons DL, Siegel ER, Midathada MV, Kim L, et al. Thiazolidinediones and the risk of lung, prostate, and colon cancer in patients with diabetes. *J Clin Oncol* 2007; 25:1476-1481.

Han KQ, Huang G, Gao CF, Wang XL, Ma B, Sun LQ, et al. Identification of lung cancer patients by serum protein profiling using surface-enhanced laser desorption/ionization time-of-flight mass spectromety. *Am J Clin Oncol* 2008; 31:133-139.

Hasegawa M, Sone S, Takashima S, Li F, Yang ZG, Maruyama Y, et al. Growth rate of small lung cancers detected on mass CT screening. *Br J Radiol* 2000; 73:1252-1259.

Hayes JH, Anderson KE, Folsom AR. Association between nonsteroidal anti-inflammatory drug use and the incidence of lung cancer in the Iowa women's health study. *Cancer Epidemiol Biomarkers Prev* 2006; 15:2226-2231.

Henschke CI, McCauley DI, Yankelevitz DF, Naidich DP, McGuinness G, Miettinen OS, et al. Early Lung Cancer Action Projecrt: overall design and findings from baseline screening. *Lancet* 1999; 354:99-105.

Hirsch FR, Lippman SM. Advances in the biology of lung cancer chemoprevention. *J Clin Oncol* 2005; 23:3186-3197.

Hocker JR, Peyton MD, Lerner MR, Mitchell SL, Lightfoot SA, Lander TJ, et al. Serum discrimination of early-stage lung cancer patients using electrospray-ionization mass spectrometry. *Lung Cancer* 2011; 74:206-211.

Hocking WG, Hu P, Oken MM, Winslow SD, Kvale PA, Prorok PC, et al. Lung cancer screening in the randomized Prostate, Lung, Colorectal, and Ovarian (PLCO) Cancer Screening Trial. *J Natl Cancer Inst* 2010; 102:722-731.

Humphrey LL, Teutsch S, Johnson M, U.S. Preventive Services Task Force. Lung cancer screening with sputum cytologic examination, chest radiography, and computed tomography: an update for the U.S. Preventive Services Task Force. *Ann Intern Med* 2004; 140:740-753.

Hung RJ, McKay JD, Gaborieau V, Boffetta P, Hashibe M, Zaridze D, et al. A susceptibility locus for lung cancer maps to nicotinic acetylcholine receptor subunit genes on 15q25. *Nature* 2008; 452:633-637.

Hwang SJ, Lozano G, Amos CI, Strong LC. Germline p53 mutations in a cohort with childhood sarcoma: sex differences in cancer risk. *Am J Hum Genet* 2003; 72:975-983.

Infante M, Cavuto S, Lutman FR, Brambilla G, Chiesa G, Ceresoli G, et al. A randomized study of lung cancer screening with spiral computed tomography: three-year results from the DANTE trial. *Am J Respir Crit Care Med* 2009; 180:445-453.

International Early Lung Cancer Action Program Investigators, Henschke CI, Yankelevitz DF, Libby DM, Pasmantier MW, Smith JP, et al. Survival of patients with stage I lung cancer detected on CT screening. *N Engl J Med* 2006; 355:1763-1771.

Jemal A, Bray F, Center MM, Ferlay J, Ward E, Forman D. Global cancer statistics. *CA Cancer J Clin* 2011; 61:69-90.

Jett JR, Midthun DE. Screening for lung cancer: for patients at increased risk for lung cancer, it works. *Ann Intern Med* 2011; 155:540-542.

Jiang F, Todd NW, Qiu Q, Liu Z, Katz RL, Stass SA. Combined genetic analysis of sputum and computed tomography for noninvasive diagnosis of non-small-cell lung cancer. *Lung Cancer* 2009; 66:58-63.

Jiang F, Todd NW, Li R, Zhang H, Fang H, Stass SA. A panel of sputum-based genomic marker for early detection of lung cancer. *Cancer Prev Res (Phila).* 2010; 3:1571-1578.

Johansson M, Relton C, Ueland PM, Vollset SE, Midttun Ø, Nygård O, et al. Seurm B vitamin levels and risk of lung cancer. *JAMA* 2010; 202:2377-2385.

Jonsson S, Thorsteinsdottir U, Gudbjartsson DF, Jonsson HH, Kristjansson K, Arnason S, et al. Familial risk of lung carcinoma in the Icelandic population. *JAMA* 2004; 292:2977-2983.

Kelley MJ, McCrory DC. Prevention of lung cancer: summary of published evidence. *Chest* 2003; 123:50S-59S.

Khuder SA, Herial NA, Mutgi AB, Federman DJ. Nonsteroidal antiinflammatory drug use and lung cancer: a metaanalysis. *Chest* 2005; 127:748-754.

Kim H, Kwon YM, Kim JS, Lee H, Park JH, Shim YM, et al. Tumor-specific methylation in bronchial lavage for the early detection of non-small-cell lung cancer. *J Clin Oncol* 2004; 22:2363-2370.

Kim DH, Park SE, Kim M, Ji YI, Kang MY, Jung EH, et al. A functional single nucleotide polymorphism at the promoter region of cyclin A2 is associated with increased risk of colon, liver, and lung cancers. *Cancer* 2011; 117:4080-4091.

Klein EA, Thompson IM Jr, Tangen CM, Crowley JJ, Lucia MS, Goodman PJ, et al. Vitamin E and the risk of prostate cancer: the Selenium and Vitamin E Cancer Prevention Trial (SELECT). *JAMA* 2011; 206:1549-1546.

Kohler BA, Ward E, McCarthy BJ, Schymura MJ, Ries LA, Eheman C, et al. Annual report to the nation on the status of cancer, 1975-2007, featuring tumors of the brain and other nervous system. *J Natl Cancer Inst.* 2011; 103:714-736.

Korte JE, Brennan P, Henley SJ, Boffetta P. Dose-specific meta-analysis and sensitivity analysis of the relation between alcohol consumption and lung cancer risk. *Am J Epidemiol* 2002; 155:496-506.

Koshiol J, Rotunno M, Consonni D, Pesatori AC, De Matteis S, Goldstein AM, et al. Chronic obstructive pulmonary disease and altered risk of lung cancer in a population-based case-control study. *PLoS One* 2009; 4:e7380.

Krewski D, Lubin JH, Zielinski JM, Alavanja M, Catalan VS, Field RW, et al. Residential radon and risk of lung cancer: a combined analysis of 7 North American case-control studies. *Epidemiology* 2005; 16:137-145.

Kubik AK, Parkin DM, Zatloukal P. Czech Study on Lung Cancer Screening: post-trial follow-up of lung cancer deaths up to year 15 since enrollment. *Cancer* 2000; 89:2363-2368.

Lam S, Boyle P, Healey GF, Maddison P, Peek L, Murray A, et al. EarlyCDT-Lung: an immunobiomarker test as an aid to early detection of lung cancer. *Cancer Prev Res* 2011; 4:1126-1134.

Lam TK, Cross AJ, Consonni D, Randi G, Bagnardi V, Bertazzi PA, et al. Intakes of red meat, processed meat, and meat mutagens increase lung cancer risk. *Cancer Res* 2009; 69:932-939.

Lam TK, Gallicchio L, Lindsley K, Shiels M, Hammond E, Tao XG, et al. Cruciferous vegetable consumption and lung cancer risk: a systematic review. *Cancer Epidemiol Biomarkers Prev* 2009; 18:184-195.

Lamy A, Sesboüé R, Bourguignon J, Dautréaux B, Métayer J, Frébourg T, et al. Aberrant methylation of the CDKN2a/p16INK4a gene promoter region in preinvasive bronchial lesions: a prospective study in high-risk patients without invasive cancer. *Int J Cancer* 2002; 100;189-193.

Landi MT, Chatterjee N, Yu K, Goldin LR, Goldstein AM, Rotunno M, et al. A genome-wide association study of lung cancer identifies a region of chromosome 5p15 associated wtih risk for adenocarcinoma. *Am J Hum Genet* 2009; 85:679-691.

Leidinger P, Keller A, Heisel S, Ludwig N, Rheinheimer S, Klein V, et al. Identification of lung cancer with high sensitivity and specificity by blood testing. *Respir Res* 2010; 11:18 doi:10.1186/1465-9921-11-18

Li R, Todd NW, Qiu Q, Fan T, Zhao RY, Rodgers WH, et al. Genetic deletions in sputum as diagnostic markers for early detection of stage I non-small cell lung cancer. *Clin Cancer Res* 2007; 13:482-487.

Lin PY, Yu SL, Yang PC. MicroRNA in lung cancer. *Br J Cancer* 2010; 103:1144-1148.

Lindell RM, Hartman TE, Swensen SJ, Jett JR, Midthun DE, Tazelaar HD, et al. Five-year lung cancer screening experience: CT appearance, growth rate, location, and histologic features of 61 lung cancers. *Radiology* 2007; 242:555-562.

Linseisen J, Rohrmann S, Miller AB, Bueno de Mesquita, B, Buchner FL, Agudo A et al. Fruits and vegetable consumption and lung cancer risk: Updated information from the European Prospective Investigation into Cancer and Nutrition (EPIC). Int J Cancer 2007; 121: 1103-1114.

Lubin JH. Environmental factors in cancer: radon. *Rev Environ Health* 2010; 25:33-38.

Machado RF, Laskowski D, Deffenderfer O, Burch T, Zheng S, Mazzone PJ, et al. Detection of lung cancer by sensor array analyses of exhaled breath. *Am J Respir Crit Care Med* 2005; 171:1286-1291.

MacMahon H, Austin JH, Gamsu G, Herold CJ, Jett JR, Naidich DP, et al. Guidelines for management of small pulmonary nodules detected on CT scans: a statement from the Fleischner Society. *Radiology* 2005; 237:395-400.

Männistö S, Smith-Warner SA, Spiegelman D, Albanes D, Anderson K, van den Brandt PA, et al. Dietary carotenoids and risk of lung cancer in a pooled analysis of seven cohort studies. *Cancer Epidemiol Biomarkers Prev* 2004; 13:40-48.

Manser RL, Irving LB, Stone C, Byrnes G, Abramson M, Campbell D. Screening for lung cancer. *Cochrane Database Syst Rev.* 2004:CD001991.

Mao JT, Roth MD, Fishbein MC,Aberle DR, Zhang ZF, Rao JY, et al. Lung cancer chemoprevention with celecoxib in former smokers. *Cancer Prev Res (Phila)* 2011; 4:984-993.

Marcus PM, Bergstralh EJ, Zweig MH, Harris A, Offord KP, Fontana RS. Extended lung cancer incidence follow-up in the Mayo Lung Project and overdiagnosis. *J Natl Cancer Inst* 2006; 98:748-756.

Matakidou A, Eisen T, Houlston RS. Systematic review of the relationship between family history and lung cancer risk. *Br J Cancer* 2005; 93:825-833.

Matthews AW. WllPoint to Cover Lung Ct Scans for Heavy Smokers. Health Blog. *Wall Street Journal.* December 1, 2011. Available at: blogs.wsj.com/health/2011/12/01/wellpoint-to-cover-lung-ct-scans-for-heavy-smokers/.

Mattson ME, Pollack ES, Cullen JW. What are the odds that smoking will kill you? *Am J Public Health* 1987; 77:425-431.

Mayne ST, Buenconsejo J, Janerich DT. Previous lung disease and risk of lung cancer among men and women nonsmokers. *Am J Epidemiol* 1999; 149:13-20.

Mazzone PJ. Analysis of volatile organic compounds in the exhaled breath for the diagnosis of lung cancer. *J Thorac Oncol* 2008; 3:774-780.

Mazzone PJ, Hammel J, Dweik R, Na J, Czich C, Laskowski D, et al. Diagnosis of lung cancer by the analysis of exhaled breath with a colorimetric sensor array. *Thorax* 2007; 62:565-568.

Mazzone PJ, Wang XF, Xu Y, Mekhail T, Beukemann MC, Na J, Kemling JW, et al. Exhaled breath analysis with a colorimetric sensor array for the identification and characterization of lung cancer. *J Thorac Oncol* 2012; 7:137-142.

McCullough A, Fisher M, Goldstein AO, Kramer KD, Ripley-Moffitt C. Smoking as a vital sign: prompts to ask and assess increase cessation counseling. *J Am Board Fam Med* 2009; 22:625-632.

McFarlane MJ, Feinstein AR, Wells CK. Necropsy evidence of detection bias in the diagnosis of lung cancer. *Arch Intern Med* 1986; 146:1695-1698.

McMahon PM, Kong CY, Bouzan C, Weinstein MC, Cipriano LE, Tramontano AC, et al. Cost-effectiveness of computed tomography screening for lung cancer in the United States. *J Thorac Oncol* 2011; 6:1841-1848.

Melamed MR, Flehinger BJ, Zaman MB, Heelan RT, Perchick WA, Martini N. Screening for early lung cancer. Results of the Memorial Sloan-Kettering study in New York. *Chest* 1984; 86:44-53.

Menezes RJ, Roberts HC, Paul NS, McGregor M, Chung TB, Patsios D, et al. Lung cancer screening using low-dose computed tomography in at-risk individuals: the Toronto experience. *Lung Cancer* 2010; 67:177-183.

Miller AB, Altenburg HP, Bueno-de-Mesquita B, Boshuizen HC, Agudo A, Berrino F, et al. Fruits and vegetables and lung cancer: Findings from the European Prospective Investigation into Cancer and Nutrition. *Int J Cancer* 2004; 108:269-276.

Murray A, Chapman CJ, Healey G, Peek LJ, Parsons G, Baldwin D, et al. Technical validation of an autoantibody test for lung cancer. *Ann Oncol* 2010; 21:1687-1693.

Nadich DP, Marshall CH, Gribbin C, Arams RS, McCauley DI. Low-dose CT of the lungs: preliminary observations. *Radiology* 1990; 175:729-731.

Naruke T, Goya T, Tsuchiya R, Suemasu K. Prognosis and survival in resected lung carcinoma based on the new international staging system. *J Thorac Cardiovasc Surg* 1988; 96:440-447.

National Lung Screening Trial Research Team, Aberle DR, Berg CD, Black WC, Church TR, Fagerstrom RM, et al. The National Lung Screening Trial: overview and study design. *Radiology* 2011a; 258:243-253.

National Lung Screening Trial Research Team, Aberle DR, Adams AM, Berg CD, Black WC, Clapp JD, et al. Reduced lung-cancer mortality with low-dose computed tomographic screening. *N Engl J Med* 2011b; 365:395-409.

Naurath N, Jones JM. Smoking rates around the world – how do Americans CompareF? *Gallup News Service*. August 17, 2007. Available at: http://www.gallup.com/poll/28432/smoking-rates-around-world-how-american-compare.aspx.

NCCN Clinical Practice Guidelines in Oncology, Lung Cancer Screening, Version 1.2012, http://www.nccn.org/professionals/physician_gls/f_guidelines.asp

Neuberger JS, Field RW. Occupation and lung cancer in nonsmokers. *Rev Environ Health* 2003; 18:251-267.

Oken MM, Hocking WG, Kvale PA, Andriole GL, Buys SS, Church TR, et al. Screening by chest radiograph and lung cancer mortality: the Prostate, Lung Colorectal, and Ovarian (PLCO) randomized trial. *JAMA* 2011; 306:1865-1873.

Omenn GS, Goodman G, Thornquist M, Grizzle J, Rosenstock L, Barnhart S, et al. The beta-carotene and retinol efficacy trial (CARET) for chemoprevention of lung cancer in high risk populations: smokers and asbestos-exposed workers. *Cancer Res* 1994; 54:2038s-2043s.

Omenn GS, Goodman GE, Thornquist MD, Balmes J, Cullen MR, Glass A, et al. Effects of a combination of beta carotene and vitamin A on lung cancer and cardiovascular disease. *N Engl J Med* 1996; 234:1150-1155.

Ostrow KL, Hoque MO, Loyo M, Brait M, Greenberg A, Siegfried JM, et al. Molecular anlaysis of plasma DNA for the early detection of lung cancer by quantitative methylation-specific PCR. *Clin Cancer Res* 2010; 16:3463-3472.

Paci M, Maramotti S, Bellesia E, Formisano D, Albertazzi L, Ricchetti T, et al. Circulating plasma DNA as diagnostic biomarker in non-small cell lung cancer. *Lung Cancer* 2009; 64:92-97.

Palmisano WA, Divine KK, Saccomanno G, Gilliland FD, Baylin SB, Herman JG, et al. Predicting lung cancer by detecting aberrant promoter methylation in sputum. *Cancer Res* 2000; 60:5954-5958.

Pastorino U, Bellomi M, Landoni C, De Fiori E, Arnaldi P, Picchio M, et al. Early lung-cancer detection with spiral CT and positron emission tomography in heavy smokers: 2-year results. *Lancet* 2003; 362:593-597.

Patz EF Jr, Campa MJ, Gottlin EB, Kusmartseva I, Guan XR, Herdon JE 2nd. Panel of serum biomarkers for the diagnosis of lung cancer. *J Clin Oncol* 2007; 25:5578-5583.

Pedersen JH, Ashraf H, Dirksen A, Bach K, Hansen H, Toennesen P, et al. The Danish randomized lung cancer CT screening trial--overall design and results of the prevalence round. *J Thorac Oncol* 2009; 4:608-614.

Pegna AL, Picozzi G, Mascalchi M, Maria Carozzi F, Carrozzi L, Comin C, et al. Design, recruitment and baseline results of the ITALUNG trial for lung cancer screening with low-dose CT. *Lung Cancer* 2009; 64:34-40.

Peng G, Tisch U, Adams O, Hakim M, Shehada N, Broza YY, et al. Diagnosing lung cancer in exhaled breath using gold nanoparticles. *Nat Nanotechno* 2009; 4:669-673.

Phillips M, Gleeson K, Hughes JM, Greenberg J, Cataneo RN, Baker L, et al. Volatile organic compounds in breath as markers of lung cancer: a cross-sectional study. *Lancet* 1999; 353:1930-1933.

PHS Guideline Update Panel 2008, Liaisons, and Staff. Treating tobacco use and dependence: 2008 update U.S. Public Health Service Clinical Practice Guideline executive summary. *Respir Care*. 2008; 53:1217-1222.

Pine SR, Mechanic LE, Enewold L, Chaturvedi AK, Katki HA, Zheng YL, et al. Increased levels of circulating interleukin 6, interleukin 8, C-reactive protein, and risk of lung cancer. *J Natl Cancer Inst* 2011; 103:1112-1122.

Pirkle JL, Bernert JT, Caudill SP, Sosnoff CS, Pechacek TF. Trends in the exposure of nonsmokers in the U.S. population to secondhand smoke: 1988-2002. *Environ Health Perspect* 2006; 114:853-858.

Piper ME, Fiore MC, Smith SS, Jorenby DE, Wilson JR, Zahner ME, et al. Use of the vital sign stamp as a systematic screening tool to promote smoking cessation. *Mayo Clin Proc* 2003; 78:716-722.

Pope CA 3rd, Burnett RT, Thun MJ, Calle EE, Krewski D, Ito K, et al. Lung cancer, cardiopulmonary mortality, and long-term exposure to fine particulate air pollution. *JAMA* 2002; 287:1132-1141.

Prorok PC, Andriole GL, Bresalier RS, Buys SS, Chia D, Crawford ED, et al. Design of the Prostate, Lung, Colorectal and Ovarian (PLCO) Cancer Screening Trial. *Control Clin Trials* 2000; 21:273E-309S.

Qiu J, Choi G, Li L, Wang H, Pitteri SJ, Pereira-Faca SR, et al. Occurrence of autoantibodies to annexin I, 14-3-3 theta and LAMR1 in prediagnostic lung cancer sera. *J Clin Oncol* 2008;26:5060-5066.

Reid ME, Duffield-Lillico AJ, Garland L, Turnbull BW, Clark LC, Marshall JR. Selenium supplementation and lung cancer incidence: an update of the nutritional prevention of cancer trial. *Cancer Epidemiol Biomarkers Prev* 2002; 11:1285-1291.

Rodriguez C, Spencer Feigelson H, Deka A, Patel AV, Jacobs EJ, Thun MJ, et al. Postmenopausal hormone therapy and lung cancer risk in the cancer prevention study II nutrition cohort. *Cancer Epidemiol Biomarkers Prev* 2008; 17:655-660.

Samet JM, Humble CG, Pathak DR. Personal and family history of respiratory disease and lung cancer risk. *Am Rev Respir Dis* 1986; 134:466-470.

Satia JA, Littman A, Slatore CG, Galanko JA, White E. Long-term use of beta-carotene, retinol, lycopene, and lutein supplements and lung cancer risk: results from the VITamins And Lifestyle (VITAL) study. *Am J Epidemiol* 2009; 169:815-828.

Seale JP, Shellenberger S, Velasquez MM, Boltri JM, Okosun I, Guyinn M, et al. Impact of vital signs screening & clinician prompting on alcohol and tobacco screening and intervention rates: a pre-post intervention comparison. *BMC Fam Pract* 2010; 11:18 doi:10:1186/1471-2296-11-18

Shen J, Todd NW, Zhang H, Yu L, Lingxiao X, Mei Y, et al. Plasma microRNAs as potential biomarkers for non-small-cell lung cancer. *Lab Invest* 2011; 91:579-587.

Shiels MS, Albanes D, Virtamo J, Engels EA. Increased risk of lung cancer in men with tuberculosis in the alpha-tocopherol, beta-carotene cancer prevention study. *Cancer Epidemiol Biomarkers Prev* 2011; 20:672-678.

Showe MK, Vachani A, Kossenkov AV, Yousef M, Nichols C, Nikonova EV, et al. Gene expression profiles in peripheral blood mononuclear cells can distinguish patients with non-small cell lung cancer from patients with nonmalignant lung disease. *Cancer Res* 2009; 69:9202-9210.

Siegel R, Ward E, Brawley O, Jemal A. Cancer statistics 2011: the impact of eliminating socioeconomic and racial disparities on premature cancer deaths. *CA Cancer J Clin* 2011; 61:212-236.

Silvestri GA. Screening for lung cancer: it works, but does it really work? *Ann Intern Med* 2011; 155:537-539.

Skillrud DM, Offord KP, Miller RD. Higher risk of lung cancer in chronic obstructive pulmonary disease. A prospective, matched, controlled study. *Ann Intern Med* 1986; 105:503-507.

Slatore CG, Au DH, Littman AJ, Satia JA, White E. Association of nonsteroidal anti-inflammatory drugs with lung cancer: results from a large cohort study. *Cancer Epidemiol Biomarkers Prev* 2009; 18:1203-1207.

Slatore CG, Chien JW, Au DH, Satia JA, White E. Lung cancer and hormone replacement therapy: association in the vitamins and lifestyle study. *J Clin Oncol* 2010; 28:1540-1546.

Smith JR, Barrett-Connor E, Kritz-Silverstein D, Wingard DL, Al-Delaimy WK. Hormone use and lung cancer incidence: the Rancho Bernardo cohort study. *Menopause* 2009; 16:1044-1048.

Sobue T, Moriyama N, Kaneko M, Kusumoto M, Kobayashi T, Tsuchiya R, et al. Screening for lung cancer with low-dose helical computed tomography: anti-lung cancer association project. *J Clin Oncol* 2002; 20:911-920.

Sone S, Li F, Yang ZG, Honda T, Maruyama Y, Takashima S, et al. Results of three-year mass screening programme for lung cancer using mobile low-dose spiral computed tomography scanner. *Br J Cancer* 2001; 84:25-32.

Sozzi G, Conte D, Leon M, Ciricione R, Roz L, Ratcliffe C, et al. Quantification of free circulating DNA as a diagnostic marker in lung cancer. *J Clin Oncol* 2003; 21:3902-3908.

Sozzi G, Roz L, Conte D, Mariani L, Andriani F, Lo Vullo S, et al. Plasma DNA quantification in lung cancer computed tomography screening: five-year results of a prospective study. *Am J Respir Crit Care Med* 2009; 179:69-74.

Spitz MR, Hong WK, Amos CI, Wu X, Schabath MB, Dong Q, et al. A risk model for prediction of lung cancer. *J Natl Cancer Inst* 2007; 99:715-726.

Sun S, Schiller JH, Gazdar AF. Lung cancer in never smokers--a different disease. *Nat Rev Cancer* 2007; 7:778-790.

Steenland K, Loomis D, Shy C, Simonsen N. Review of occupational lung carcinogens. *Am J Ind Med* 1996; 29:474-490.

Swensen SJ, Jett JR, Hartman TE, Midthun DE, Mandrekar SJ, Hillman SL, et al. CT screening for lung cancer: five-year prospective experience. *Radiology* 2005; 235:259-265.

Tammemagi CM, Pinsky PF, Caporaso NE, Kvale PA, Hocking WG, Church TR, et al. Lung cancer risk prediction: Prostate, Lung, Colorectal And Ovarian Cancer Screening Trial models and validation. *J Natl Cancer Inst* 2011; 103:1058-1068.

Taylor KL, Cox LS, Zincke N, Mehta L, McGuire C, Gelmann E. Lung cancer screening as a teachable moment for smoking cessation. *Lung Cancer* 2007; 56:125-134.

Thun MJ, Hannan LM, DeLancey JO. Alcohol consumption not associated with lung cancer mortality in lifelong nonsmokers. *Cancer Epidemiol Biomarkers Prev* 2009; 18:2269-2272.

Thun MJ, Henley SJ, Calle EE. Tobacco use and cancer: an epidemiologic perspective for geneticists. *Oncogene* 2002; 21:7307-7325.

Tockman MS. Survival and mortality from lung cancer in a screened population. The Johns Hopkins study. *Chest* 1986; 89(Supp 4):324S-325S.

Tockman MS, Frost JK, Stitik FP, Levin ML, et al. *Screening and detection of lung cancer.* Vol. 3, in *Contemporary Issues in Clinical Oncology*, Aisner JA Ed. Philadelphia, PA; Churchill Livingstone, 1985.

Toh CK, Gao F, Lim WT, Leong SS, Fong KW, Yap SP, et al. Never-smokers with lung cancer: epidemiologic evidence of a distinct disease entity. *J Clin Oncol* 2006; 24:2245-2251.

Tokuhata GK, Lilienfeld AM. Familial aggregation of lung cancer among hospital patients. *Public Health Rep* 1963; 78:277-283.

Topaloglu O, Hoque MO, Tokumaru Y, Lee J, Ratovitski E, Sidransky D, et al. Detection of promoter hypermethylation of multiple genes in the tumor and bronchoalveolar lavage of patients with lung cancer. *Clin Cancer Res* 2004; 10:2284-2288.

Townsend CO, Clark MM, Jett JR, Patten CA, Schroeder DR, Nirelli LM, et al. Relation between smoking cessation and receiving results from three annual spiral chest computed tomography scans for lung carcinoma screening. *Cancer* 2005; 103:2154-2162.

Toyoda Y, Nakayama T, Kusunoki Y, Iso H, Suzuki T. Sensitivity and specificity of lung cancer screening using chest low-dose computed tomography. *Br J Cancer* 2008; 98:1602-1607.

Tsou JA, Hagen JA, Carpenter CL, Laird-Offringa IA. DNA methylation analysis: a powerful new tool for lung cancer diagnosis. *Oncogene* 2002;21:5450-5461.

Turner MC, Chen Y, Krewski D, Callee EE, Thun MJ. Chronic obstructive pulmonary disease is associated with lung cancer mortality in a prospective study of never smokers. *Am J Respir Crit Care Med* 2007; 176:285-290.

Turner MC, Krewski D, Pope CA 3rd, Chen Y, Gapstur SM, Thun MJ. Long-term Ambient Fine Particulate Matter Air Pollution and Lung Cancer in a Large Cohort of Never-Smokers. *Am J Respir Crit Care Med* 2011; 184:1374-1381.

U.S. Department of Health and Human Services, Public Health Service. Treating Tobacco Use and Dependence. *Quick Reference Guide for Clinicians: 2008 Update.* April 2009. ISSN-1530-6402. Available at: http://www.ahrq.gov/clinic/tobacco/tobaqrg.pdf.

U.S. Preventive Services Task Force. Lung cancer screening: recommendation statement. *Ann Intern Med* 2004; 140:738-739.

van den Brandt PA, Goldbohm RA, van't Veer P, Bode P, Dorant E, Hermus RJ, et al. A prospective cohort study on selenium status and the risk of lung cancer. *Cancer Res* 1993; 53:4860-4865.

Van Dyke AL, Cote ML, Prysak G, Claeys GB, Wenzlaff AS, Schwartz AG. Regular adult aspirin use decreases the risk of non-small cell lung cancer among women. *Cancer Epidemiol Biomarkers Prev* 2008; 17:148-157.

van Iersel CA, de Koning HJ, Draisma G, Mali WP, Scholten ET, Nackaerts K, et al. Risk-based selection from the general population in a screening trial: selection criteria, recruitment and power for the Dutch-Belgian randomised lung cancer multi-slice CT screening trial (NELSON). *Int J Cancer* 2007; 120:868-874.

van Klaveren RJ, Oudkerk M, Prokop M, Scholten ET, Nackaerts K, Vernhout R, et al. Management of lung nodules detected by volume CT scanning. *N Engl J Med* 2009; 361:2221-2229.

Varella-Garcia M, Schulte AP, Wolf HJ, Feser WJ, Zeng C, Braudrick S, et al. The detection of chromosomal aneusomy by fluorescence in situ hybridization in sputum predicts lung cancer incidence. *Cancer Prev Res (Phila)* 2010; 3:447-453.

Wakelee HA, Chang ET, Gomez SL, Keegan TH, Feskanich D, Clarke CA, et al. Lung cancer incidence in never smokers. *J Clin Oncol* 2007; 25:472-478.

Wang Y, Broderick P, Webb E, Wu X, Vijayakrishnan J, Matakidou A, et al. Common 5p15.33 and 6p21.33 variants influence lung cancer risk. *Nat Genet* 2008; 40:1407-1409.

Welch HG, Black WC. Overdiagnosis in cancer. *J Natl Cancer Inst* 2010; 102:605-613.

Welch HG, Woloshin S, Schwartz LM, Gordis L, Gotzsche PC, Harris R, et al. Overstating the evidence for lung cancer screening; the International Early Lung Cancer Action Program (I-ELCAP) study. *Arch Intern Med* 2007; 167:2289-2295.

Wiener RS, Schwartz LM, Woloshin S, Welch HG. Population-based risk for complications after transthoracic needle lung biopsy of a pulmonary nodule: an analysis of discharge records. *Ann Intern Med* 2011; 155:137-144.

Wilson DO, Weissfeld JL, Fuhrman CR, Fisher SN, Balogh P, Landreneau RJ, et al. The Pittsburgh Lung Screening Study (PLuSS): outcomes within 3 years of a first computed tomography scan. *Am J Respir Crit Care Med* 2008; 178:956-961.

Wright ME, Park Y, Subar AF, Freedman ND, Albanes D, Hollenbeck A, et al. Intakes of fruit, vegetables, and specific botanical groups in relation to lung cancer risk in the NIH-AARP Diet and Health Study. *Am J Epidemiol* 2008; 168:1024-1034.

Xie Y, Todd NW, Liu Z, Zhan M, Fang H, Peng H, et al. Altered miRNA expression in sputum for diagnosis of non-small cell lung cancer. *Lung Cancer* 2010; 67:170-176.

Xing L, Todd NW, Yu L, Fang H, Jiang F. Early detection of squamous cell lung cancer in sputum by a panel of microRNA markers. *Mod Pathol* 2010; 23:1157-1164.

Yang P, Sun Z, Krowka MJ, Aubry MC, Bamlet WR, Wampfler JA, et al. Alpha1-antitrypsin deficiency carriers, tobacco smoke, chronic obstructive pulmonary disease, and lung cancer risk. *Arch Intern Med* 2008; 168:1097-1103.

Yang WS, Va P, Wong MY, Zhang HL, Xiang YB. Soy intake is associated with lower lung cancer risk: results from a meta-analysis of epidemiologic studies. *Am J Clin Nutr* 2011; 94:1575-1583.

Yildiz PB, Shyr Y, Rahman JS, Wardwell NR, Zimmerman LJ, Shakhtour B, et al. Diagnostic accuracy of MALDI mass spectrometric analysis of unfractionated serum in lung cancer. *J Thorac Oncol* 2007; 2:893-901.

You M, Wang D, Liu P, Vikis H, James M, Lu Y, et al. Fine mapping of chromosome 6q23-25 region in familial lung cancer families reveals RGS17 as a likely candidate gene. *Clin Cancer Res* 2009; 15:2666-2674.

Yu YY, Pinsky PF, Caporaso NE, Chatterjee N, Baumgarten M, Langenberg P, et al. Lung cancer risk following detection of pulmonary scarring by chest radiography in the prostate, lung, colorectal, and ovarian cancer screening trial. *Arch Intern Med* 2008; 168:2326-2332.

Yuan JM, Koh WP, Murphy SE, Fan Y, Wang R, Carmella SG, et al. Urinary levels of tobacco-specific nitrosamine metabolites in relation to lung cancer development in two prospective cohorts of cigarette smokers. *Cancer Res* 2009; 69:2990-2995.

Zander T, Hofmann A, Staratschek-Jox A, Classen S, Debey-Pascher S, Maisel D, et al. Blood-based gene expression signatures in non-small cell lung cancer. *Clin Cancer Res* 2011; 17:3360-3367.

Zhang JJ, Smith KR. Household air pollution from coal and biomass fuels in China: measurements, health impacts, and interventions. *Environ Health Perspect* 2007; 115: 848-855.

Zhuo H, Smith AH, Steinmaus C. Selenium and lung cancer: a quantitative analysis of heterogeneity in the current epidemiological literature. *Cancer Epidemiol Biomarkers Prev* 2004; 13:771-778.

Ziegler A, Zangemeister-Wittke U, Stahel RA. Circulating DNA: a new diagnostic gold mine? *Cancer Treat Rev* 2002; 28:255-271.

Chapter 24
Early Detection of Cancer in Asia (Including Australia)

Robert Burton, Cheng-Har Yip, and Marilys Corbex

24.1 Introduction

Early detection of cancer is the diagnosis of certain solid cancers at a point in their growth when they remain localized and have a better chance of being cured with effective treatment. Early detection is only possible for some cancers. Those include breast, cervix, colon and rectum, oral cavity, nasopharynx, larynx, stomach, bladder, prostate, retinoblastoma, testis, and skin cancers (Baade and Coory 2005; WHO 2007). For other cancers like liver, esophagus, pancreas, or ovary, neither the screening tools developed to date nor surveillance for early symptoms can ensure that the disease will be detected early enough to be cured (WHO 2007). Early detection can only be successful in decreasing cancer mortality when linked to effective diagnosis and treatment. It is unethical to initiate an early detection program in the absence of adequate follow-up diagnostic and treatment facilities.

The two approaches to early detection are early diagnosis and screening. Early diagnosis (also named "clinical downstaging") means increasing the proportion of early-stage more curable cancers detected in patients presenting with symptoms (WHO 2007). Screening consists in applying a diagnostic test in an asymptomatic,

R. Burton, MD, PhD(✉)
School of Public Health and Preventive Medicine, Monash University
Victoria Australia, Melbourne, Vic, Australia
e-mail: robert.burton@monash.edu

Department of Epidemiology and Preventive Medicine,
Epidemiology & Preventative Medicine Monash Medical School Building,
The Alfred Hospital, Level 6 The Alfred Centre (Alfred Hospital), 99 Commercial Road,
Melbourne, Vic 3004, Australia

C. Yip, FRCS
Department of Surgery, University of Malaya, Kuala Lumpur, Malaysia

M. Corbex, PhD
Institute of Tropical Medicine, Antwerp, Belgium

A.B. Miller (ed.), *Epidemiologic Studies in Cancer Prevention and Screening*, Statistics for Biology and Health 79, DOI 10.1007/978-1-4614-5586-8_24,

but at risk, population in order to detect possible cancers or precancers before the appearance of symptoms. Detecting precancers should reduce incidence and thereby reduce mortality, and detecting early cancers should reduce mortality.

Population-based and hospital cancer registries are required for measuring the cancer burden (incidence, stage at diagnosis, and/or mortality) in a population and monitoring the impact that earlier diagnosis of symptomatic cancer and/or screening for cancers in asymptomatic populations can have on this burden. The two critical health system determinants for successful early diagnosis and screening programs are a primary healthcare system which is available, affordable, and competent and a secondary healthcare system which is also available, affordable, and competent, where patients detected with possible cancers can be referred for effective diagnosis and treatment. In the absence of primary and secondary healthcare systems which meet these criteria, it is usually impossible to implement effective population-based early diagnosis or screening programs for cancer (WHO 2007). Indeed, attempts to do so may cause more harm than good and thus fail to meet the ethical criterion of "Primum nil nocere" (first do no harm), attributed to Hippocrates (Wikipedia 2011).

24.2 The Burden of Cancer in Asia

Asia contains over half the world's population, about 4 billion people in 2008, and the International Agency for Research on Cancer (IARC) estimate of the cancer burden in Asia for 2008 was 6.1 million new cancer cases and 4.1 million cancer deaths (Table 24.1), or almost half of all new cancer cases (12.7 million) and more than half of all cancer deaths (7.6 million) worldwide in 2008 (Globocan 2008). This means an incidence to mortality ratio of 0.66, indicating that about two-thirds of Asians who get cancer will currently die of it. The 7 commonest Asian cancers, each with more than 300,000 cases in 2008, are cancers of the lung, stomach, liver, breast, colorectum, esophagus, and cervix (Fig. 24.1).

These data are estimates, since only a minor proportion of the 4 billion people in Asia are covered by population-based cancer registries. Four countries in Asia report on cancer incidence for their whole populations, Australia, Korea, New Zealand, and Singapore, and seven countries have regional cancer registries endorsed by IARC: China (5 registries), India (7), Japan (8), Malaysia (2), Pakistan

Table 24.1 Asia: demographics and cancer incidence and mortality (Globocan 2008)

	Male	Female	Both sexes
Population (thousands)	2097629	2000037	4097667
Number of new cancer cases (thousands)	3241.2	2851.1	6092.4
Age-standardized rate (ASR)	170.6	139.6	153.6
Number off cancer deaths (thousands)	2353.6	1718.7	4072.3
Age-standardized rate (W)	124.2	83.2	102.6
Mortality: incidence ratio (%)	78%	60%	67%

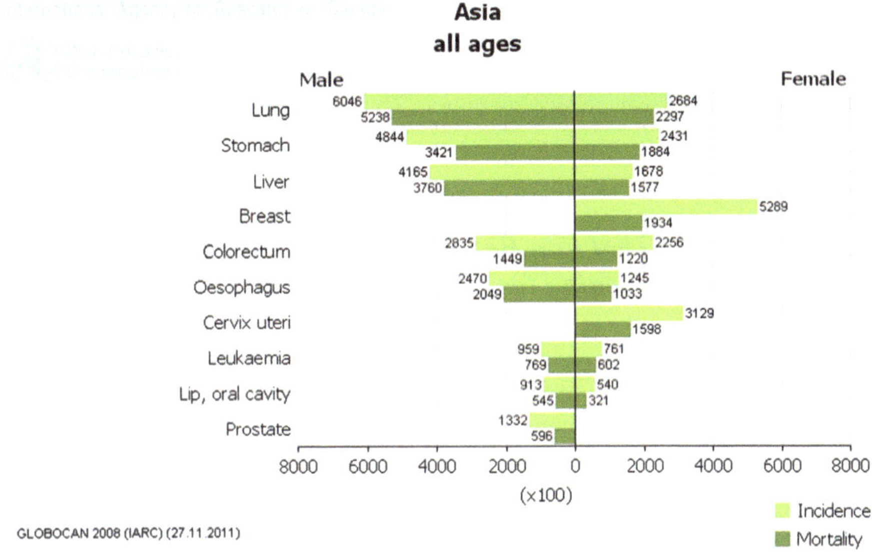

Fig. 24.1 Top 10 cancers in Asia among males and females (Globocan 2008)

(1), Philippines (1), and Thailand (2) (IARC 2008). Useful estimates for planning cancer control for regional or national populations can usually be made from regional registry data, and so total national population coverage is not generally needed.

24.3 Early Detection and Screening of Cancers in Asia (Excluding Australia and New Zealand)

The majority of countries in Asia are low- and middle-income (LMI) countries; the exceptions are the high-income countries of Singapore, Hong Kong, Japan, South Korea, and Taiwan (World Bank 2011). The commonest cancers in those countries are stomach, colon, lung, liver, and prostate in men and breast, colon, thyroid, stomach, and lung in women. In the LMI countries of Southeast and Central Asia, the commonest cancers are lung, stomach, liver, esophagus, and colorectum in men and breast, cervix, lung, stomach, and colon in women (Globocan 2008).

The majority of cancers in LMI countries present at advanced stages with low 5-year survival, high mortality, and therefore high mortality to incidence ratios. Evidence for efficacy of screening for breast and colorectal cancer comes from randomized screening trials (RST) done in high-income countries (IARC 2002; Towler et al. 2007), and the effectiveness of cervical cancer screening has been established by population-based Papanicolaou (Pap) smear screening programs in these countries (Cervical Cancer Screening 2004). With the exception of screening for cervical cancer (Sankaranarayanan et al. 2007; 2009), there is very little information available from LMI countries about screening for these cancers. There is evidence from RST in Asia that screening for primary liver cancer in hepatitis B virus (HBV)- and hepatitis C virus (HCV)-positive adults and for oral cancer in adults who use tobacco and alcohol heavily can reduce mortality (Zhang et al. 2004; Sankaranarayanan et al. 2006).

24.3.1 Lessons That Can Be Learned from Australia About Screening for Cancer

Australia is a high-income country with a small population, 22 million in 2010, and is very different from most of Asia. It has the fundamental structural prerequisites for the early diagnosis and screening for cancer: efficient population-based cancer registries, high-quality primary and secondary healthcare systems, and tertiary referral cancer units and institutes, which are available to the entire population at no direct cost to patients. The population is highly educated, and there has been mass media and other population education programs about early diagnosis of cancer for about half a century and population education about cancer screening for at least two decades. Australia has organized free population-based cancer screening programs for cervical, breast, and colorectal cancers, while opportunistic screening for skin and prostate cancer is very common. Breast and cervical cancer mortality have both fallen significantly in Australia since the free national breast and cervical cancer screening programs began in 1991 (AIHW 2010), but it is far too early yet to judge whether screening for colorectal cancer, which began in 2008,will be effective in practice.

There is convincing evidence that the Australian national cervical cancer Pap smear screening program, which aims to detect precancers and commenced in 1991, has been effective in reducing incidence and mortality from cervical cancer (Table 24.2). This Australian experience was preceded by the success of population-based Pap smear screening programs in Scandinavia, which began in the 1960s.

In the Australian program, 25 lifetime 2-yearly Pap smears beginning at age 18 years are recommended, compared with 15 lifetime 3-yearly Pap smears beginning at age 25 years in Norway. The mortality reduction to date in the Australian program (55%) is no greater than in the Norwegian program (63%) which began slightly later in 1995 (Table 24.2). So cost effectiveness and the age of beginning screening are issues for the Australian cervical cancer screening program. The efficacy of screening for cervical cancer using the Pap smear had never been tested until it was found in an RST that took place in India that a once-in-a-lifetime Pap smear did not reduce mortality from cervical cancer after nine years of follow-up (Sankaranarayanan et al. 2009).

The Australian free biennial mammography screening program for breast cancer, which targets women aged 50–69 years, has been associated with a 28% fall in breast cancer mortality since it began in 1991, with participation of this age group currently about 55% (Burton et al. 2011). However, the balance of evidence in

Table 24.2 Pap test screening for cervical cancer (Cervical Cancer Screening 2004; Entre Nous 2007; AIHW 2010)

	Australia	Iceland	Finland	Sweden	Denmark	Norway
Start of organized screening	1991	1964	1963	1964	1962	1995
Target age groups since 1985	18–69	20–69	30–69	23–60	23–75	25–69
Screening interval (years)	2	2–3	5	3–5	3–5	3
Lifetime Pap screening tests	25	16–24	7	7–12	10–17	15
Outcomes to 2000–2004:						
Reduction in overall world adjusted incidence rate	49%	64%	72%	60%	64%	50%
Reduction in overall world adjusted mortality rate	55%	83%	82%	71%	68%	63%

Australia, as in other high-income countries like the United Kingdom (UK), Norway, Denmark, and Belgium, is that most of the reductions in breast cancer mortality which have occurred after their national mammography screening programs began are not attributable to screening but to improved treatment (Autier et al. 2011; Burton et al. 2011; Jorgensen et al. 2010, Kalager et al. 2010, Gotzsche and Jorgensen 2011, and see Miller, this volume). The dilemma in high-income countries now is whether the balance between the benefits of mammography screening is not now outweighed by the harms of false-positive screening mammography and overdiagnosis of cancers, with unnecessary invasive diagnostic tests and treatments (McPherson 2010; Burton et al. 2011, Jorgensen and Gotzsche 2009; Jorgensen et al. 2011; Bell and Burton 2012). An inquiry into the benefits and harms of screening mammography has just been announced for the UK (Richards 2011). This debate has important implications for all countries using or introducing mammography screening for breast cancer and emphasizes the importance of concentrating on programs which educate women and healthcare professionals so that early diagnosis of breast cancer improves.

Australia is one of 17 countries beginning colorectal cancer screening programs, inviting adults aged 55–70 years to self-screen by mail, using a self-administered fecal occult blood test (FOBT) with follow-up colonoscopy for those screening positive, which started with ages 50, 55, and 65 years (Towler et al. 2007; Benson et al. 2008). Australia, like all the other16 countries including Japan and Taiwan, is still evaluating the feasibility of population-based screening, and so far only a small proportion of eligible adults have been screened. There are no generalizations possible yet about these screening programs, and the International Colorectal Cancer Screening Network will follow and report on them (Benson et al. 2008).

Screening for prostate cancer is leading to a great amount of overdiagnosis and unnecessary treatment, as was predicted by the RST which found that 49 men must be diagnosed via the prostate-specific-antigen (PSA) blood test to prevent one prostate cancer death (Schröder et al. 2009, and see Miller, this volume). In Australia, opportunistic screening began more than 20 years ago, and to date there is no convincing evidence that PSA testing has had a significant impact on prostate cancer mortality, while there is evidence of considerable harm to men who screen positive and of misinformation in the Australian news media: The benefit of screening is overrated (Mackenzie et al. 2007). The US Preventive Task Force (2011) has recently reviewed the evidence on benefits and harms of PSA screening for prostate cancer in the USA and recommended against routine PSA testing of low-risk men. This recommendation should be followed in all countries currently screening or contemplating screening for prostate cancer.

Self and opportunistic skin cancer screening is very common in Australia for malignant melanomas (malignant moles), potentially fatal pigmented skin cancers that are common in white-skinned people exposed to excessive ultraviolet radiation (UVR). Since this screening began about half a century ago, mortality from melanoma has fallen significantly in Australia (Baade and Coory 2005), but about 20 benign moles (brown or black skin lesions) are currently removed by family practitioners for each melanoma detected (English et al. 2004). Dermoscopy has been successfully evaluated by family practitioners and has the potential to make this opportunistic screening program much more cost effective (Menzies et al. 2009). This has relevance to higher latitude Asian countries where people do not have heavily pigmented skin that is protective against UVR exposure, for example, Japan.

24.3.2 Early Detection of Cervical Cancer in Asia

More than 80% of women who develop cervical cancer are from LMI, and the global burden of the disease is highest in Africa, Latin America, and South and Southeast Asia (Ferlay et al. 2010). Prevention of cervical cancer by safe sexual practices and immunization against the common causative strains of the human papillomavirus (HPV) is addressed by Bosch (this volume). There are three methods for screening of cervical cancer currently available (IARC 2004), and a fourth (below) is in advanced field trials in China.

1. The Pap test, a smear or brushing for liquid-based cytology taken from the cervix for cytological examination, is the current gold standard cervical screening test.
2. Direct visualization of the cervix after the use of a chemical (dilute acetic acid, VIA, or iodine, VILI) to look for patches of abnormal cells visible as white (VIA) or yellow (VILI) areas adjacent to the squamocolumnar junction at the cervical os.
3. A DNA test of cervical cells for the presence of oncogenic strains of HPV, particularly HPV 16 and HPV 18.

All these tests display high false-positive rates, with the Pap test having the least and DNA testing for HPV having the most. For example, in a recent prevalence survey of sexually active women in Mongolia, 13% of all women had a positive Pap test, and 35% of all women were positive for one or more HPV strains using the DNA test (Dondog et al. 2008). However, only 42/969 (4.3%) of the tested women had a cervical cytology result of CIN 2 or CIN 3, indicating that they were at risk of cervical cancer (Dondog et al. 2008). False-positive results increase the costs of screening, the burden of anxiety for women, and morbidity from unnecessary diagnostic and treatment procedures. The presence of oncoproteins, produced by oncogenic HPV strains, is a necessary condition for the development of cervical cancer in chronically infected women. A new test for the detection of the specific E6 oncoproteins of HPV strains 16, 18, and 45 is close to government certification for use in China (Sellors et al. 2011). This approach shows considerable promise in reducing high false-positive rates and could help triage women positive with any of the three other currently available screening tests for better targeted diagnosis and treatment.

Certain standards of care are required after a positive screening result. For example, if the Pap smear is positive, a colposcopy is required for biopsy, and if the biopsy is positive, excision or cryotherapy of the abnormal area is usually carried out. In resource-poor settings, this sequence, requiring 3 visits at least, may not be feasible and requires specialized care (pathology and gynecology) which may not be available.

VIA or VILI can be carried out by nurses or midwives, and VIA has been shown to have a similar or higher sensitivity but lower specificity compared with the Pap smear for CIN 2, CIN 3, or invasive cancer (Cervix cancer screening 2004). Cryotherapy of cervical lesions detected by VIA or VILI can be carried out by health workers immediately, hence reducing the number of visits that the woman has to make (Sankaranarayanan et al. 2007). This has been termed the "see and treat" approach and has proven to be efficacious in an Indian RST, where a single VIA followed by cryotherapy for women screening positive significantly reduced mortality compared with non-screened controls (Sankaranarayanan et al. 2007). This approach is particularly suited to cervical cancer screening in resource poor settings.

Screening for HPV by DNA assays has a sensitivity of about 95% for detecting CIN 2 or more severe lesions in women older than 30 years, making it more sensitive than cytology (IARC 2004). A recent RST in India, which compared a single DNA, or Pap or VIA screening test followed by referral for colposcopy of women screening positive, showed that only the HPV DNA screening test significantly reduced mortality when compared to the non-screened controls (Sankaranarayanan et al. 2009). A single HPV test identifies almost all women who are chronically infected with oncogenic strains of the HPV and hence are at risk of cervical cancer at the time of the test (Cervix cancer screening 2004; Sankaranarayanan et al. 2009). Effective management of these women would be expected to impact on population mortality from cervical cancer.

A once-in-a-lifetime Pap test was of unknown efficacy until this RST. Modeling had produced an estimate that 3 lifetime Pap tests could reduce cervical cancer incidence by about 60% (Cervix cancer screening 2004). Repeated Pap testing is recommended because of the nature of the test; it is only a surrogate for the causative agent and the possibilities of not getting sufficient abnormal cells with a single smear and/or false-negative readings (quality control). In contrast it was not surprising that a single VIA "see and treat" could reduce mortality while VIA and refer did not. VIA "see and treat" leads to overtreatment, but minimizes or abolishes loss to follow up for diagnosis and treatment, which VIA and refer involves and which can be a major obstacle to the impact of screening in LMI countries (Pisani et al. 2006). Also it depends on nurses trained to "see and treat" being trained to be "over treaters," since this maybe the women's only chance of secondary prevention of cervical cancer.

24.3.3 Early Detection of Breast Cancer in Asia

Breast cancer is the commonest cancer of women in Asia with 530,000 new cases in 2008 (Ferlay et al. 2010). Due to population aging and changes in reproductive patterns, breast cancer incidence is increasing rapidly and the number of new cases is estimated to reach 690,000 in 2020 (Ferlay et al. 2010). Mammography screening programs have been developed in many of the high-income Asian countries. However, screening is not systematically provided free of charge; for example, within the national screening program of Singapore, a mammogram costs US$40 for Singaporean citizens and US$79 for others (BreastScreen Singapore 2011). Coverage is not optimal, for example, participation is only 30% in South Korea (Suh and Park 2009). As previously indicated (Section 3.1), the effectiveness of mammography screening is now being seriously questioned in a number of high-income countries, so Asian countries implementing or planning to begin mammography screening would be wise to wait on the outcome of the UK enquiry (Richards 2011) before proceeding with their programs.

Screening for breast cancer, the commonest cancer in women worldwide, is a particular challenge in LMI countries (Corbex et al. 2012). Screening based on clinical breast exam (CBE) has been tested in Asia: A cluster randomized trial was initiated in Manila (The Philippines) involving 151,168 women aged 35–64 years (Pisani et al. 2006). After the first round of screening, screen-detected cases were less advanced than the others, but the difference did not reach statistical significance. However, among the 3479 women detected positive with a breast lump and referred for diagnosis in this first round, only 18% initially completed follow-up for diagnosis, and another 17% completed it only after a home visit by the intervention staff. Almost half (42.4%) actively refused further investigation even with home visits. This behavior was not attributable to logistic or economic barriers since in this trial all diagnosis and treatment services were offered for free, including transportation. This unexpected outcome resulted in the trial being stopped prematurely (Pisani et al. 2006) and illustrates the need to ensure that women who accept the invitation to screen commit to complete the follow-up diagnosis and treatment if the screening test is positive.

A second trial, involving CBE breast cancer screening and cervical cancer screening, is currently being conducted in Mumbai (India) on 150,000 women aged 35–64 years. This study has now entered its tenth year and more than 3 rounds of screening have taken place. Early results show that the stage distribution is significantly better in the screened group than in the control groups. (Mittra et al. 2010). However, this trial has also raised questions about the degree of persuasion required to induce women to participate in screening and to attend for follow-up diagnostic procedures. It is reported that nearly 100 full-time personnel were engaged to screen the 75,000 women. Door-to-door visits, usually more than once, were required not only to persuade women to attend screening tests but also to induce them to comply with others steps related to diagnosis and treatment once screened positive. The manpower cost involved has been described as "formidable" (Mittra 2008). Strong sociocultural barriers to screening appear to exist in many Asian countries, and this raises questions about the feasibility of screening whatever screening tool is used.

The "clinical downstaging" program developed in Sarawak, Malaysia, represents an interesting alternative to screening. This program focused on symptomatic patients only and aimed at detecting breast cancer in women with the earliest symptoms. It consisted in training first- and second-level healthcare staff to improve their skills in early cancer diagnosis and in raising public awareness. In four years, the proportion of breast cancers diagnosed in stage III and IV were reduced from 60% (1994) to 35% (1998) [$p<0.0001$] (Devi et al. 2007). The cost was minimal and the approach has been cited as an example of effective clinical downstaging by the WHO (2007). Such relatively easy-to-implement and cost-effective programs are indeed a promising approach for LMI countries (Corbex et al. 2012).

However, this clinical downstaging program was successful in Malaysia because this country has a well-organized and efficient health system which is accessible and affordable to all inhabitants. All cancer patients are offered up-to-date and free-of-charge treatment. This is not the case in most of the low-income countries of Asia. For example, in Cambodia and Laos, cancer treatment departments have existed since only 2003 and 2009, respectively, and are not yet in a position to offer much more than palliative care free of charge (Buisson 2011).

24.3.4 *Early Detection of Other Common Cancers in Asia*

24.3.4.1 Gastrointestinal Cancers

Gastric cancer is the second commonest cause of cancer death in Asia. Although screening by endoscopy seems to be the most accurate method for early detection of gastric cancer, the availability of endoscopic services in Asia for mass screening remains a major barrier. Serum pepsinogen testing can be used as an initial screening tool where patients with abnormal results are then screened by endoscopy. The role of eradication of H pylori, the commonest cause of gastric cancer, which is endemic in Asia, remains to be defined. At present there is a paucity of data from Asia to lend support for population-based screening for gastric cancer (Leung et al. 2008). In Japan, where gastric cancer is the leading cause of cancer death, gastric cancer screening has been advocated for all residents aged 40 and above (Leung et al. 2008). An RST-utilizing barium meal as a screening test in 1050 patients (364 in the screened group and 686 in the non-screened group) showed that the cancers diagnosed in the screened group were smaller with fewer metastatic lymph nodes than in the control group (Kunisaki et al. 2006). Disease-specific survival was also significantly better in the screened cases among all registered and curatively resected patients as compared to controls (Kunisaki et al. 2006).

The incidence of colorectal carcinoma (CRC) is rapidly increasing in Asian countries such as China, Japan, Korea, and Singapore due to changes in lifestyle. As reviewed above, population-based colorectal cancer screening has begun in Australia, Japan, and Taiwan using the FOBT test (Towler et al. 2007); however, these programs are in their infancy and it is far too early to draw any conclusions on their effectiveness (Benson et al. 2008). The Asia Pacific Consensus on colorectal screening recommends fecal occult blood test (FOBT, guaiac-based and immunochemical tests), flexible sigmoidoscopy, and colonoscopy for CRC screening (Sung et al. 2008). In resource-limited countries, FOBT is the first choice for CRC screening (Sung et al. 2008). The Asia Pacific colorectal working group has developed and validated the Asia Pacific Colorectal Screening (APCS) score, which stratifies individuals into three tiers of risk (average, moderate, and high risk) based on age, sex, family history, and smoking, to select people for priority of colorectal screening (Yeoh et al. 2011).

24.3.4.2 Liver Cancer

Liver cancer (hepatocellular carcinoma – HCC) is among the top three causes of cancer deaths in many Asian and African countries (Ferlay et al. 2010), with 75% of deaths from HCC occurring in countries of the Asia Pacific region. Chronic HBV infection from birth and early childhood causes 80% of the liver cancers, with HCV accounting for most of the remaining cases. In Japan, the majority of HCC are associated with HCV, unlike the rest of Asia (Kudo et al. 2010). Vaccination against HBV infection has the potential to prevent up to 80% of cases of liver cancer in Asia, but will take decades to have an impact on population mortality. Late diagnosis means that the average survival after diagnosis is often quoted as 3–6 months. An RST in Qidong, China, during 1989–1995, in men aged 30–69 who were chronic carriers of hepatitis B virus (HbSAg positive), showed that screening with 6-monthly measurement of alpha-fetoprotein (AFP) resulted in earlier diagnosis of hepatocellular carcinoma but there was no reduction in mortality (Chen et al. 2003; Kudo et al. 2010). However, another RST in Shanghai, using screening with 6-monthly AFP and ultrasound, did show a significantly reduced HCC mortality of 37% during the follow-up period (Zhang et al. 2004).

At present, Korea, Taiwan, and Japan have established surveillance programs for early detection of HCC, targeting people at risk because of liver cirrhosis and/or a HBV or HCV infections. These programs utilize a combination of ultrasonography and AFP at 6-month intervals. To improve the detection rate of early-stage HCC, the benefit of additional tests and a shorter surveillance interval should be confirmed by an RST in Asia. The application of an individualized prediction model to surveillance programs may improve the cost effectiveness by focusing on the high-risk group (Kudo et al. 2010).

24.3.4.3 Head and Neck Cancers

Oral cancer ranks as one of the top ten cancers worldwide, and the majority of cases are seen in Asia. These are attributed to the widespread habit in some communities of chewing Areca (betel) nut which has a high carcinogenic potential and is usually mixed with tobacco. In low-resource regions with high-risk populations, a combination of lack of public awareness about the disease and inadequate resources and expertise for screening leads to long delays in diagnosis, resulting in high morbidity and mortality. Early detection of oral premalignant lesions and early neoplastic changes by visual inspection of the mouth may be the best and most cost-effective means to improve survival and quality of life for oral cancer patients from all socio-economic communities. A RST of oral visual inspection for cancer or premalignant lesions in Kerala, South India, showed a nonsignificant 21% reduction in mortality from oral cancer compared with the control group. In high-risk groups, that is, users of alcohol, tobacco, or both, there was a significant 34% reduction (relative risk=0.66, 95% confidence interval 0.45–0.95) in mortality in the follow-up period of the RST (Sankaranarayanan et al. 2006).

Nasopharyngeal carcinoma (NPC) is a rare malignancy in most parts of the world, but is one of the commonest cancers in Southeast Asia. Both genetic and environmental factors contribute to the causation of NPC, and Epstein-Barr virus (EBV) infection is involved in all cases (Busson et al. 2004). NPC is difficult to detect in the early stages because the symptoms are not specific. Use of radiology modalities such as PET scan and MRI is not justified in screening (Tabuchi et al. 2011). EBV antibody has been investigated as an early marker of NPC, and repeated screening of high-risk individuals (i.e., with family history) showed early promising results (Ji et al. 2007).

24.4 Barriers to the Early Detection of Cancers in Asia

In Asia as in many other LMI countries, late diagnosis of cancer is attributable to several factors including:

1. Education and awareness – literacy rates in parts of Asia are low, and hence people are not aware of the signs and symptoms of cancer. There is also a belief that cancer is invariably fatal, and hence treatment is futile.
2. Belief in alternative therapy – alternative therapy is seen to be more holistic and alternative practitioners are preferable to what is seen to be a hostile hospital environment.
3. Decision making – for most women, the decision for consulting doctors/get treatment is in the hands of their husbands or parents.
4. Financial constraints – in many parts of Asia, the treatment is not subsidized by the government and patients have to pay out of pocket which can lead to financial catastrophe.
5. Access to healthcare facilities – in isolated areas, there may be no cancer facilities, and traveling for early detection or follow-up with a positive screening test may be impossible for many people.

References

Australian Institute of Health and Welfare (AIHW) 2010, ACIM (Australian Cancer Incidence and Mortality) books, AIHW, Canberra.

Autier P, Boniol M, Gavin A, Vatten LJ. Breast cancer mortality in neighbouring countries with different levels of screening but similar access to treatment: trend analysis of WHO database. *BMJ* 2011; 343: doi: 10.1136/bmj.d44111.

Baade P, Coory M. Trends in melanoma mortality in Australia: 1950-2002 and their implications for melanoma control.*Australian & New Zealand Journal of Public Health* 2005;29:383-386.

Bell R, Burton R. Do the benefits of screening mammography outweigh the harms of over diagnosis and unnecessary treatment? *Med J. Australia* 2012; 196:17.

Benson VS, Patnick, J, Davies AK, Nadel MR, Smith RA, on behalf of the International Colorectal Cancer Screening Network. Colorectal cancer screening: A comparison of 35 initiatives in 17 countries. *Int. J. Cancer* 2008; 122:1357–1367.

BreastScreen Singapore.2011 Singapore government web-site about breast cancer screening. http://www.hpb.gov.sg/programmes/article.aspx?id=3324

Buisson PY. 2011. Compte-rendu du séminaire "Cancers et agents infectieux en Asie du Sud-Est": http://www.ifmt.auf.org/article.php3?id_article=475

Burton RC, Bell RJ, Thiagarajah G, Stevenson, C. Adjuvant therapy, not mammographic screening, accounts for most of the observed breast cancer specific mortality reductions in Australian women since the national screening program began in 1991 *Breast Cancer Res Treat* 2011; DOI 10.1007/s10549-011-1794-6.

Busson P, Keryer C, Ooka T, Corbex M. EBV-associated nasopharyngeal carcinomas: from epidemiology to virus-targeting strategies. *Trends Microbiol.* 2004; 12:356-360.

Chen JG, Parkin DM, Chen QD, Lu JH,Shen QJ, Zhang BC et al. Screening for liver cancer: results of a randomised controlled trial in Qidong, China. *J Med Screen* 2003; 10: 204-209.

Corbex M, Burton R, Sancho-Garnier H. Breast cancer early detection methods for low and middle income countries, a review of the evidence. *Breast* 2102; http://dx.doi.org/10.1016/j.breast.2012.01.002

Devi B, Tang TS, Corbex M. Reducing by half the percentage of late-stage presentation for breast and cervix cancer over 4 years: a pilot study of clinical downstaging in Sarawak, Malaysia. *Ann Oncol* 2007; 18:1172-1176.

Dondog B, Clifford GM, Vaccarella S, Waterboer T, Unurjargal D, Avirme D et al. Human papillomavirus infection in Ulaanbaatar, Mongolia: a population-based study. *Cancer Epidemiol Biomarkers Prev* 2008; 17:1731-1738.

English DR, Del Mar C, Burton RC. Factors influencing the number needed to excise: excision rates of pigmented lesions by primary care doctors in Perth, Western Australia. *Med J Australia* 2004; 180:16-19.

Entre Nous. The European Magazine for Sexual and Reproductive Health, Vol 64, No 6, 2007, WHO Regional Office for Europe.

Ferlay J, Shin HR, Bray F, Forman D, Mathers C, Parkin DM. Estimates of worldwide burden of cancer in 2008: GLOBOCAN 2008. *Int J Cancer* 2010; 127: 2893–2917.

Globocan 2008,*http://globocan.iarc.fr IARC, www.IARC.fr*

Gotzsche PC, Jorgensen KJ. The Breast Screening Programme and misinforming the public. *J R Soc Med* 2011; 104:361-369.

IARC. *Breast Cancer Screening*. IARC Handbooks of Cancer Prevention Vol 7, 2002, Lyon, France.

IARC Cervix cancer screening. IARC Handbooks of Cancer Prevention Vol 10, 2004, Lyon, France.

IARC. Cancer Incidence in Five Continents, vol 9, 2008 http://www.iarc.fr/en/publications/pdfs-online/epi/sp160/CI5vol9-1

Ji MF, Wang DK, Yu YL,Guo YQ,Liang JS,Cheng WM et al. Sustained elevation of Epstein-Barr virus antibody levels preceding clinical onset of nasopharyngeal carcinoma. *Br J Cancer* 2007; 96: 623-630.

Jørgensen KJ, Gøtzsche PC. Overdiagnosis in publicly organised mammography screening programmes: systematic review of incidence trends. *BMJ* 2009; 339:b2587 doi:10.1136/bmj.b2587

Jorgensen KJ, Zahl P-H, Gotzsche PC. Breast cancer mortality in organised mammography screening in Denmark: comparative study. *BMJ* 2010; 340:c1241. doi:10.1136/bmj.c1241

Jørgensen, KJ, Keen, JD, Gøtzsche, PC. Is Mammographic Screening Justifiable Considering Its Substantial Overdiagnosis Rate and Minor Effect on Mortality? *Radiology* 2011; 260:621-627.

Kalager M, Zelen M, Langmark F, Adami H-O. Effect of Screening Mammography on Breast-Cancer Mortality in Norway. N Engl J Med 2010;363:1203-1210.

Kudo M, Han KH, Kokudo N, Cheng AL, Choi BI, Furuse J et al. Liver Cancer Working Group report. *Jpn J Clin Oncol* 2010; 40 (Suppl 1): i19-27

Kunisaki C, Ishino J, Nakajima S, Motohashi H, Akiyama H, Nomura M et al. Outcomes of mass screening for gastric carcinoma *Ann Surg Oncol* 2006; 13:221-228.

Leung WK, Wu MS, Kakugawa Y, Kim JJ, Yeoh KG, Goh KL, et al. Screening for gastric cancer in Asia: current evidence and practice. *Lancet Oncol* 2008; 9:279-287

MacKenzie R, Chapman S, Barratt A, Holding S. "The news is [not] all good": misrepresentations and inaccuracies in Australian news media reports on prostate cancer screening. *Med J Australia* 2007; 187:507–510.

McPherson K. Screening for breast cancer–balancing the debate. *BMJ* 2010; 340:c3106. doi:10.1136/bmj.c3106

Menzies S, Emery J, Staples M, Davies S, McAvoy B, Fletcher J et al. Impact of dermoscopy and short-term sequential digital dermoscopy imaging for the management of pigmented lesions in primary care: a sequential intervention trial. *Br J Dermatol* 2009; 161:1270-1277.

Mittra I. Screening for breast cancer: is it globally applicable? *Nat Clin Pract Oncol.* 2008; 5:60-61.

Mittra I, Mishra GA, Singh S, Aranke S, Notani P, Badwe R et al, A cluster randomized, controlled trial of breast and cervix cancer screening in Mumbai, India: methodology and interim results after three rounds of screening. *Int J Cancer* 2010; 126:976–984.

Pisani P, Parkin DM, Ngelangel C, Esteban D, Gibson L, Munson M et al. Outcome of screening by clinical examination of the breast in a trial in the Philippines. *Int J Cancer* 2006; 118:149-154.

Richards M. An independent review is under way. *BMJ* 2011; 343:d6843.

Sankaranarayanan, R, Dinshaw K, Nene BM, Pulikattil KR, Esmy O, Jayant, K et al. Cervical and oral cancer screening in India. *J Med Screen* 2006; 13 (Suppl 1): S35-38.

Sankaranarayanan R, Esmy PO, Rajkumar R, Swaminanathan R, Shanthakumari S, Fayette J-M et al. Effect of visual screening on cervical cancer incidence and mortality in Tamil Nadu, India: a cluster-randomised trial. *Lancet* 2007; 370:398-406.

Sankaranarayanan R, Nene BM, Shastri SS, Jayant K, Muwonge R, Atul M et al. HPV screening for cervical cancer in rural India. *N Engl J Med* 2009; 360:1385-1394.

Schröder FH, Hugosson J, Roobol MJ, Tammela TLJ, Ciatto S, Nelen V, et al, Mortality Results from a Randomized Prostate-Cancer Screening Trial. *N Engl J Med* 2009; 360:1320-1328.

Sellors J, Schweizer, JG, Lu PS, Liu B, Weigl, BH, Cui, JF et al. Association of Elevated E6 Oncoprotein With Grade of Cervical Neoplasia Using PDZ Interaction Mediated Precipitation of E6. *J Low Genit Tract Dis* 2011; 15:159-176.

Suh EE, Park S. Mammography use and its demographic correlates among women in South Korea. *Asian Nursing Research* 2009; 3:71-80.

Sung J, Lau JY, Young GP, Sano Y, Chiu H, Byeon J et al. Asia Pacific consensus recommendations for colorectal cancer screening. *Gut* 2008; 57:1166-1176.

Tabuchi K, Nakayama M, Nishimura B, Hayashi K, Akira Hara A. Early detection of nasopharyngeal carcinoma.Int J Otolaryngol 2011: doi:10.1155/2011/638058

Towler BP, Irwig L, Glasziou P, Weller D, Kewenter J. Screening for colorectal cancer using the faecal occult blood test, hemoccult. *Cochrane Database Syst Rev.* 2007; (1):CD001216.Tabuchi K, Nakayama M, Nishimura B, Hayashi K, Akira Hara A. Early detection of nasopharyngeal carcinoma. *Int J Otolaryngol* 2011: doi:10.1155/2011/638058

U.S. Preventive Services Task Force. 2011. http://www.uspreventiveservicestaskforce.org/draftrec3.htm

WHO Guide for effective programmes; Cancer control: knowledge into action; module 3: Early detection. 2007
http://www.who.int/cancer/modules/en/index.html
Wikipedia 2011.wikipedia.org/wiki/Primum_non_nocere#Origin
World Bank 2011 *www.worldbank.org*
Yeoh KG, Ho KY, Chiu HM, Zhu F, Ching JY, Wu DC et al. The Asia-Pacific Colorectal Screening score: a validated tool that stratifies risk for colorectal advanced neoplasia in asymptomatic Asian subjects. *Gut* 2011; 60:1236-1241.
Zhang, B. H., B. H. Yang, Tang ZY. Randomized controlled trial of screening for hepatocellular carcinoma. *J Cancer Res Clin Oncol* 2004; 130:417-422.

Chapter 25
Prevention and Screening for Cancer in Primary Health Care

Alan Katz and Jennifer Enns

25.1 Introduction

Even though the delivery of primary health care varies significantly between different jurisdictions based on the socioeconomic and political environment, prevention and screening are universally accepted as fundamental components of primary health care (Starfield 2003). There are many challenges to the delivery of cancer prevention and screening in primary care; some based in the organization and delivery of primary care services while others are more specific to the content to be delivered. The fundamental challenge is that primary health care involves a diffuse array of services, including prevention, screening, diagnosis, treatment, and rehabilitation, delivered by a variety of professionals, none of whom are dedicated specifically to either prevention or screening.

25.2 Cancer Prevention

While we still have much to learn about cancer prevention, the scientific basis of what can be done to prevent cancer has been presented in previous chapters of this book. The prevention focus in this chapter will be on the translation of that knowledge into clinical practice within primary health care. While a population-based approach to cancer prevention is critical to address issues like environmental, nutritional, and occupational exposure to known or suspected carcinogens, there is a place for prevention at the individual level in primary care.

A. Katz, MB ChB MSc CCFP (✉) • J. Enns, MSc
Family Medicine Research Unit, Faculty of Medicine, University of Manitoba,
P228-770 Bannatyne Ave, Winnipeg MBR3E0W, Canada
e-mail: Alan_Katz@cpe.umanitoba.ca

A.B. Miller (ed.), *Epidemiologic Studies in Cancer Prevention and Screening*,
Statistics for Biology and Health 79, DOI 10.1007/978-1-4614-5586-8_25,

There are four potential roles primary care practitioners can play in cancer prevention: (1) educating and supporting patients to reduce exposure to cancer risk factors, (2) providing immunizations to develop immunity to protect against specific cancers, (3) detecting and treating precancerous conditions (screening), and lastly (4) administering chemoprophylaxis to prevent the development of cancer. There is strong evidence supporting the potential impact of the first role, while the limited opportunities for the third and the fourth have been addressed by Dr. Marshall in a previous chapter.

There are currently only two commercially available vaccines that have been shown to be effective in preventing cancer. Immunization against specific subtypes of the human papillomavirus (HPV) has been shown to be effective in preventing approximately 70 % of cervical cancers (IARC 2007). While use of the vaccine in girls has been widely supported by departments of public health and widespread vaccination programs, its use in adolescent girls remains controversial among the public (Agosti and Goldie 2007; Klug et al. 2008; Markowitz et al. 2007; Mays et al. 2004). Use of the vaccine in boys has not been widely supported. The vaccine against the hepatitis B virus is promoted for its effects in preventing hepatitis as well as cancer and is more readily accepted than the HPV vaccine, as the hepatitis B virus is spread by other routes as well as by sexual activity (Shepard et al. 2006). The role of primary health-care practitioners is in promoting these vaccines and delivering them to the target populations (Hontelez et al. 2010; Mele et al. 2008).

25.2.1 Reducing Exposure to Cancer Risk Factors

The potential impact of dietary interventions, tobacco control, and exercise has also been addressed in general in this book, but not within the context of primary health care. All of these cancer risk factors involve behavioral change, and many are shared with other major diseases like cardiovascular and respiratory disease. Counseling to avoid tobacco use, keep physically active, maintain a healthy weight, and eat a healthy diet is therefore not seen as a specific cancer prevention intervention in primary care. As a result, the outcomes reported in the literature rarely include cancer prevention because of the long time lag between behavior change (implementation of a healthy behavior) and cancer onset.

Multiple studies in primary care have attempted to address the challenge of behavior change (Lin et al. 2010). First, the clinician needs to address the issue. Second, the information exchange needs to result in a response from the patient, and third, the patient needs to sustain the behavior change for ongoing benefit. Many of the studies demonstrating the effectiveness of lifestyle counseling use more intensive interventions (multiple sessions with follow-up) that are provided by professionals other than physicians (Lin et al. 2010). While most other studies show varied success, motivational interviewing has shown promise as a technique to facilitate behavior change specific to tobacco use (Lai et al. 2010).

25.3 Practice Organization: Facilitators and Barriers

The most common barriers to the delivery of recommended preventive care (screening and prevention) are found within the organization of health-care delivery and in practice, such as the absence of financial incentives for preventive service delivery and the lack of a reminder system to offer these services in the office (Anderson et al. 2006; Guerra et al. 2007; Klabunde et al. 2007; Hudson et al. 2007; Hung et al. 2006; Sarfaty and Wender 2007) and the lack of time. Yarnall et al. (2003) calculated the time it would take to address the recommended prevention counseling for an average 55-year-old patient. For the average practitioner, it would take over seven hours per day for a year to address all the recommended prevention issues with each patient on an annual basis thus leaving little time for anything else!

Using specially trained prevention experts who work as facilitators to support prevention initiatives has been shown to be a promising solution to the challenge of increasing prevention activities (Hogg et al. 2008). The addition of staff with the specific goal of increasing prevention results in additional cost to the system but is consistent with the current recognition of need for team-based approaches to primary care service. It is in keeping with the recognition that physicians are not necessarily the best providers to deliver many services currently provided in primary care, and if physician resources are redirected to providing other necessary medical services, the use of alternative providers may prove to be cost effective (Gilfillan et al. 2010; Moran et al. 2011; Rosenthal 2008; Sarfaty et al. 2011).

25.4 Cancer Screening

Cancer screening is traditionally offered either within the context of routine care (so-called opportunistic screening) or within specific population-based screening programs. Primary health-care providers have a role in supporting and promoting screening within both contexts (Weller and Campbell 2009). Once again, the evidence supporting the efficacy of specific screening tests has been addressed in previous chapters, and the focus here will be on the promotion and delivery of screening tests in primary care settings. Because there is significant room for improvement in the rates of cancer screening (U.S. Department of Health and Human Services 2009; Canadian Cancer Society et al. 2011), the following discussion will address the role of primary health care in improving rates of cancer screening. Efforts at increasing screening may be directed at the target population, the health-care provider, or both (Ornstein et al. 2010). Screening uptake rates differ between different cancers and between subpopulations; for example, immigrant and lower-income women have been shown to have lower screening rates (Downs et al. 2008; Moser et al. 2009). This has lead to screening interventions targeted at specific populations as well as more general interventions aimed at increasing the rates of opportunistic screening. Low-income women in particular have been targeted in multiple interventions to increase screening uptake for cervical and breast cancer (Dietrich et al. 2006; Spadea et al. 2010; Tu et al. 2006). While the success of both types of intervention is dependent on the health service context and the characteristics of the screening program (Weller et al. 2009), targeted interventions have been shown to more effective (Luckmann et al. 2003; Myers et al. 2007; Rawl et al. 2008; Sohl and Moyer 2007; Vernon et al. 2008).

Because screening exposes healthy people to interventions that might be more harmful than beneficial (like further testing), efforts to improve uptake in cancer screening should take care not to mislead invitees (Weller et al. 2009). Primary health-care practitioners need to be aware of both the potential benefits and harms of the screening tests they recommend and provide patients with the opportunity for informed choice to participate in screening (Trevena et al. 2008).

25.4.1 Interventions to Remind Providers to Offer Screening

There is extensive literature on prevention and screening of both cancer and chronic disease. While much of the literature focuses on specific interventions, such as those that encourage physicians to provide more prevention counseling or the encouragement of screening by their patients, or on patients to engage in screening more consistently, ultimately the most successful interventions are multifaceted approaches that address multiple issues simultaneously (Arroyave et al. 2011). Several organizational approaches have been shown to increase screening rates, including the establishment of separate clinics for prevention/screening, use of planned prevention visits, use of continuous quality improvement techniques, and allocation of specific prevention responsibilities to nonphysician staff (e.g., nurses and clerical staff) (Arroyave et al. 2011). In addition, electronic reminders for practitioners with electronic medical records have shown some success in increasing screening uptake in general (Wei et al. 2005; Ling et al. 2009).

25.5 Cancer Genetics in Primary Care

Cancer genetic services have proven to benefit high-risk patients (Collins 2004) and, as such, are powerful tools for cancer prevention or treatment at an early stage, offering insight into surgical and chemopreventive risk management options, as well as genetically targeted cancer treatment therapies. As the prevalence and marketing of genetic tests for cancer increase and public awareness of the heredity of cancer rises, primary care providers will be called upon to evaluate their patients' genetic risk. So what is the primary care physician's role in counseling about hereditary cancer?

25.5.1 DNA-Based Genetic Risk Assessment

None of the cancer tests that are currently available are appropriate for screening of asymptomatic individuals (American Society of Clinical Oncology 2003), so initiating genetic testing is typically done with patients who present with symptoms matching a defined cancer susceptibility syndrome or suggestive individual cancer family histories. In primary care, the first step in this process is the collection of a complete family history or pedigree (3–4 generations of medical history in both lineages, including current ages and ages at death), which is required for interpreting the results of DNA-based testing (Scheuner and Gordon 2002). In patients with symptoms suggestive of a cancer susceptibility syndrome, the family history and the physical examination can be used to estimate the mutation probability, using modeling tools to estimate the probability of an individual carrying suspected mutations. If genetic testing is indicated by the results of the risk estimate model and evaluation of the family history, DNA samples are obtained from the patient. The genetic counselor and primary care physician may jointly discuss the results of the DNA testing with the patient and provide counseling on appropriate preventative measures and/or early detection.

25.5.2 Risk Perceptions and Health Behavior

Gathering family history data and assessing cancer risk allow patients to make more informed decisions about prevention. In many cases, patients will have developed interpretations of their family histories and their personal risk of a disease before consulting with a physician or other health-care provider, which may affect their perceived susceptibility and actions taken to prevent it (Acheson et al. 2010). In some cases, patients may overestimate their risk for getting cancer and experience considerable anxiety. Some patients may be motivated to adopt preventive behaviors, but for others, inherited risk may be perceived as unavoidable and could therefore result in fatalistic attitudes and lack of motivation to instigate lifestyle changes (Senior et al. 2000). Primary care providers need to be aware of their patients' attitudes and preconceptions about their family histories and perceived cancer risk and of their readiness to adopt preventive lifestyle behaviors.

References

Acheson LS, Wang C, Zyzanski SJ, Lynn A, Ruffin 4th MT, Gramling R et al. Family history and perceptions about risk and prevention for chronic diseases in primary care: A report from the family healthware impact trial. *Genetics in Medicine* 2010; 12:212–218.

Agosti JM, Goldie SJ. Introducing HPV vaccine in developing countries--key challenges and issues. *New Engl J Med* 2007; 356:1908–1910.

American Society of Clinical Oncology. American society of clinical oncology policy statement update: Genetic testing for cancer susceptibility. *J Clin Oncol* 2003; 21:2397–2406.

Anderson KK, Sebaldt RJ, Lohfeld L, Burgess K, Donald FC, Kaczorowski J. Views of family physicians in southwestern ontario on preventive care services and performance incentives. *Family Practice* 2006; 23:469–471.

Arroyave AM, Penaranda EK, Lewis CL. Organizational change: A way to increase colon, breast and cervical cancer screening in primary care practices. *J Commun Hlth* 2011; 36:281–288.

Canadian Cancer Society's Steering Committee on Cancer Statistics. *Canadian Cancer Statistics 2011*. Toronto, ON: Canadian Cancer Society; 2011.

Collins F. Genomics and the family physician: Realizing the potential. *American Family Physician* 2004; 70:1637–1642.

Dietrich AJ, Tobin JN, Cassells A, Robinson CM, Greene MA, Sox CH et al. Telephone care management to improve cancer screening among low-income women: A randomized, controlled trial. *Ann Int Med* 2006; 144:563–571.

Downs LS, Smith JS, Scarinci I, Flowers L, Parham G. The disparity of cervical cancer in diverse populations. *Gynecologic Oncology* 2008; 109(2 Suppl):S22–30.

Gilfillan RJ, Tomcavage J, Rosenthal MB, Davis DE, Graham J, Roy JA et al. Value and the medical home: Effects of transformed primary care. *The American Journal of Managed Care* 2010; 16:607–614.

Guerra CE, Schwartz JS, Armstrong K, Brown JS, Halbert CH, Shea JA. Barriers of and facilitators to physician recommendation of colorectal cancer screening. *J Gen Int Med* 2007; 22:1681–1688.

Hogg W, Lemelin J, Moroz I, Soto E, Russell G. Improving prevention in primary care: Evaluating the sustainability of outreach facilitation. *Canadian Family Physician* 2008; 54:712–720.

Hontelez JA, Hahne S, Koedijk FH, de Melker HE. Effectiveness and impact of hepatitis B virus vaccination of children with at least one parent born in a hepatitis B virus endemic country: An early assessment. *J Epidemiol Commun Hlth* 2010; 64:890–894.

Hudson SV, Ohman-Strickland P, Cunningham R, Ferrante JM, Hahn K, Crabtree BF. The effects of teamwork and system support on colorectal cancer screening in primary care practices. *Cancer Detection and Prevention* 2007; 31:417–423.

Hung DY, Rundall TG, Crabtree BF, Tallia AF, Cohen DJ, Halpin HA. 2006. Influence of primary care practice and provider attributes on preventive service delivery. *Am J Prev Med* 2006; 30:413–422.

IARC. *Human papillomaviruses*. IARC Monographs on the evaluation of carcinogenic risks to humans Vol 90. Lyon; International Agency for Research on Cancer, 2007.

Klabunde CN, Lanier D, Breslau ES, Zapka JG, Fletcher RH, Ransohoff DF, Winawer SJ. Improving colorectal cancer screening in primary care practice: Innovative strategies and future directions. *J Gen Intern Med* 2007; 22:1195–1205.

Klug SJ, Hukelmann M, Blettner M. Knowledge about infection with human papillomavirus: A systematic review. *Preventive Medicine* 2008; 46:87–98.

Lai DT, Cahill K, Qin Y, Tang JL. Motivational interviewing for smoking cessation. *Cochrane Database of Systematic Reviews (Online)* 2010; 1:CD006936.

Lin JS, O'Connor E, Whitlock EP, Beil TL. Behavioral counseling to promote physical activity and a healthful diet to prevent cardiovascular disease in adults: A systematic review for the U.S. preventive services task force. *Ann Int Med* 2010; 153:736–750.

Ling BS, Schoen RE, Trauth JM, Wahed AS, Eury T, Simak DM et al. Physicians encouraging colorectal screening: A randomized controlled trial of enhanced office and patient management on compliance with colorectal cancer screening. *Arch Int Med* 2009;169:47–55.

Luckmann R, Savageau JA, Clemow L, Stoddard AM, Costanza ME. A randomized trial of telephone counseling to promote screening mammography in two HMOs. *Cancer Detection and Prevention* 2003; 27:442–450.

Markowitz LE, Dunne EF, Saraiya M, Lawson HW, Chesson H, Unger ER. Quadrivalent human papillomavirus vaccine: Recommendations of the advisory committee on immunization practices (ACIP). *MMWR.Recommendations and Reports : Morbidity and Mortality Weekly Report. Recommendations and Reports / Centers for Disease Control* 2007; 56:1–24.

Mays RM, Sturm LA, Zimet GD. 2004. Parental perspectives on vaccinating children against sexually transmitted infections. *Social Science & Medicine* 2004; 58:1405–1413.

Mele A, Tosti ME, Mariano A, Pizzuti R, Ferro A, Borrini B et al. 2008. Acute hepatitis B 14 years after the implementation of universal vaccination in italy: Areas of improvement and emerging challenges. *Clinical Infectious Diseases* 2008; 46:868–875.

Moran K, Burson R, Critchett J, Olla P. Exploring the cost and clinical outcomes of integrating the registered nurse-certified diabetes educator into the patient-centered medical home. *The Diabetes Educator* 2011; 37:780–793.

Moser K, Patnick J, Beral V. 2009. Inequalities in reported use of breast and cervical screening in great britain: Analysis of cross sectional survey data. *BMJ* 2009; 338:b2025.

Myers RE, Sifri R, Hyslop T, Rosenthal M, Vernon SW, Cocroft J et al. A randomized controlled trial of the impact of targeted and tailored interventions on colorectal cancer screening. *Cancer* 2007; 110:2083–2091.

Ornstein S, Nemeth LS, Jenkins RG, Nietert PJ. Colorectal cancer screening in primary care: Translating research into practice. *Medical Care* 2010; 48:900–906.

Rawl SM, Champion VL, Scott LL, Zhou H, Monahan P, Ding Y et al. A randomized trial of two print interventions to increase colon cancer screening among first-degree relatives. *Patient Education and Counseling* 2008; 71:215–227.

Rosenthal TC. The medical home: Growing evidence to support a new approach to primary care. *Journal of the American Board of Family Medicine* 2008; 21:427–440.

Sarfaty M, Wender R. How to increase colorectal cancer screening rates in practice. *CA* 2007; 57:354–366.

Sarfaty M, Wender R, and R. Smith. Promoting cancer screening within the patient centered medical home. *CA* 2011; 61:397–408.

Scheuner MT, Gordon OK. Genetic risk assessment for common diseases. In *Emery and Romoin's principal and practice of medical genetics, 4th ed.* London: Churchill-Livingstone 2002; pp 654–674

Senior V, Marteau T, Weinman J. Impact of genetic testing on causal models of heart disease and arthritis: An analogue study. *Psychol Health* 2000; 14:1077–1088.

Shepard CW, Simard EP, Finelli L, Fiore AE, Bell BP. Hepatitis B virus infection: Epidemiology and vaccination. *Epidemiologic Reviews* 2006; 28:112–125.

Sohl SJ, Moyer A. Tailored interventions to promote mammography screening: A meta-analytic review. *Preventive Medicine* 2007; 45:252–261.

Spadea T, Bellini S, Kunst A, Stirbu I, Costa G. The impact of interventions to improve attendance in female cancer screening among lower socioeconomic groups: A review. *Preventive Medicine* 2010; 50:159–164.

Starfield B. The effectiveness of primary health care. In *A celebration of general practice.*, ed. M. Lakhani. Oxon, UK: Radcliffe. 2003.

Trevena LJ, Irwig L, Barratt A. Randomized trial of a self-administered decision aid for colorectal cancer screening. *Journal of Medical Screening* 2008; 15:76–82.

Tu SP, Taylor V, Yasui Y, Chun A, Yip MP, Acorda E et al. Promoting culturally appropriate colorectal cancer screening through a health educator: A randomized controlled trial. *Cancer* 2006; 107:959–966.

U.S. Department of Health and Human Services. *National healthcare quality report 2008.* Agency for Healthcare Research and Quality, 09-0001, 2009.

Vernon SW, del Junco DJ, Tiro JA, Coan SP, Perz CA, Bastian LA et al. 2008. Promoting regular mammography screening II. results from a randomized controlled trial in US women veterans. *J Natl Cancer Inst* 2008; 100:347–358.

Wei EK, Ryan CT, Dietrich AJ, Colditz GA. Improving colorectal cancer screening by targeting office systems in primary care practices: Disseminating research results into clinical practice. *Arch Int Med* 2005; 165:661–666.

Weller DP, Campbell C. Uptake in cancer screening programmes: A priority in cancer control. *Br J Cancer* 2009a; 101 Suppl 2:S55–59.

Weller DP, Patnick J, McIntosh HM, Dietrich AJ. Uptake in cancer screening programmes. *Lancet Oncology* 2009b; 10:693–699.

Yarnall KS, Pollak KI, Ostbye T, Krause KM, Michener JL. 2003. Primary care: Is there enough time for prevention? *Am J Pub Hlth* 2003; 93:635–641.

Chapter 26
Finale: What Can We Expect from Cancer Prevention and Screening?

Anthony B. Miller

Theoretically, it should be possible to prevent at least 50 % of cancer cases and deaths from them occurring by applying what we know about causation of cancer and at least a further 10 % of cancer deaths by screening. Yet, we seem unable to achieve this, though remarkable success has been achieved in preventing smoking-attributable cancers from occurring. The success for smoking was largely due to the application of a fiscal weapon, combined with restrictions on smoking in public places. This has led to calls for taxing unhealthy foods, yet governments have been remarkably resistant to that suggestion.

In Part I of this book, the authors have attempted to show the way forward for prevention. Cameron and Kerner propose three strategies for reducing disease incidence. These include scaling up preventive maneuvers in primary care settings, introducing high-reach low-cost programs (using print and electronic media), and creating environments that promote healthy behavior patterns. Collishaw and Callard, in discussing tobacco control, suggest that in the future, in addition to more effective measures that will influence individual behavior, tobacco control will need to be expanded to include measures directed at changing the ways tobacco suppliers do business, in effect by ensuring that governments take control of supply. Blair et al. document that controlling occupational exposures leads to a reduction in cancer risk, but point out that information is needed to identify and characterize successful exposure-reduction approaches so as to reduce the cancer burden on working populations in a timely manner. Bosch, after reviewing the developments relating to human papillomavirus (HPV) vaccines, suggests that comprehensive strategies of HPV vaccination and HPV-based screening tests could eliminate cervical cancer in defined populations, thus profiting on the knowledge that infection with oncogenic types of HPV is a necessary cause of cancer of the cervix. Tanaka, after reviewing the evidence that, the world over, infections are responsible for 15 % of

A.B. Miller (✉)
Dalla Lana School of Public Health, University of Toronto,
155 College Street, Ontario M5T 3 M7, Canada
e-mail: ab.miller@sympatico.ca

A.B. Miller (ed.), *Epidemiologic Studies in Cancer Prevention and Screening*,
Statistics for Biology and Health 79, DOI 10.1007/978-1-4614-5586-8_26,

cancers, suggests that some behavioral changes in infected individuals, such as smoking cessation, alcohol abstinence (in patients with chronic hepatitis B and C), and reduction of salt intake (in *H. pylori* carriers), can reduce the corresponding cancer risks. Friedenreich et al. show that physical activity is a modifiable lifestyle risk factor associated with a decreased risk of several cancers, especially of the breast and colon, though sedentary behavior is emerging as a risk factor for cancer that should be considered independently from physical activity. Brawley and Kramer agree that cancer prevention interventions, if fully implemented, could potentially prevent several hundred thousand cancer deaths per year, but if this is to be achieved, much of the emphasis should be on children as most prevention interventions are most useful when deployed early in life. Effective interventions must be applied at the individual, clinical, community, and policy levels, a public health challenge at national and local levels. James points out that evidence is growing that the contribution of diet in the causation of cancer has previously been underestimated. So an emphasis on biomarker studies of both intake and the carcinogenic process is needed as are dietary trials in cancer survivors. Reid and Marshall conclude that formal testing of chemopreventive agents in randomized, placebo-controlled trials has indicated that their preventive effects are modest to negligible or that their toxicities are unacceptable for use in average-risk populations. Thomas emphasizes that women should be informed that early age at the birth of one's first child protects against breast cancer and that risk of both breast and ovarian cancers declines with increasing duration of breast feeding. Vineis points out that controlling the environmental causes of cancer requires a coordinated effort for the identification of exposed populations, particularly in low-income countries, and for effective primary prevention policies. Finally, in this part, Ulrich reviews how the World Health Organization has integrated cancer control within its approach to the increasing burden of noncommunicable diseases, the world over.

In Part II, the possible role of screening is critically reviewed. Miller discusses approaches to the evaluation of screening, especially how we can approach the evaluation of new screening tests. Broutet reviews the contributions of WHO to cervical cancer control. There are many challenges for cervical cancer control programs. They include the need to reform health-care systems in many countries and ensure the availability of human resources, because of a shortage of trained health workers for vaccinating, screening, and treating. Hakama concludes that screening for cervical cancer can be relatively inexpensive even if coverage of the total target population is achieved. An important future determinant of screening for cervix cancer will be vaccination against HPV infection, though screening for cervix cancer will continue to have an important role. Patel and Ahnen conclude that although colon screening can be expensive, depending on the test used, any type of screening appears to be cost effective. However, Miller concludes that we may have reached the point of negligible benefit in screening for invasive breast cancer, largely because of improvements in cancer therapy. Similarly, he finds no justification for the introduction of population-based organized screening for prostate cancer at any age, while in view of the potential harms associated with screening, physicians should generally recommend against PSA testing for asymptomatic men. In many respects, these contrasting conclusions on screening reflect the fact that when screening for a precursor, as for cervix and colon cancer, removal of the precursor results in reduction in both incidence and mortality from the cancer, whereas when screening for the cancer when a precursor is not known, the absolute benefit in terms of mortality reduction declines drastically as treatment improves. Finally, in this part of the book, Patnick describes how operating a service paid from public funds allows a population approach to be taken which can have many advantages in terms of the ability to quality assure a program, to use the program to develop knowledge about screening and for which the cancer or its precursor is screened, to have an equitable approach to screening across all groups in society, and to operate a highly efficient and cost-effective service.

In Part III, the authors consider evidence on the impact of prevention and screening in populations and how this can be improved. Autier concludes that incidence rates of advanced cancer in populations where screening is widespread may inform on the effectiveness and public health relevance of cancer screening methods. However, he finds little evidence that the incidence of advanced breast cancer has fallen in populations where mammography screening has been widespread, presumably because of the impact of effective therapy. Stout et al. describe the use of mathematical modeling to aid the design of the national cervical cancer screening program in the Netherlands, to develop a package of tobacco control policies in the United States, and to evaluate the contributions of cancer screening and treatment to observed trends in breast cancer mortality. That some of the conclusions drawn, especially on breast screening, conflict with those of Autier and Miller largely reflect the assumptions built into the models, especially on the background trends in the absence of screening and improved treatment of breast cancer and the natural history of the disease. It is likely in the next few years that there will be further work both using the models described by Stout et al. and others being developed elsewhere. Hryniuk takes the discussion to a different level by suggesting an innovative way oncologists could lead the development of a comprehensive survivorship care plan for each cancer survivor. Hryniuk suggests this new role would involve them in more comprehensive cancer prevention and rehabilitation by focusing on their own patients who have already overcome the first attack of the disease. Hocking takes up the challenge of the continuing burden of lung cancer and suggests that the combination of low-dose computerized tomography and the future biomarkers should help improve the accuracy and clinical utility of lung screening programs, though all screening programs should incorporate access to tobacco cessation resources. Burton et al. focus on Asia which has the largest cancer burden of any region in the world and show how knowledge on cancer prevention and early detection could make major inroads into the cancer burden. Finally, Katz and Enns highlight the role of primary care practitioners in educating patients and supporting lifestyle changes to reduce exposure to cancer risk factors. They emphasize the key role that family practice has in cancer prevention and the targeting of specific populations for screening.

There is therefore a great deal that can be done to raise the profile of cancer prevention and to ensure that approaches to early detection and screening do not consume resources that could be more effectively used for cancer prevention.

Too frequently National Cancer Control Plans are initiated without the benefit of prior strategic planning to ensure that available resources are appropriately used, as recommended nearly two decades ago by the World Health Organization. Governments need to take a longer-term view as to what is possible and can be accomplished. All components of government are potentially involved, not just ministries of health but those concerned with agriculture, finance, and social security. We trust that this book will play its part in facilitating appropriate planning and action.

Index

A.B. Miller (ed.), *Epidemiologic Studies in Cancer Prevention and Screening*, Statistics for Biology and Health 79, DOI 10.1007/978-1-4614-5586-8_1,

D

FSC
www.fsc.org
MIX
Papier aus verantwortungsvollen Quellen
Paper from responsible sources
FSC® C105338

If you have any concerns about our products,
you can contact us on
ProductSafety@springernature.com

In case Publisher is established outside the EU,
the EU authorized representative is:
Springer Nature Customer Service Center GmbH
Europaplatz 3, 69115 Heidelberg, Germany

Printed by Libri Plureos GmbH
in Hamburg, Germany